# THE
# VIRGIN DIET
# COOKBOOK

Also by JJ Virgin, CNS, CHFS

*The Virgin Diet*
*Six Weeks to Sleeveless and Sexy*

# THE VIRGIN DIET COOKBOOK

## 150 Easy and Delicious Recipes to Lose Weight and Feel Better Fast

## JJ Virgin, CNS, CHFS

GRAND CENTRAL

Life&Style

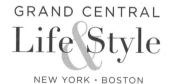

NEW YORK • BOSTON

Neither this diet nor any other diet program should be followed without first consulting a health-care professional. If you have any special conditions requiring attention, you should consult with your health-care professional regularly regarding possible modification of the program contained in this book.

Copyright © 2014 by JJ Virgin
All rights reserved. In accordance with the U.S. Copyright Act of 1976, the scanning, uploading, and electronic sharing of any part of this book without the permission of the publisher is unlawful piracy and theft of the author's intellectual property. If you would like to use material from the book (other than for review purposes), prior written permission must be obtained by contacting the publisher at permissions@hbgusa.com. Thank you for your support of the author's rights.

Grand Central Life & Style
Hachette Book Group
237 Park Avenue
New York, NY 10017

www.GrandCentralLifeandStyle.com

Printed in the United States of America

RRD-C

First Edition: February 2014
10 9 8 7 6 5 4 3 2 1

Grand Central Life & Style is an imprint of Grand Central Publishing.
The Grand Central Life & Style name and logo are trademarks of Hachette Book Group, Inc.

The Hachette Speakers Bureau provides a wide range of authors for speaking events. To find out more, go to www.HachetteSpeakersBureau.com or call (866) 376-6591.

The publisher is not responsible for websites (or their content) that are not owned by the publisher.

Library of Congress Cataloging-in-Publication Data
Virgin, JJ, author.
    The virgin diet cookbook: 150 easy and delicious recipes to lose weight and feel better fast/JJ Virgin.
        pages cm.
    Summary: "The companion to the New York Times bestseller *The Virgin Diet* brings the groundbreaking health and weight-loss program into your kitchen. With more than 100 delicious and practical recipes, THE VIRGIN DIET COOKBOOK is designed to show you how to incorporate anti-inflammatory, healing foods into your diet to reclaim your health and reset your metabolism, while avoiding the 7 foods that are most likely to cause food intolerance. These tasty, easy-to-make recipes are free of gluten, soy, dairy, eggs, corn, peanuts, and added sugar and artificial sweeteners. With mouthwatering suggestions for breakfast, lunch, dinner, dessert, and snacks, you'll lose weight fast while enjoying what you eat! THE VIRGIN DIET COOKBOOK will also help you to stock your kitchen, provide delicious substitutes for common ingredients, and offer easy swaps for eating out and on-the-go"—Provided by publisher.
    Includes bibliographical references and index.
    ISBN 978-1-4555-7779-8 (hardback)
    1. Weight loss.   I. Title.
    RM222.2.V5278 2014
    613.2'65—dc23

*While it's wonderful to hear "I love you," there's nothing quite like having someone tell you, "You changed my life." To those of you who've had the courage and commitment to change your lives, you are my inspiration.*

# Contents

# Acknowledgments

With *The Virgin Diet* I learned that it takes a village to get a book out to the world. And with a cookbook, we're talking an even bigger village, because there are recipes to create and test on top of everything else!

Of course, it all starts with my awesome rock-star literary agent, Celeste Fine. I trust Celeste's insight implicitly; she is always spot-on with her guidance. I've had a blast working with Ellyne Lonergan, who produces my PBS shows and book trailers and co-writes my scripts, videos, and books. Alan Foster, thank you for believing in me and convincing PBS stations to give my show a chance. My team writer/blogger and researcher Jason Boehm has been invaluable in adding his input to the mix.

When we decided to do a cookbook, I knew I would need some real foodies to make sure everything was extra delicious, so I brought Marge Perry and David Bonom onto the team. Jonathan Heindemause, your photos made everything look as good as it tastes! And of course my team tested all of the recipes, because I wanted to make sure everyone found meals that spoke to them and set them up for success.

And speaking of team—I have the most amazing group of people who work with me to help spread the message of the Virgin Diet, including Travis Houston, Mary Agnes Antonopoulos, Lacy Kirkland, Traci Knoppe, Patsy Wallace, Mary Ann Guillory, and Michelle Santo. And big special hugs to Susan Tafralis, who has been in the trenches with me now for over twelve years! My president and COO, Camper Bull, saved the day with *The Virgin Diet* and is instrumental in ensuring that everything I think up actually happens. Camper, I promise you a week free of, "I've got an idea!"

Thanks to my legal eagles, Darryl Sheetz and Peter Hoppenfeld; and my pubbies, Barbara Teszler of Teszler PR, and Mike Danielson of Media Relations. And to my stylist, Liana Chaouli—thank you for coming over and dumping half my closet (no, I really mean it ☺), and teaching me how to dress for any situation.

## Acknowledgments

Lesley Bohm, photographer extraordinaire, you make taking pictures fun... something I didn't think possible! And I'll never take photos without the other half of my photo dream team: makeup artist and stylist Tamara Gold. You two actually make me want to take photos more often just so I can hang out with you!

It goes without saying (I hope) that when you're cooking, you need to start with great ingredients, and for this book we needed the best. Naturally it was no surprise to me that my pals came through with amazing goodie packages. Thanks to Randy Hartnell and the crew at Vital Choice—you've ruined me for being able to eat any other seafood! And to the team at Carolina Bison: I've cleared out more of my freezer so I can keep your products well stocked! Hilary Martin and Mike Murray over at So Delicious Dairy Free: I adore working with you and love being involved in the product testing (but quit sending me the ice creams—I can't control myself!). Kara Goldin, I am totally addicted to Hint water; thanks for supplying it for all of our shoots and events. And Betsy Foster and Marci Frumkin at Whole Foods, you gals are the best. Whenever I need a store to tape in or products to demo, you come to the rescue. If Whole Foods sold condos, I would move in!

Brendon Burchard, your strategy is beyond brilliant; thank you for helping me get this message out on a grand scale. And Frank Kern, your advice is flat-out epic—I so get the big reputation you have! And to our "red gals pack"—Dr. Sara Gottfried, Dr. Jen Landa, Dr. Anna Cabeca, Dr. Hyla Cass, Jackie Wicks, and Leanne Ely—our first gathering for my fiftieth was one of the best times ever and it must be an annual event!

How lucky am I to have landed my dream publisher, Grand Central, and to work with such a talented team? To my editor, Diana Baroni, you had me at Hello! It is such an honor to work with you. And big thanks to Sonya Safro, who heads up my PR; Elizabeth Connor for such incredible art direction; and Amanda Englander for her editorial assistance.

And of course, the most important acknowledgment of all goes to my two sons, Grant and Bryce. Thank you for being my inspiration and motivation. Grant, you are such a warrior; you amaze me daily with your strength, tenacity, and winning attitude. And Bryce, I am so impressed with who you are and the man you are becoming. Beyond your amazing athleticism, creativity, and brilliance, I love seeing how kind, empathetic, and supportive you are. I wake up every day with huge gratitude that I have you both as sons.

*Introduction*

# DROP 7 FOODS, LOSE 7 POUNDS, JUST 7 DAYS

Does it seem like trying to lose weight has cast a shadow over your life and robbed you of the joy you should be experiencing when you eat? Has the torrent of information on nutrition become so overwhelming, it's paralyzing? It doesn't have to be that way. If you're looking for the key to feasting freedom, you're reading the right book! I've made it clear and simple, and best of all, I promise you that it can actually be easy and delicious to ditch the foods that hurt you, so that you can finally lose weight and feel better—fast!

My *New York Times* bestselling book, *The Virgin Diet*, has helped hundreds of thousands of people break free from the grip of stubborn weight gain more quickly than they ever dreamed was possible. I get amazing testimonials on Facebook every day from people losing anywhere from two to twelve pounds...in the first week!

More important, this type of fast weight loss can actually be *healthier*: Research shows that people who lose weight fast have the greatest long-term success with weight loss. A study in the *International Journal of Behavioral Medicine* found that people who burned fat fast lost more weight and kept it off better than slow burners. And a more recent study in the *New England Journal of Medicine* reinforced that with the news that fast fat loss can become *permanent* fat loss. That means when you lose a lot of weight after just a few weeks on my plan, you're more likely to continue to lose weight and then maintain that loss than people who try to lose pounds slowly. Which makes sense, right? After all, it's pretty tough to stay motivated when weight is dribbling off you at the rate of a pound a month!

For more than twenty-five years, I've been helping people break through their weight loss resistance, get rid of cravings, and look and feel better. Over that time I've discovered that many of the foods we consider to be "healthy" or "dietetic" can actually put the brakes on weight loss and even cause weight gain. Yes, you heard that right: "Healthy foods" could be causing you to *gain weight*. How unfair is that?

The good news is that just by making some simple changes to what you eat and what you buy at the grocery store, you'll finally drop weight fast, reverse belly bloat and inflammation, and feel and look better than ever before.

## FOOD VS. CALORIES

Shifting the foods in your diet is the number one way to move the needle on weight loss and health. We've all spent years demonizing calories, carbs, and fat (believe me, I've been there, too), but science has finally helped us figure out that we've been doing it wrong. It's not about any of those things; it's about the foods you eat, and the foods you don't eat.

If it seems like your body is fighting back every time you try to lose weight, it could be because it is. You may be suffering from food intolerances you've developed over time. Food intolerances aren't life-threatening, like food allergies, but they can be misery-inducing. Food intolerances can be genetic, immunological, or hormonal, but most of the time they are very "stealth." Rather than an outright immediate reaction, the body reacts negatively to food in a subtler, more drawn-out way, creating unpleasant symptoms and conditions like weight gain, eczema, cravings, achy joints, and digestive unrest. And since food intolerance usually comes on gradually, it can be especially hard to connect the dots between what you eat, how you feel, and what you weigh. I've intentionally kept the science in this cookbook to a minimum for simplicity, but if you just can't get enough, check out *The Virgin Diet* for more in-depth explanations and studies.

## THE "HEALTHY" FOODS THAT HURT YOU

You probably never suspected "health" foods as the stealth attackers in your creeping weight gain, fatigue, brain fog, and other chronic symptoms. After all, you're eating the same way you always have, and you used to weigh less and feel better, right?

So here's the headline: Faux "health foods" may not only be stalling your weight loss, they may actually be hurting you. No doubt you've been eating them with abandon, believing all the well-funded hype about them. Which means you're trapped—

feeling like you're doing everything right but not knowing why the weight just won't come off. It's because these foods are not what they pretend to be. And they're taking their toll on your weight, your looks, your health, and your life expectancy.

The obesity epidemic in this country is a public health crisis, and obesity-related illnesses like heart disease, cancer, and diabetes are skyrocketing. But even if you're not dealing with full-blown disease, the foods you eat may be pushing you in that direction, and along the way manifesting as everything from dangerous fat around your middle to low-grade anxiety to brain fog. These masquerading "health foods" can also be the culprit in joint discomfort and gastrointestinal problems like painful gas and bloating...things that most of us are led to believe are the normal by-products of aging. I'm here to tell you *nothing* could be further from the truth.

## 7 FOODS TO FREEDOM

I've discovered the 7 common foods literally holding your health hostage. When you pull these 7 foods out of your diet for just three weeks, miracles happen. The weight falls off, your energy soars, your skin looks younger, your pain is gone, and your cravings are in the rearview mirror. Imagine not being a prisoner to that afternoon cookie or evening sweet. Imagine looking and feeling great in a few weeks by eliminating just 7 foods from your diet. I've helped thousands of my clients experience dramatic results, and I want them for you, too!

So, drumroll, please....Here are the 7 foods:

Gluten
Dairy
Peanuts
Eggs
Corn
Soy
Sugar and artificial sweeteners

Don't panic. I make it so easy to live without them, and it's just three weeks. You can do anything for three weeks! But I'm going to bet that once you've finally cleared that weight loss hurdle, you'll look and feel so great you won't even want these 7 foods anymore. Most people who eliminate these foods for three weeks want to stay off of them for life. And that's where this cookbook comes in.

## PREPARE FOR POWER

You may start my program to lose weight, but you'll stay on it because you'll feel so much better! Simply put, your diet is where healing begins. Eating the right foods and eliminating the wrong foods can work wonders even beyond weight loss—it's the soothing medicine that increases energy, brightens looks, evens out hormones, detoxifies your system, balances blood sugar, reduces inflammation, and slows down the aging process. Who doesn't want all that?

Avoiding the foods that cause weight gain and hurt your health can be easy if you know what to do. And in this cookbook I've done all the work for you (well, except the cooking!). No other cookbook eliminates all 7 problem foods for you and still offers delicious, easy meals that are fun to make and will eliminate your cravings. I've even included three-week meal plans for numerous lifestyle scenarios, so everyone can benefit from the plan, including:

- extra-fast weight loss;
- managing blood sugar;
- vegetarians and vegans;
- travel;
- feeding a family;
- Paleo followers; and
- eating on a budget.

Taking control of what you eat—from what you buy at the grocery store to making sure it's prepared to fuel your health—is completely empowering. It should not be a hobby; it should be a way of life. And if you're serious about losing weight and feeling great, it's the only way to know for sure what's in the food you're eating. Besides, cooking your own food is not only an elixir for your body and soul, it's also easier on your wallet. It costs less than eating out and can take less time, too. You just have to be prepared—and getting prepared is half the fun. You'll feel healthier just shopping for the ingredients in these recipes!

## GET EXCITED!

Think of what's in store for you when your cravings are gone and you've retrained your taste buds to appreciate the natural sweetness of fruit, cinnamon, and vanilla; the zest of fresh lemon; and the savory taste of turmeric…and when you've finally lost that unwelcome extra weight, have the energy you used to have, and are not plagued with the roller coaster of blood sugar spikes and crashes. Oh yeah, and your skin looks younger and you're thinking clearly again!

My plan has helped thousands of people, and I promise you will have amazing results if you follow the recipes and meal plans in this book.

If you've already read *The Virgin Diet*, you know I'll be with you every step of the way and be your biggest cheerleader. But if you're finding my plan through this cookbook and you'd like even more help with the program, and additional tools and resources, *The Virgin Diet* book is your answer. It offers all that and more.

So here are 150 scrumptious recipes that will put you in control of what you're eating, and not only will you love (love!) them, they're just the beginning for you. They're the springboard for discovery in your own kitchen—tweak to your tummy's content and make easy swaps in your own favorite recipes! These recipes were carefully crafted to be easy, delicious, and fulfilling, so you'll never feel that you're missing anything or being deprived. Plus, you'll find answers to the most frequently asked questions I receive through my website and social media: Can I do this program and eat out? Can I do it when I travel? Can I do it as a vegetarian? Yes! Yes! Absolutely! I've created meal plans for all those scenarios—and others—and included them in this cookbook. You'll be amazed at how easy it is to keep the weight off, no matter where you are or what your eating style.

Processed ingestibles that pass as food have had their day. It's time to get back to food—real food—so we can all enjoy the complete health, life, family gatherings, and good times that come with it.

Enjoy!

# PART I

# DROP 7 FOODS, FEEL BETTER FAST

# FOOD INTOLERANCE IS THE HIDDEN CAUSE OF WEIGHT GAIN

1

You're on your way! And you're going to do great. What I love about having you start my program is knowing how excited you're going to be after the first 7 days, when you've dropped the weight, look younger, and feel so much better! But don't settle for that! Just wait. By the end of 3 weeks, you'll never go back. Even beyond 3 weeks, as you continue to eat the foods that work with your body's chemistry, your body will be steadily healing and getting stronger.

Three weeks is just a place to start—an in-range target that can quickly show you how the foods you eat affect you and that gives you power and control over what you eat, how much you weigh, and how you feel. It shows you—and fast—how much food choices matter. Because guess what? Food is not just for pleasure (though there is that). It's here to fuel you. It's information. And based on the choices you make, it creates responses in your body, for better or worse.

Sadly, what most people accept as feeling normal is anything but, and you could be tolerating being less than your best without even realizing it. Too many of us were taught to tough it out, to push through discomfort and accept common symptoms as the inevitable signs of aging. So instead of asking some basic questions and choosing not to put up with your growing waistline and fatigue, you may be suffering, and worse yet, counting calories and endlessly dieting in ways that only exacerbate the problem.

You may think weight gain, gas and bloating, headaches, joint pain, moodiness, skin problems, and brain fog are normal signs of aging, because that's what we're told. Well, who wants that person staring back in the mirror if you can help it? It's time to throw out the old playbook. It's time to realize that weight gain, lack of sleep, and feeling lousy are not the result of aging, they're *the culprits* that make us look and feel older than our years.

People who've used my plan to drop that clingy weight around the middle and get rid of debilitating symptoms feel liberated when they discover they're not doomed to suffer with any of that. It's simply not their fate; it's a choice. The body is an elastic, dynamic system, and it will respond, make changes, and rebound according to the direction it's given. This cookbook will help you make great choices to finally lose the weight and change the way you look and feel (you've already made one—you're here!).

## FOOD INTOLERANCE: WHAT SETS THE VIRGIN DIET APART

The Virgin Diet is unique and effective because it does what other diets don't: It targets food intolerance. Food intolerance could very well be the thorn in the side of your efforts to lose weight and feel better. Why? Many foods that cause intolerance cloak themselves in a faux health halo, and you may be eating them believing you're doing everything right. And because they're not the usual suspects, they're hard to spot—they can hide in plain sight in vegetable egg white omelets, nonfat Greek yogurt, and soy burgers on whole-grain buns. No wonder you can't figure out where the weight is coming from! But the weight gain is only one clue. How you feel is another huge one.

While it's true that you may notice you don't feel so well right after eating certain foods, other times it may take awhile for you to have symptoms because the response takes place over hours or even days. This makes it tougher to sleuth out what's made you feel crummy. If you've been eating a lot of a certain food your system doesn't like, you eventually exceed your sensitivity threshold (i.e., you overdose), and antibodies build up to fight that food and send your body a message. By then, you may have been living with adverse effects—including inflammation that causes you to hold on to weight and age faster—for a long time.

Inflammation is the body's healing response to injury, whether that wound is on the inside or the outside. We couldn't live without the swift response of acute inflammation. But when that red, hot, swollen response is turned on chronically, it can create far-reaching problems, from mild discomfort to life-changing disease. Among them, it causes you to hold on to fat by releasing chemicals that make you resistant to your body's routine messages that dictate appetite and satiety, mood, and calorie burning. Inflammation contributes to insulin resistance, putting you at risk for diabetes; it makes you retain fluid and endure digestive problems; and it diminishes your energy.

It can contribute to a syndrome called "leaky gut" (pretty much what it sounds like), which in turn escalates intolerance to certain foods. But wait, there's more—the fat that inflammation causes you to hold on to creates its own inflammation, causing you to hold on to even more fat. And around it goes.

## FOOD INTOLERANCE VS. FOOD ALLERGIES

A food intolerance is not the same as a food allergy, and it's worth clarifying the distinction between the two so you have a clear understanding of the connection between what you eat, what you weigh, and how you feel, and how to best address it (hint: if it's an intolerance, the answer is this cookbook!).

Food allergies are very different and fairly rare (though they're becoming more common). They trigger an immediate immune system response to a protein in the offending food. Think of a peanut allergy and how the slightest sniff of a peanut can close up someone's throat. When you have a food allergy, your body sprays your system with an antibody called immunoglobulin E (IgE), which in turn triggers the release of copious amounts of histamine and chemicals to fight the enemy.

"Food intolerance," on the other hand, is an umbrella term used to describe negative reactions to certain foods—everything from a medical condition like lactose intolerance to unpleasant issues that affect your central nervous system, your respiratory system, your digestive system, and your skin. It can manifest as headaches, irritability, upset tummy, joint aches, eczema, and more.

So you can see that food intolerances are much more common than food allergies. And there are a lot of ways we end up with them. Here are several:

■ You could have inherited it. A common example of genetic food intolerance is the intolerance to gluten. What you've inherited is the absence of certain enzymes or chemicals needed to digest what's in the food. And if that's the case, there's not much you can do other than to avoid the food in order to avoid the reaction. Another example of this kind of intolerance is lactose intolerance, a result of lactase deficiency.

■ Your body may not be able to absorb certain nutrients. One such abnormality that's fairly common is fructose malabsorption. When you can't absorb fructose, gas, cramping, diarrhea, and even bad breath are the result. Not fun!

▪ You could have a chemical, or hormonal, interaction with the food. These are among the most common reasons food intolerance may be padding your middle, robbing you of energy, and making you look older than your years. But they're also the most easily addressed because the reaction—and the result—can be reversed by removing my 7 high-FI (high–Food Intolerance) foods—those foods most likely to cause the health issues we associate with "intolerance." For example, soy (and foods made from soy, like tofu and tempeh) *and* gluten contain goitrogens, naturally occurring compounds that can impair thyroid function by interfering with iodine uptake. Soy also contains phytoestrogens that can mimic estrogen, which can lower testosterone in men. Similarly, sugar and processed carbs can drive up both cortisol and insulin: Your body responds to the arrival of sugar with an insulin surge to reduce the amount of sugar in your blood. When sugar drops, the body calls cortisol to the scene to make sure you have enough sugar to get up and go when you need to. Frequent spikes in those hormones create metabolic havoc that results in weight gain and devastated energy.

▪ You might have increased gut permeability, or leaky gut. When your gut leaks, it lets bacteria and undigested food particles slip into your bloodstream. Your body responds to these invaders with an immune reaction that results in a wide range of gastrointestinal problems and inflammation. Leaky gut can be caused by fructose and gluten, certain artificial sweeteners, GMO foods, toxins, chronic stress, and even certain medications.

▪ You might have a microbial imbalance in your gut. A high-functioning metabolism and your health depend on harmony between the good and the bad in your gut. When the balance is tipped in favor of the bad guys, food intolerance, digestive unrest, and other unpleasant conditions are the likely result. How does your gut bacteria get out of balance? First and foremost, by what you eat. If you're eating antibiotic-fed animals, genetically modified foods, and artificial sweeteners, or if you generally adhere to the Standard American Diet (SAD)—which is high in refined sugar and low in fiber and fresh vegetables—you're a perfect candidate for food intolerance.

▪ One of the most common ways your body may react to problem foods is through your immune system, with an IGG response. IGG stands for immunoglobulin G, another antibody. The activation of these IGG antibodies is known as a delayed immune response, and it keeps your immune system revved, in constant gear. These IGG responses are chronic, low-grade, and develop over time, often without your realizing they're happening.

■ Antibiotics may increase the chance of developing food intolerance, possibly because of their role in upending the balance of gut flora and their impact on the immune system in general.

■ You might be reacting to genetically modified organisms, or GMOs. More than 80 percent of the soy and corn grown in the U.S. comes from seeds that have had their DNA altered. And soy and corn are in an endless number of processed foods, from chips to dips. There is a growing body of evidence to suggest GMOs can contribute to immune system and digestive disorders, especially leaky gut.

The ways we know we can be intolerant to food are disconcerting enough. But to be honest, we really don't know all the reasons people react negatively to food. Beyond what I've already mentioned, some intolerances could be a result of cross-contamination, which happens when allergenic proteins from a problem food come in contact with food you would otherwise tolerate. Obviously that's a huge issue if you have an actual allergy.

To compound the issue, there's no single global test to determine whether you have an intolerance as a result of all these factors. And because we don't even know all of the ways we can become intolerant to food, the best test is—you guessed it—your own body. After all, food intolerance reactions are chemical, and your body chemistry is unique to you.

## THE BIG PICTURE

I've identified 7 problem foods that are the top candidates for food intolerance. I am willing to go out on a limb and bet that you are reacting to at least some of these (and possibly all of them). And if that's happening to you, you're hanging on to weight like it's your BFF and you're experiencing health issues you're probably not connecting to what you're eating. When you eliminate these foods you'll not only lose weight, you'll have more energy, sleep better, and have clearer skin—bonus!

I've laid out my program in three easy-to-follow cycles to help you be your own guinea pig. I'm going to give you the highlights here, but if you want or need more information, there's plenty more detail in my first book, *The Virgin Diet*. The three cycles are designed to provide these fundamentals to help you reach your goals:

1. Identify the best foods for your body to lose fat fast
2. Weigh and measure each week
3. Get support; be accountable
4. Rechallenge and customize
5. Plan for maintenance

In Cycle 1, you'll cut out these 7 high–Food Intolerance (high-FI) foods I've identified:

Gluten
Dairy
Peanuts
Eggs
Corn
Soy
Sugar and artificial sweeteners

In Cycle 2, you'll test your system each week with one of the four most reactive high-FI foods: soy, dairy, eggs, and gluten. This cycle will tell you if you can tolerate some of these once your system has healed (though I don't want artificial sweeteners back into your diet ever again, okay?), or whether you might have to wait longer while you continue to heal your gut or even let them go forever. We won't be rechallenging the other three high-FI foods. Instead, I advise keeping corn and peanuts out 95 percent of the time and limiting sugar to no more than 5 added grams per 100 calories in any given food item.

In Cycle 3, I'll give you the tips and tools you need to experience the benefits of the Virgin Diet and maintain the fabulous new you for life, because *losing* and *maintaining* your weight require very different strategies.

If you have any worries about where to start or how to understand what a label is really telling you, rest easy. This cookbook holds your hand every step of the way. Plus, my recipes are free of these top high-FI foods...so cook and eat worry-free. And lose weight and feel great in the process.

Following these three cycles just as they're laid out will shine a spotlight on your food intolerances and clear the path to fast weight loss and healing. And here's a bit of joy before you get started: None of these cycles, and no part of this program, involve counting calories!

You have to eat food to lose weight, so I'm going to make sure you eat well. Where your calories come from matters a whole lot more than how closely you're counting them, because a slice of cake and its calorie equivalent in kale (that's a lot of kale!) are not going to send your body the same messages about blood sugar and insulin, fullness and hunger, or mood and energy.

So, fear not! I'm not going to turn you into an obsessive calorie counter or point collector. But I do want to at least acknowledge that calories count. And that means even too much healthy food can be, well, unhealthy. The shortest route to fast weight loss and reclaiming your energy and health is eating the right balance of clean, lean protein; healthy fats; non-starchy veggies; and slow low carbs—unrefined or less-refined carbohydrates that are high in fiber, digested slowly, and have a limited impact on your blood sugar, like beans, legumes, and quinoa.

And of course the other factor—and this is a biggie—is knowing your triggers. I can tell you I know mine! I lose my mind with nut butter. Lose. My. Mind. I can't do a spoonful; I keep going back to "clean up the jar" until the next thing I know, it really *is clean*. So if you have a trigger food that you're prone to overeat (e.g., 10 to 20 nuts passes as nutritious; a cup is over the top), then consider it the enemy and keep it out of the house!

The big *aha!* you'll have on this program is that you'll lose weight, look younger, and feel better fast, without feeling hungry or deprived. I know that from where you sit, this hardly seems possible. Prepare to become a believer!

## SYMPTOMS QUIZ

Did you ever go on WebMD to check your symptoms, only to leave there pretty sure you're going to die? This is not that. This is the opposite of that. The symptoms quiz I've made for you is designed to identify things you're experiencing and to track your healing and weight loss throughout this program. It's especially helpful to determine if you need additional gut support during the process. So to make sure you have a base-line to measure your progress, take the symptoms quiz before you start, again after 3 weeks (the end of Cycle 1), and then daily during Cycle 2, the challenge phase.

# Quiz: What Are You Tolerating?

Are you still not sure whether food intolerance is the cause of your weight gain and premature aging? Take this quiz and find out.

## Is Food Intolerance Holding You Hostage?

- If you have 1 or more of the symptoms listed below 1 to 2 times a week at a mild or moderate level—even if you barely notice it—score 2 points each.
- If you have mild or moderate symptoms 3 or more times a week, or severe symptoms 2 or more times a week, score 4 points each.

| | |
|---|---|
| ___Abdominal cramping | ___Fatigue |
| ___Acne/rosacea | ___Food cravings |
| ___ADD and hyperactivity | ___Gas and bloating |
| ___Arthritis (osteo or rheumatoid) | ___Headaches |
| ___Asthma | ___Inability to lose weight |
| ___Brain fog | ___Joint pain |
| ___Chronic mucus/stuffy nose | ___Moodiness |
| ___Congestion | ___Muscle pain |
| ___Constipation and/or diarrhea | ___Psoriasis |
| ___Dark circles under the eyes | ___Sinusitis |
| ___Depression | ___Skin rashes |
| ___Eczema | ___Throat clearing |

Total points: _____

## Your Food Intolerance Score:

**0 to 5: Low FI.** Currently you seem to suffer from few food allergies or intolerances, if any. I've found that most people feel and look better while removing high-FI foods and often are reacting to one or more of them whether or not they have any overt symptoms. You're reading this book because you want to make sure you eat the best diet so you can keep feeling and looking lean and young.

**6 to 14: Mid FI.** You consistently suffer mild or moderate discomfort and bloating with certain foods, but you do experience periods of relief. Over time, you've probably noticed weight gain even though your diet hasn't changed. Your skin and hair may look somewhat dull, and you tend to feel more tired or stressed than you used to.

**15+: High FI.** Help! You can't remember the last time you felt light and lean after a meal, and it feels as though your stomach is constantly bloated. You've done everything you can think of to lose weight, and it just hasn't worked. Every time you look in the mirror, you think, *How did I get so old? Why do I look so tired?*

## THE CYCLES

The three cycles of the Virgin Diet are specifically designed to shepherd you through your weight loss journey with all the support and information you need, to ensure you come out the other side doing the Snoopy dance in celebration of a lighter, healthier, and happier you.

## CYCLE 1

Cycle 1 covers 21 days. For those 21 days, I want you to cut out all the top 7 high-FI foods—gluten, soy, dairy, eggs, corn, peanuts, and sugar and artificial sweeteners. All of them, 100 percent of the time. The only exception here is sugar, as there's sugar in some of the foods on the plan, including low-glycemic fruits and veggies. You'll also be allowed up to 5 grams of added sugar in other foods—more on this later.

The length of Cycle 1 is intended to give enough time for the fire in your immune system to die out. Allowing even a little bit of any of the 7 high-FI foods to sneak in during these 21 days matters; it can trigger the antibody response to that food and reignite your immune system. So if you cheat, it's back to the starting line. That's incentive, right?

To begin, get in the right frame of mind. Consider grocery shopping as a health pilgrimage. Instead of these 7 foods, you'll be eating foods that are healing. So whenever you can, buy organic, especially when it comes to thin-skinned fruits and vegetables. Check out ewg.org for a list of the "Dirty Dozen" that you will absolutely want to buy organic. And be sure to buy humanely raised, antibiotic-free, no-hormones-added lean meats and poultry.

You may be concerned that these foods will be more expensive than the ones you're used to buying; that's not necessarily true. Even so, this is not the time to jump over nickels to pick up pennies. When you intentionally choose food only because it's cheap, you very well could be adding to a bill that will come due on your health and cost you much more in health care in the long term. Besides, when you quit buying all that processed junk, you may actually save some money!

If you have 30 or more pounds to lose or are suffering from many of the symptoms on the symptoms quiz, I recommend extending Cycle 1 until you are within 5 pounds of your goal weight or your symptoms have reduced dramatically. You can actually live the rest of your life on Cycle 1, and to be honest, once you see how much better you feel and how easy it is to maintain your weight, you may want to. But I do want you to know which foods you need to be vigilant about—because they create extreme reactions—and which foods you can let sneak in here and there without wreaking havoc on your system.

Of course, more than anything I don't want to scare you off by telling you that you have to give up these 7 foods forever—because you don't. But I find that once people have the first 3 weeks behind them, they're locked in: They've lost the weight, which was the reason for starting the program, but they also know that the way they're eating is responsible for how good they look and feel, and they don't want to go back. Ever.

It helps that on average my clients lose 7 pounds in the first 7 days—and you can, too, just by following the recipes and guidelines in this cookbook.

The 3 weeks of Cycle 1 break out this way:

- Week 1—Jump-Start Week: You'll have 2 shakes, 1 meal, and an optional snack every day.
- Weeks 2 and 3—Healing Weeks: You'll have 1 shake, 2 meals, and an optional snack every day.

If you prefer to do 2 shakes a day during the entire time you're on Cycle 1, that's fine, too. Quite often—when I'm busy—I'll do 2 shakes during the day.

When you dive into Cycle 1 for the first time, here are some words of wisdom: For the first few days, stay focused on the benefits to come. Because I'm not going to lie to you—those first few days may be tough. You'll probably experience your body's withdrawal tantrums as cravings, hunger, and possibly headaches and fatigue. This is a good thing. Remember I said that! The worse the reaction, the more your body is letting you know it was reacting to those foods, because lots of antibodies are screaming for a food to fight. You're craving the very foods that hurt you. Think of it as your body's war against addiction. (Spoiler alert: The good guys win.) Once you come out the other side, your path to weight loss and healing has been cleared. In 7 days, fuggeddaboutit. You'll see and feel a big difference.

Remember, you didn't get here overnight, and you won't get fixed overnight, either. Still, you'll be happy to know it happens pretty darn quickly. You'll see dramatic shifts in the first 7 days and great improvement over 3 weeks. Give your body time to heal. It's worth earning back!

## MAKING THE CASE

To make the case even stronger, let's take a closer look at the 7 high-FI offenders.

### *Eggs*

Many people are sensitive to eggs; it's very common. But most people who have this intolerance aren't aware of it because the symptoms are often delayed for a couple of days and show up as gas, bloating, and heartburn, and possibly eczema and psoriasis. And it's not just about eating eggs themselves—eggs live in a lot of places. Omelets, quiches, and other breakfast foods are obvious, but eggs are also baked into pastries, pancakes, breads, and salads (the picnic kind), and are often hidden in meat loaf, crab cakes, soups (egg drop, of course, and matzo ball), crepes, zucchini fritters (they sound so healthy!), stuffing, noodles, and meatballs. Bye-bye to all.

So you can be vigilant, I'm going to help you become an educated label reader. Know the ingredients in your food. You'll be surprised how many foods contain egg. Now, you may be tempted to use an egg substitute to get your fix, but that will only give you a substance with the same gluey texture as eggs, not the nutrition (even "Egg Beaters" are made only of the whites). Choose a real protein replacement like fish, chicken, or grass-fed beef. And of course, if eggs have been your go-to breakfast choice, my Virgin Diet Shakes (pages 92–97) or my Hot Quinoa Flake Cereal with Warm Berry Compote (page 90) is the perfect swap.

**Where They Hide**

| | | |
|---|---|---|
| Baked goods | Flan | Meringues |
| Batter mixes | French toast | Noodles |
| Bavarian cream | Fritters | Pancakes |
| Boiled dressings | Frosting | Puddings |
| Bouillon | Hollandaise sauce | Quiche |
| Breaded foods | Ice cream | Salad dressings |
| Breads | Macaroons | Sauces |
| Cake flours | Malted drinks | Sausages |
| Creamy fillings | Marshmallows | Soufflés |
| Custards | Mayonnaise | Tartar sauce |
| Egg drop soup | Meat loaf | Waffles |

## EGGS MAY BE LISTED ON FOOD LABELS AS . . .

- Albumin
- Egg protein
- Egg white
- Egg yolk
- Globulin
- Livetin

### Gluten

You've been hearing a lot about gluten these days. It affects a huge number of people negatively (30 to 40 percent of Americans), whether they're gluten intolerant or have actual celiac disease. And I'll be honest with you, I find that 90 percent of the people I pull off of gluten feel better without it (I'm convinced the other 10 percent didn't really get it all out). Intolerance symptoms are similar to the symptoms of egg sensitivity: weight gain, digestive upset, headaches, joint pain, anxiety, depression, and especially leaky gut.

If you haven't identified gluten as a problem for you yet, you might still be confused by all that's swirling out there about it. Gluten is a protein in grains like wheat, barley, and rye. The food business is a mega machine, and gluten has become their go-to ingredient in everything that sits on a shelf. P.S.: This does not mean gluten-free processed foods get a pass as healthy—do not pretend to hear angels sing when you see this label on food you know is not good for you (I'm talking to you, gluten-free cupcakes!). During Cycle 1, I would also like you to keep out oatmeal; it turns out it is similar in structure to gluten and although it doesn't contain gluten, it can often trigger a similar response.

### Where It Hides

Alcoholic drinks (such as beer, ale, lager)
All-Bran
Anything cooked with breadcrumbs
Baked beans (there may be gluten in the tomato sauce)
Biscuits and cookies
Blue cheeses (may be made with bread)
Bread and bread rolls
Brown rice syrup
Bulgur wheat
Cakes
Cheap brands of chocolate
Chutneys and pickles

Couscous

Crispbreads

Crumble toppings

Curry powder and other spices (can be bulked out with flour)

Durum wheat

Farina

Gravy powders and stock cubes, such as OXO cubes

Hydrolyzed vegetable protein (HVP)

Imitation crabmeat

Instant coffee (may be bulked out with flour)

Licorice

Luncheon meat (may contain fillers)

Malted drinks

Malt vinegar

Matzo flour/meal

Meat and fish pastes

Muesli

Muffins

Mustard (dry mustard powder contains gluten)

Pancakes

Pasta (macaroni, spaghetti)

Pastry or pie crust

Pâtés

Pizza

Potato crisps/chips (some are okay—read the ingredients!)

Pretzels

Pumpernickel

Rye bread

Salad dressings

Sauces (often thickened with flour)

Sausages (often contain rusk—and the machines used to make them are often cleaned out with bread)

Scones

Seitan (doesn't contain gluten, it *is* gluten!)

Self-basting turkeys

Semolina

Shredded suet in packs (flour is normally used to keep the strands separate)

Some breakfast cereals

Soups—may be roux-based (made with flour)

Soy sauce

Stuffings

Waffles

White pepper (gluten is sometimes added to improve flow)

Yorkshire pudding

## Soy

Let me be blunt—there's no joy in soy! In fact, the news is bad. It's been pushed as a health food—mostly by soy companies—but nothing could be further from the truth. Here's its rap sheet: Soy has been linked to impaired thyroid function, reproductive disorders, cognitive decline, digestive problems, and lower sperm count. It's a relative newcomer to our food supply, so many people's systems respond to it as an allergen. It contains phytates, which can block mineral absorption, leading to nutrient deficiencies. Soy also contains lectins, which can cause leptin resistance and result in increased hunger (leptin is a hormone that regulates appetite). And nearly all soy has been genetically modified, a process that creates a whole host of other issues and also means that it is likely to contain high amounts of pesticides.

### Where It Hides

| | |
|---|---|
| Asian foods | Soy sauce |
| Energy bars and shakes | Tempeh |
| Miso | Teriyaki sauce |
| Prepared foods | Tofu |
| Soy protein powders | Vegetable burgers |

## Peanuts

You already know peanuts are one of the most common food allergens. That's because they have a high risk for aflatoxin mold, which can be carcinogenic as well. But they're not even nuts—they're legumes. So they don't contain as many good fatty acids as nuts like almonds, walnuts, cashews, and hazelnuts. Stock up on those instead. And here's something else: Other legumes offer more nutrients per calorie.

### Where They Hide

| | |
|---|---|
| Candy | Peanut butter |
| Cookies | Peanut oil |
| Food toppings | Snacks |

## Dairy

Allergies and sensitivity to dairy—especially cow's milk—are also pretty common. But growing up, we couldn't get through the day without being told to drink milk because dairy was a great source of calcium for our growing bones. The truth is that cow's milk can make you fat, promote insulin resistance, and foster acne and rosacea, and it may actually be bad for your bones due to its high acid load! There are many other calcium-rich foods—like salmon, sardines, broccoli, and leafy greens—that are much healthier and don't cause any of the GI distress or carry the same potential aller-genicity as dairy.

### Where It Hides

Anything in a container that says "milk proteins," "milk solids," "casein," or "whey" on it

Butter and many margarines

Canned foods (soups, spaghetti, ravioli)

Chocolate (except some dark chocolate products)

Cottage cheese

Cow, goat, and sheep milk yogurts and cheeses

Cream soups and chowders

Creamy cheese or butter sauces (often on vegetables or meats)

Desserts

Ice cream

Macaroni and cheese

Many baked goods (breads, crackers, desserts)

Many baking mixes (pancake mix)

Many "non-dairy" products (coffee creamer, whipped topping)

Many salad dressings (ranch, blue cheese, creamy, Caesar)

Mashed potatoes (often prepared with butter and/or milk)

Shakes and hot chocolate mixes and drinks

Whey protein powder

---

## DAIRY MAY BE LISTED ON LABELS AS . . .

- Buttermilk or buttermilk solids
- Butter or artificial butter flavor
- Casein, caseinate, sodium caseinate
- Cheese, cream cheese, cottage cheese
- Cream, sour cream, half-and-half, whipped cream
- Lactose, lactalbumin
- Milk, milk solids, nonfat milk solids
- Whey
- Yogurt, kefir

---

### Corn

In addition to helping you pack on the pounds (after all, this is what we feed cows and pigs to fatten them up), corn is a pro-inflammatory food that causes your blood sugar to spike and crash. Corn sensitivity can show up as rashes and hives, migraines, joint pain, mood disorders, temporary depression, insomnia, eczema, fatigue, hyperactivity in children, night sweats, dark circles around the eyes, recurring ear and urinary tract infections, and frustrating battles with sinus problems. Wow! It's in a ton of processed food in various forms, such as cornstarch, corn syrup (you know how damaging that can be), and corn oil, because, like soy, it's cheap. And it's one of the most genetically modified crops on the market, which (again) may bring with it another set of health risks altogether.

### Where It Hides

| | |
|---|---|
| Breakfast cereals (such as cornflakes) | Corn syrup |
| Corn chips (tortilla chips, Fritos) | Corn tortillas |
| Corn fritters | Grits |
| Cornmeal | Hominy |
| Corn oil | Maize |
| Cornstarch | Margarine |
| Corn sugars (dextrose, Dyno, Cerelose, Puretose, Sweetose, glucose) | Popcorn |
| | Vegetable oil |

## Sugar and Artificial Sweeteners

The news for sugar is less than sweet. The average American eats about 140 pounds of sugar a year. Yikes! And besides landing on their hips and waistline, it's wreaking havoc on their health. Here are some of its unwelcome gifts to your body: Sugar spikes and crashes your blood sugar, it disrupts your insulin metabolism, it raises your stress hormones so you burn less fat, it feeds bad gut bacteria and candida, it depresses your immune system, it makes you better at storing fat, it depletes nutrients, and like any good drug, it creates cravings for more.

If you've got a mad love for sugar, you'll go through a few days of withdrawal in Cycle 1. But soon after that, when true sensitivity returns to your taste buds, you'll have a whole new appreciation for the delicious, natural sweetness of berries, vanilla, and cinnamon in the recipes throughout this cookbook. Your new rule of thumb is to limit added sugar to 5 grams or less.

As for artificial sweeteners, ban them completely, forever. They're toxic chemicals that only help you pack on pounds and may contribute to the low-grade maladies plaguing you every day. They might even be raising your insulin, so break free from the grip of these fake sugars—ditch the diet sodas and the sweeteners in your coffee, and pass on any foods that have artificial sweeteners as an ingredient.

The many names for sugar:

| | | |
|---|---|---|
| Barley malt | Dextrin | Lactose |
| Beet sugar | Dextrose | Maltodextrin |
| Blackstrap molasses | Diastatic malt | Maltose |
| Brown sugar | Diatase | Malt syrup |
| Cane juice crystals | D-mannose | Maple syrup |
| Cane sugar | Evaporated cane juice | Molasses |
| Caramel | Fructose | Raw sugar |
| Carob syrup | Fruit juice concentrate | Rice syrup |
| Castor sugar | Galactose | Sucrose |
| Confectioners' sugar | Glucose | Syrup |
| Corn sweeteners | High-fructose corn | Table sugar |
| Corn syrup | syrup (HFCS) | Treacle |
| Date sugar | Honey | Turbinado sugar |
| Demerara sugar | Invert sugar | |

Other names for artificial sweeteners:

| | |
|---|---|
| Acesulfame potassium | Neohesperidine dihydrochalcone |
| Alitame | NutraSweet |
| Aspartame | Saccharin |
| Aspartame–acesulfame salt | Splenda |
| Cyclamate | Sucralose |
| Isomalt | |

## VIRGIN DIET SUCCESS

### Robin Brown—Eaton, CO

My husband, Scott, is the real winner. Scott's father passed away when Scott was in his early twenties, and around the holidays he was feeling sad that his father had not been around to take part in his adult years with his children. As he was thinking about that, he realized he had been struggling with his weight. He sat in his chair and thought about his mother with type 2 diabetes, his sister who was struggling with obesity, and his son who was in a size 44 pants and only 21. He looked at me and said, "I honestly think I am going to bury my mom, sister, and son before I die." I didn't know what to say.

Scott had been trying all these different things to lose weight. He is a total self-help reader and has looked into so many different diets. Yes, even the worst…fasting for 2 weeks with just water. That one actually made me mad because in my mind all I thought was, "If you can have the dedication to not eat for 2 weeks, then get up off your butt and get on the treadmill!"

He is 6' 2" and was approaching 230 pounds—and his frame isn't big at all. One day, the television was on and on comes this lady talking about losing weight if you take 7 things out of your diet. He immediately pushes the record button on the DVR and all I thought was, "Great! Another damn diet!" He asked me to buy the book and I did.

When he got close to wanting to begin this diet, he looked at me and said, "Robin, you have to do this with me because I can't cook like you and I really like sugar!" I said, "Okay," and we set the date for January 2, 2013. We both took our weights and started the diet. At first, it was fine because I really like to cook. The biggest constraint was getting my meals prepared for the evening. I work in a town about an hour away, so I started thinking about quick 30-minute meals. We spent a long time in the store looking at labels. I was amazed at how much corn is in things. My grocery bill may have changed a little, but the food tastes better. Anyway, after a week the pounds were coming off Scott. I was getting jealous because he kept saying, "Lost another pound," and I would shoot him one of those evil stares. We kept going and I will admit that after 2 weeks I was ready to quit because I had only dropped about 7 pounds or so. Scott was, of course, doing the happy dance because he had lost about 20 pounds.

By the end of week 3, though, we were shrinking in inches big-time. Scott went to put on his pants and the belt couldn't be notched anymore. We had lost more than we thought. After week 5, we were in total disbelief!

"JJ Virgin" is now a common family word. Scott went from 230 to 182, and I went from 168 to 135. The big thing was the clothing size difference. Yes, JJ! Thank you for my new wardrobe! I went from a size 12 to a 4 and Scott from a 38/40 to a 33/34. We have also participated in a couple of 5Ks with ease. We have lots more energy and feel wonderful.

Let's just say our family and friends are becoming "Virginized," too. Once the weight came off and seemed to be staying off, we went nuts. We had to tell everyone!

This is just amazing. I totally don't understand why in the world *The Virgin Diet* book isn't in every person's house! You are amazing!

### *My Original Virgin Diet Recipe*

## SPRING HALIBUT SPICY SOUP

*Serves 2 as a main course, or as a starter*

3 stalks celery, chopped into bite-sized pieces
½ red onion, finely chopped
1 head garlic, chopped (I love *garlic*!)
1 jalapeño, seeded and chopped
3 tablespoons Malaysian red palm fruit oil
2 cups organic vegetable stock
3 cups water
1 acorn squash, cut into bite-sized pieces
½ teaspoon ground cumin
3 teaspoons sea salt
½ teaspoon black pepper
½ teaspoon dried basil
1 sprig rosemary, leaves chopped
12 to 16 ounces halibut, cut into 2-inch pieces
Fresh cilantro leaves

Sauté the celery, onion, garlic, and jalapeño in the palm fruit oil in a 2-quart pot for 5 to 7 minutes. Add the vegetable stock and water to the pot. Next add the cut-up acorn squash and bring to a low boil. Cook until the squash is tender.

Add the cumin, sea salt, pepper, basil, and rosemary. Then add the fish and cook for 2 to 3 minutes, until cooked through. Place in bowls and top with the fresh cilantro.

To see Robin's interview, visit thevirgindietcookbook.com/bonus.

## RINSE AND REPEAT—REDO CYCLE 1 EVERY YEAR

Like the cathartic and energizing effects of a good spring cleaning, your system benefits from a fresh start, a purging of the clutter of bad habits that may have crept in and a return to the basics that springboarded your success. So I want you to redo Cycle 1 every 12 months as a purifying exercise. Don't forget, it's only 3 weeks!

## DO I HAVE TO LEAVE?

Since my book *The Virgin Diet* came out, many people have asked if there's a limit to how long they can stay in Cycle 1. The answer is—nope! You can stay in Cycle 1 the rest of your life, and why wouldn't you if you've lost the weight, you feel great, you look younger, and you don't miss any of those 7 foods (I told you you wouldn't!). You'll be much better off and there's no downside.

Whether or not you choose to live the full-out Virgin Diet for life, I still want you to go through Cycle 2. It's important that you find out which of the most potentially reactive foods, my high-FI four—gluten, soy, dairy, and eggs—require you to be hypervigilant, and which you can sneak back in here and there. You may learn that eggs can be rotated back into your diet, that you can use organic fermented soy occasionally, or that you can even have a little goat cheese on your salad. Fingers crossed!

Gluten may be another story since it's such a common irritant, so you will soon figure out how cautious you have to be with gluten. Personally, I believe you'll be better off with no gluten in your diet, but depending on your tolerance to it, you may be able to handle the occasional splash of soy sauce with wheat in it without repercussions. And let me beat this drum again, for good reason: Even if you showed no reactions to gluten and soy, I believe you're better off keeping them out of your diet 95 percent of the time, for the rest of time. Corn and peanuts don't even need to be retested because there's no question they should also stay out of your diet 95 percent of the time.

If you struggle with congestion or skin issues, you can probably connect those to dairy and keep it out long-term, too. Artificial sweeteners are a goner; banish them 100 percent, forever. And finally, my rule for sugar is to avoid obvious sugar traps, including energy bars, bagels, muffins, pasta sauce, frozen pizza, and salad dressings, and limit any prepared foods to 5 grams or less of added sugar, with less always being best (that goes for your smoothies, too!).

If you're specifically plagued by GI issues—indigestion, heartburn, gas and bloating, cramping or constipation—you could really benefit from additional support. To expedite your gut healing, I recommend some high-quality probiotics, digestive enzymes, and supportive nutrients including glutamine, n-acetyl glucosamine, quercetin, and ginger (see the Resources section, under "Virgin Diet Supplements").

If you're struggling with constipation, here are a few tips: Increase the amount of fiber you get every day, but be sure to do it over time, not overnight. Your goal should be 50 grams per day. This may take you several weeks to build up to—go slowly and increase your water intake as you do (drink throughout the day, including between meals). An easy place to start is to throw some extra fiber into your smoothies. And I've had amazing success in tackling constipation with magnesium citrate—a combination of magnesium and vitamin C. Both have laxative effects and are nutrients people are often deficient in.

## CYCLE 2

Cycle 2 covers 28 days. During each week of the cycle, you'll reintroduce one of those four potentially most reactive foods—gluten, soy, dairy, and eggs—back into your diet. The beauty of this cycle is that you're painting a picture of what a customized diet will look like for you going forward.

Who knows? Maybe only one food is an issue for you and you can eat the others worry-free. Eggs and dairy do have some health benefits. Wouldn't it be great to find out you can have them once in a while? Or that you don't have to be in DEFCON 5 worrying about gluten and soy 100 percent of the time?

But this is where the rubber meets the road: You're going to find out—and quickly—which ones are causing you problems, so you'll know which are out for good and which you can tolerate in small amounts.

Testing is the key step in identifying which food or foods are holding your weight hostage, draining your energy, and may even be hurting you. So I especially want to make sure that if you're reacting severely to something, it happens in a controlled environment where you can immediately know the culprit.

Of course, as with most things in life, timing matters. Since your body has healed, a reaction to one of these foods should be pretty easy to ferret out. And you already know that food intolerance responses can be immediate or take as long as 72 hours to show up. The minute they do show up, however, you're done. There's no need to keep the experiment going if you're reacting. The key is to tune in and track the symptoms you're having, because your body is sending you a message. The message is either "You can't have this now" (in which case you will rechallenge in 3 to 6 months to see if more gut healing fixes the issue) or "You can never have it," but either way, if you continue to eat the offender, weight will pile back on and your symptoms will be back in full force as your immune system kicks into chronic gear.

One final note on Cycle 2: When you're reintroducing, make healthy choices, such as organic eggs, Greek yogurt, sprouted breads, organic fermented soy, and the like. You can find more details on reintroduction in *The Virgin Diet*.

## CYCLE 3

Once you're lean and feeling great, you'll never want to go back. Cycle 3 is all about helping you stay in your new happy place; it's the road map for your new lifestyle. I call it your lifetime cycle.

It's also the cycle that rewards you for all the hard work you've done to get here! Sure, the way you look and feel is a reward in itself, but you can treat yourself once in a while now, too. You've earned it.

Of course, that doesn't mean all your rewards have to be about food! Pamper yourself occasionally with a mani-pedi or a massage, or take an afternoon off and go see a movie.

But 5 percent of the time you *can* splurge on forbidden foods—something that's really worth it—as long as you abide by my three-bite rule. Once or twice a week you can have something you wouldn't eat on this plan, as long as it isn't one of the foods you reacted badly to. But that's the limit: three polite bites and put the fork down. Otherwise, you're undoing a lot of good work and you're going to hate the view when you're at the starting line again. But when you do it right, you can indulge without any reason for guilt. This includes alcohol, which I get asked about frequently. Keep it out during Cycle 1, of course (sugar!), but long-term feel free to have a glass of wine (red is best) with dinner. I don't recommend you make a habit of it, though. Your health and weight are better off if you save it for that special evening out or dinner with friends rather than making it a nightly ritual.

Remember, the other 95 percent of the time, avoid gluten, soy, corn, peanuts, and sugar and artificial sweeteners, especially if you want to continue to lose weight and feel better. And here's some reason for hope if you're mourning the loss of a food that didn't agree with you in Cycle 2: Rechallenge any potentially healthy high-FI foods that you reacted to in Cycle 2 after 3 to 6 months, especially organic dairy and eggs. There's a possibility you'll be able to tolerate them after that much time has passed and your system has healed.

## KEEP A JOURNAL

I think I heard you groan when you read that. If you're fitful about this, you're not alone. But it's nonnegotiable. Why? Because I'm here to make sure you succeed, and keeping a journal of what you eat is an essential part of making that happen. A study in *Science Daily* in 2008 showed that participants who kept a food diary lost twice as much weight as those who didn't, and my own experience bears that out, too. Writing it down makes it real. You can download journal pages at www.thevirgindietcookbook .com/bonus. And here's an easy way to ensure that you actually do it: Hook up with an accountability partner. If there's someone in your family or a friend who can help, great. If not, connect with someone at thevirgindietcoach.com. We've created a great community and have pulled together support tools to amplify your success. See, easy!

---

### VIRGIN DIET SUCCESS

*Susan Johnson—Gilbert, AZ*

To date I have lost 58 pounds, and I owe that to *The Virgin Diet*. I've been overweight for my entire life, and in my adult years my weight problem transitioned to outright morbid obesity. Two years ago I was diagnosed with diabetes, my blood pressure was out of control, I had arthritis in all of my joints, and to top it all off my mobility was quickly becoming more and more limited. I was forced to use the electric cart in the grocery stores, and at other times, my family had to push me around in a wheelchair. I was on four very scary medications to control the diabetes, high blood pressure, and depression. I had tried every diet known to mankind and spent 20 or more years studying food and nutrition, trying to get a handle on my compulsive overeating, but nothing worked long-term.

---

I had given up and thought I might die. I was in pain all the time and couldn't do simple tasks without sitting down. I couldn't stand in the shower. I had to sit on the edge of the tub to bathe. I couldn't reach my feet. My self-esteem was very low, and I couldn't understand why I was unable to control my eating. I thought I had an eating disorder, and my family was afraid for my life. I saw a short segment about JJ and *The Virgin Diet* on the *Rachael Ray* show in late December of 2012. I had never heard of removing 7 foods from your diet before. When I saw the show, something in my heart said, "This is the answer you've prayed for!" and I knew that this was it.

I bought the book soon after and was captivated by it. I read it in 24 hours, and I began my Virgin Diet journey on January 13, 2013. It was that day I got my life back! From that point on my health progressively improved. I started to move more. I could stand for longer periods of time, and I lost weight!

The most amazing part for me is that the horrible cravings and binge-eating episodes are gone—simply *gone*—after 40 years of struggle. What an amazing miracle! Somewhere around the fortieth day or so, JJ posted on Facebook that she would be at a Whole Foods in my city. I made up my mind that I was going to *walk* into that store and shake her hand and *thank her* for saving my life. And that's what I did!

I am feeling even better now and have much less pain. I am walking and swimming several times a week. I have quite a lot more to lose, but I know that every extra pound is going to come off in due time. My family has been so encouraged by my progress. They are happy to have their wife, mother, grandmother, sister, and daughter back. My daughter, who inherited my food intolerances, has been inspired to start her own Virgin Diet, as have many other friends and family members. We have banded together on Facebook in a group called the Virgin Diet Support Team, where members share stories of their own successes! I am so proud of them. We are doing our part to give you your "million pounds," JJ!

### *My Original Virgin Diet Recipe*

## VIRGIN STUFFED MUSHROOMS

This dish is great as an appetizer but can also be used for the main course.

*Serves 3 to 4 as a main course*

12 to 14 large button mushrooms, stems removed (chop the stems), caps
    wiped clean

1 teaspoon sea salt

1 teaspoon freshly cracked black pepper

3 tablespoons olive oil (not extra-virgin)

1 medium onion, chopped

2 garlic cloves, minced

1 box frozen chopped spinach, thawed and squeezed dry

1 bunch kale, chopped

1 tablespoon coconut aminos

¼ teaspoon red pepper flakes

1 pound wild shrimp, chopped small

¼ cup almond butter

2 tablespoons whole flaxseeds

½ cup chopped walnuts

Preheat the oven to 350°F.

Season the mushroom caps with ½ teaspoon of the salt and ½ teaspoon of the pepper. Heat 1 tablespoon of the olive oil in a frying pan, add the mushroom caps, and sauté for a few minutes. Do not cook through. Remove from the pan and let cool.

Add 1 tablespoon of the olive oil to the pan and sauté the onion and garlic. Add the greens, coconut aminos, red pepper flakes, and chopped mushroom stems. Cook until the kale is softened and the onions are translucent. Season the shrimp with the remaining ½ teaspoon salt and ½ teaspoon pepper, add them to the pan, and cook until any liquid has evaporated and the shrimp have turned pink; do not overcook. Stir in the almond butter and flaxseeds.

Stuff the mushroom caps with this mixture, and place them in a baking pan coated with the remaining 1 tablespoon of olive oil. Top the mushrooms with the chopped nuts and bake for 30 minutes, until heated through and the nuts are toasty.

To see Susan's interview, visit thevirgindietcookbook.com/bonus.

## SUCCESS TASTES SO GOOD!

After you figure out which foods you can and can't tolerate, the key to ongoing success—whether you have more weight to lose or you just want to continue to look and feel younger—is in the planning. In the next couple of chapters I'll show you how to do that well, from assembling your meals to the golden rules of meal timing.

The recipes and ways of eating outlined in this cookbook will help you lose weight and feel better no matter where you live, if you love to eat out all the time, or if you travel a lot. These results don't belong just to the lucky, to winners of the genetic lottery or to Hollywood A-listers . . . they're yours for the taking, too!

## TOP SWAPS AND THE VIRGIN PLATE  2

Now that you understand the benefits of the Virgin Diet, it's time to look under the hood. I'm going to give you a framework and some tools to help you optimize the recipes in this cookbook for the fastest weight loss, energy boost, and healing.

## TOP SWAPS

A fun, easy place to start is by making swaps.

We've all been there. Just as you're being drawn in by the tractor beam of a gooey pecan pumpkin torte made by your best friend (who just happens to be a pastry chef), you suddenly remember the little black strapless dress hanging in the closet for that special night out, and a pang of regret surges through your veins. But eating smart doesn't mean you have to constantly deprive yourself or puritanically abstain from delicious foods.

That news is often the lightbulb moment; it's when people discover the difference between the Virgin Diet and all the other diets they've bounced among most of their adult lives. Diets are usually about deprivation, with little or no other guidance. And it makes you want what you can't have so badly!

I'm all about giving you better alternatives. So rather than tell people what they can't have and leaving it at that, I've developed what I call lateral shifts: healthier, satisfying substitutes for your favorite foods without the sugar or lingering guilt. You won't feel as though you're missing a thing, and you may even like the swaps better!

Here's a great example. Say you start your day with oatmeal or a protein smoothie. You probably make them with cow's milk, right? Well, even if you're not lactose intolerant, cow's milk can trigger acne, rosacea, and other skin conditions, not to mention the fact that it can stall fast fat loss. Unsweetened coconut milk, which is loaded with fat-burning medium-chain triglycerides (MCTs), makes the perfect lateral shift. Coconut milk can give you all of dairy's pleasure without the downsides of cow's milk. Unsweetened almond milk is another smart lateral shift from cow's milk. I switch between So Delicious unsweetened coconut milk and their new protein-rich almond milk in my Virgin Diet Shake every morning.

Are you a yogurt lover? If so, this news may hurt: Many fruit-on-the-bottom yogurts have as much sugar as a candy bar! Instead, I recommend stirring organic berries into coconut milk Greek-style yogurt. You can even find dairy-free, 1-gram-of-sugar-added coconut milk ice cream to satisfy your sweet tooth. Nothing too deprived about that!

Every meal can become an opportunity for a nourishing lateral shift. If you like to nosh on a wheat wrap stuffed with sliced turkey and avocado for lunch, sub out the wheat for a romaine lettuce wrap instead. You'll save calories and boost your nutrient and fiber intake. And who needs high-fructose corn syrup–loaded condiments like ketchup or barbecue sauce when you can use flavorful salsa or marinara?

Think creatively and you can make a lateral shift with just about any food. Once you get the hang of this, it can even become fun. Here are five of my favorite lateral shifts:

1. **Swap peanuts and peanut butter for almonds and almond butter.** Peanuts are legumes, not nuts, and they're susceptible to a mold that produces aflatoxin, a potential carcinogen. Many commercial peanut butters also come loaded with trans fats and high-fructose corn syrup. Besides being more nutrient-rich, almonds and almond butter are flat-out yummier than peanuts and peanut butter.

2. **Swap potatoes for faux-tatoes or sweet potatoes.** Are your kids begging for mashed potatoes with their grilled chicken and Brussels sprouts (hooray for you if your kids eat Brussels sprouts!)? Make a healthier choice by switching to faux-tatoes, a blend of pureed cauliflower and coconut milk. Or make baked sweet potato fries so the whole family can indulge in a guiltless French fry fix.

3. **Swap pasta for spaghetti squash.** Spaghetti squash is rich in fiber and nutrients compared to regular pasta, which can be just an addictive delivery sys-

tem for empty carbohydrates. Quinoa pasta (look for a certified gluten-free one with no corn) makes another nutrient-rich pasta alternative.

4. **Swap purchased hot chocolate for a healthier homemade version.** Everyone loves hot chocolate during the holidays, but those coffee shop cocoas can pack a 600-calorie punch. An easy switch is chocolate vegan protein powder with warm So Delicious unsweetened coconut milk. It is, well, so delicious.

5. **Swap wheat flour for almond or coconut flour.** Kids love chicken strips, but frozen and fast-food varieties contain gluten and damaged fats. Almond or coconut flour is a great way to coat their chicken with a much more nutritious crunch.

This cookbook will give you loads of tasty recipes that make lateral shifts for you, but sometimes it's helpful to have an at-a-glance cheat sheet to pull the 7 high-FI foods out of your daily diet as quickly and painlessly as possible. So just stick this handy reference on your fridge and you'll never be out of options:

### Gluten

Swap pasta for no-corn quinoa pasta or spaghetti squash.
Swap whole wheat wraps for rice wraps or lettuce leaves.
Swap glutenous grains for quinoa, amaranth, buckwheat, or wild or brown rice.
Swap crackers for brown rice crackers, kale chips, or bean chips.

### Soy

Swap soy milk for unsweetened coconut milk or almond milk.
Swap soy ice cream for no-sugar-added coconut milk ice cream.
Swap soy burgers for lentil burgers.

### Dairy

Swap cow's milk for unsweetened coconut milk or almond milk.
Swap cheese for cashew cheese.
Swap creamer for coconut milk creamer.
Swap ice cream for no-sugar-added coconut milk ice cream.
Swap cream cheese for hummus.
Swap butter for avocado or coconut butter.

### Eggs

Swap your omelet for a protein shake.

Swap your hard-boiled eggs for salmon or turkey jerky.

### Peanuts

Swap peanuts for raw, dehydrated or slow-roasted almonds, walnuts, pecans, macadamia nuts, or other tree nuts.

Swap peanut butter for almond or cashew butter.

### Corn

Swap popcorn for raw veggies.

Swap corn for lentils.

Swap corn chips for kale chips.

Swap corn tortillas for rice tortillas.

### Sugar and Artificial Sweeteners

Swap sugar for pure organic stevia, xylitol (corn-free), monk fruit, or an erythritol/stevia blend with no maltodextrin or flavoring.

Swap sugary dips for guacamole or salsa.

Swap sweetened store-bought salad dressings for extra-virgin olive oil and lemon juice.

Swap chocolate for dark chocolate containing 85 percent or higher cacao (5 grams of sugar or less per serving).

## THE GOLDEN RULES OF MEAL TIMING

When you eat and how long you go between meals really matters, especially for keeping your blood sugar nice and even. Constant grazing and overindulging are obvious culprits working against your weight loss, but skipping meals can be just as bad.

When you don't eat for a long time, your blood sugar drops. Setting aside the fact that you probably won't make a healthy choice when you're starving, when you finally get around to eating again you'll likely overindulge, spiking your blood sugar and causing a big insulin surge. Guess what that excess insulin does? It makes it easier for your body to store fat. Yikes! Plus, it can lead to much bigger problems like insulin resistance and diabetes.

You may have heard that eating five or six meals throughout the day is the best way to keep blood sugar stable, boost your metabolism, and help with appetite control. That might be the case if we're talking about five small meals of wild salmon and broccoli. But let's check in with reality here. What most people reach for as a snack is usually a refined-high-carb treat that raises their blood sugar and triggers an insulin response, which in turn shuts off fat burning. The truth is, when you're eating balanced meals of clean, lean protein; healthy fats; loads of non-starchy veggies; and a small amount of slow low carbs, you need only three meals a day (and possibly a snack if you're going more than 4 to 6 hours between meals). And remember to drink water throughout the day, especially between meals; often we aren't really hungry anyway, we're actually thirsty! More meals usually just means more chances to overeat, and while I don't want you to focus on calorie counting as much as I want you to be concerned about where those calories come from, too much healthy food is also unhealthy. So even if you're making good choices, you don't need to be grazing all day long!

Three balanced, filling meals (and one optional snack) a day are enough to keep us satisfied and ensure that our bodies are fueled between feedings, so they don't go into starvation mode and start holding on to fat.

Here's how the timing of those three meals breaks out:

- Eat a substantial breakfast within an hour of waking up. If you're a skipper, remember what I said about blood sugar. You're doing yourself physical harm and impeding your weight loss efforts. Routine breakfast skippers tend to be fatter and lead a less healthy lifestyle than people who regularly eat breakfast. So I'm asking you to add a meal to your day and telling you you'll lose weight and feel better in the bargain. That can't make you too unhappy!
- Eat every 4 to 6 hours, and have a snack if you need it.
- Close the kitchen and stop eating 3 hours before bed (no, this does not mean you can just go to bed later!). Ideally, I'd like you to have at least a 12-hour span between dinner and breakfast to allow insulin to return to fasting levels so your body can use stored fat for fuel. So if you insist on skipping a meal, dinner is the one to blow off—not breakfast.

## THE VIRGIN PLATE

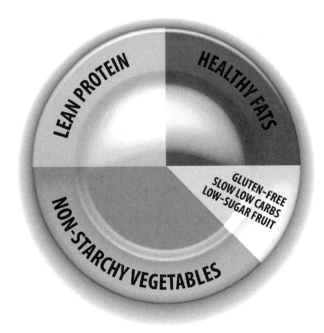

*This is the ideal balance that you are striving for on your plate at each meal.*

I designed the Virgin Plate to make sure you're getting all the nutrition you need and optimizing your fat-burning machinery at every meal. When you eat according to the Virgin Plate, as this cookbook will help you do, you'll find it easily keeps you full and happy so you can eat one of the three balanced meals every 4 to 6 hours without feeling deprived of a thing.

Specifically, each meal should include:

- 1 serving of clean, lean protein (e.g., fish, chicken, turkey, grass-fed beef)

  *Serving size:*
  - Women should eat 4 to 6 ounces at each meal; larger or more athletic women can bump it up to 6 to 8 ounces.
  - Men should eat 6 to 8 ounces at every meal, and larger or very athletic men should be closer to 10 ounces.

- Also lean toward the higher end of the ranges if you are recovering from surgery or healing from an injury, if you're very athletic, or if you're actively working to put on muscle.

■ 1 to 3 servings of healthy fats

*Serving size:*

- Examples are 1 tablespoon olive oil, ¼ small avocado, 4 ounces coldwater fish, 10 nuts, 1 tablespoon nut butter, 5 olives.
- Be sure to count fat from protein, so if you're having grass-fed beef or fish, count it as a fat serving, too.

■ 2+ servings of non-starchy vegetables

*Serving size:*

- ½ cup cooked or 1 cup raw
- More is better—eat at least 5 servings a day; you can always increase the portion size of your non-starchy vegetables. My ultimate goal for you is *10* servings a day!

■ 0 to 2 servings of high-fiber starchy carbs

*Serving size:*

- Examples are ½ cup cooked beans or rice, ½ small sweet potato, or 1 piece of fruit.
- Please keep fruit to 2 servings of low- or medium-sugar fruit per day (and avoid fruit juice entirely). Your genetics, your activity level, and your metabolism determine how many high-fiber starchy carbs you can handle before you start to feel lousy. Generally speaking, people under stress do better with a bit more of them, and those who are insulin resistant or diabetic do better with less. When in doubt, err on the side of less and gauge how you feel. This is a perfect example of why journaling is so important!

The recipes in this cookbook are designed to be as easy to make as they are delicious. So rest assured that building meals based on the Virgin Plate will become second nature in no time. But just in case you had any doubts, here are some extra tips to make sure you'll spend as little time in the kitchen as possible and more time out and about enjoying how good you look and feel!

- Make quick one-plate meals—bowls, soups, wraps, and salads.
- Keep it easy and use leftovers. Last night's chicken will be great for today's lunch.
- Make substitutions; replace a good fat with another good fat from the "optimal choices" list on page 47.
- Leftover veggies? Toss them into a soup or bowl.
- Add a salad or crudités to any meal—you can even have one or both with your smoothie; the more non-starchy veggies, the better.

## VIRGIN DIET SUCCESS

### *Laura Kiel—Auburn, WA*

I have struggled with a lifetime of weight issues, and have lost over 75 pounds many times. I have tried nearly all systems and even hypnosis. Finally, after a lifetime of struggle and being diagnosed with diabetes, I had lap band surgery and achieved my after-surgery goal weight of 175 pounds, and then lost an additional 10 pounds after that. I was able to keep the weight off for 2 years. However, my diet consisted of potatoes, pasta, and, generally, Cream of Wheat for dinner. I was unable to eat meat, vegetables, or fruit successfully. Finally I became so hungry for vegetables and fruit that I purchased a Vitamix so that I could make smoothies. They tasted fabulous. I had a smoothie every day, along with the other foods that were easy to swallow.

My band opening was approximately the size of a drinking straw. I was required to crush my medications, as it was impossible to swallow them whole. In order to be able to swallow the crushed pills, I masked them with 9 packets of Splenda. In addition to that I drank several cups of coffee a day with 2 packets of Splenda each. I even put it in my smoothies! All told, I was consuming at least 25 packets of Splenda a day.

Additionally, my weight was beginning to climb up at a rate of about a pound a week because I was experiencing extreme GERD (gastroesophageal reflux disease). The surgeon who had placed the band determined that with the amount of acid reflux I was having, it was dangerous and even life-threatening to continue to have the band tightened. So he opened the band up and said that I would gain weight, and that once my esophagus had healed a bit I could have the band retightened. Additionally, at that time my blood pressure was 189/92 and my average glucose was 189. I began studying nutrition as I had no intention of being a victim of diabetes.

My family and I began soaking up information. We eventually came upon JJ Virgin and made a 100 percent commitment to this lifestyle. If you were to see the charts of my glucose readings, and my weight loss chart, it would be easy to see exactly when we began the Virgin Diet and how it has changed my life. Last night my before-dinner glucose was 98!!!!! In addition, I have been able to eliminate one blood pressure medication and will begin eliminating a second one soon. I have every expectation I'll be off all blood pressure medication before long.

I am also completely off all artificial sweeteners. This was a big struggle for me as I was so dependent upon them. I was on two Prilosec tablets a day and now I don't take any. I took Ex-lax and Gas-X every day after having lap band surgery. These products are no longer needed in my life. I was on allergy medication and now no longer need that, either. I took 10 mg of Ambien every night for sleep, and I now sleep perfectly with no medication at all.

The change in my health is nothing short of miraculous, and my husband and daughter are both on this program as well. My daughter is a runner, and was astonished that she has lost over 20 pounds on this program and feels better than she ever has. My husband is off allergy medication and has also lost 17 pounds. What he likes best is how delicious and plentiful the beautiful foods are. He supported me completely with the lap band procedures, but eating Cream of Wheat almost every night pales in comparison to the bounty of food we eat now.

## My Original Virgin Diet Recipe

## LASAGNA

*Serves 8 generously*

It's hard to believe this lasagna recipe has *no pasta, no cheese, no dairy, no eggs,* and is packed with plenty of great nutrition. This looks, tastes, and satisfies like any delicious lasagna should. Enjoy!

2 heads cauliflower
1 spaghetti squash

*continued*

2 tomatoes

1 onion

2 red bell peppers

4 garlic cloves

8 fresh basil leaves

4 sprigs rosemary

2 tablespoons olive oil

2 pounds ground organic grass-fed beef

¼ cup chia seeds

3 tablespoons flaxseeds

Sea salt

Freshly cracked black pepper

2 packages sliced chicken breast (organic, no nitrates or antibiotics); I like Applegate

2 cups sliced mushrooms

4 tomato slices, for garnish

Preheat the oven to 435°F.

Steam the 2 heads of cauliflower, drain, and set aside. Cut the spaghetti squash in halves or quarters and place facedown in a pot containing one inch of boiling water. Steam the spaghetti squash until it easily pulls away from its shell with a fork, approximately 20 minutes, set aside, and let cool. Place the tomatoes, onion, bell peppers, garlic, basil, rosemary, and 1 tablespoon of the olive oil in a roasting pan. Roast for 30 minutes, until the vegetables are browned, and set aside. Reduce the oven temperature to 375°F.

Brown the beef in a large pot or pressure cooker using the remaining 1 tablespoon olive oil.

Remove the leaves from the rosemary sprigs. Place all the roasted vegetables and the rosemary leaves in a high-speed blender and blend into a tomato-pepper "marinara" sauce. Incorporate this marinara sauce into the ground beef and add the chia seeds and flaxseeds. Add salt and pepper to taste, and cook for desired time. (I enjoy letting the flavors meld together so I prefer a long cook time, but it is also delicious if you just incorporate the ingredients and then immediately put the lasagna together.)

Blend the cauliflower into a puree in a high-speed blender. Shred the spaghetti squash into threads by using a fork to pull the squash away from the skin. Stir the cauliflower and spaghetti squash together. (This is what I use in place of cheese.)

Begin layering your lasagna in a roasting pan (I use a pan just a bit smaller than the traditional 9 x 13-inch baking pan and it makes a very generous serving) in this order:

Layer 1: One-third of the meat marinara sauce

Layer 2: 1 package of the roasted chicken slices, spread into a layer. This becomes my "lasagna noodles."

Layer 3: 1 cup of the sliced mushrooms

Layer 4: Half of the cauliflower/spaghetti squash mixture

Repeat the layers and finish with the meat/marinara sauce as the top layer. Top with the 4 tomato slices, cut in half, for decoration. Bake in the oven for 45 minutes. Let sit for 20 minutes before serving so the lasagna can set up a bit.

To see Laura's interview, visit thevirgindietcookbook.com/bonus.

## FOOD'S EFFECT ON BLOOD SUGAR

As you begin to pay more attention to what you eat and how it impacts your weight, your energy, and how you look and feel, it's worth having a general understanding of how food affects your blood sugar levels. The traditional way to grasp those effects has been through the yardstick of the glycemic index.

You may at least be familiar with the term; maybe you've heard it in reference to certain foods that have a lower glycemic impact. Or you may even know someone who's following a low-glycemic diet recommended by a doctor.

The glycemic index determines, on a numerical scale from 0 to 100, how a particular carbohydrate affects your body's blood sugar when you consume 50 grams of it alone. Scientists assigned glucose a rating of 100, and all other foods are measured against it. The higher a food's glycemic index, the more pronounced an effect it has on your blood sugar, and the more stressful it is to your insulin system.

Here is the gist of the way macronutrients rate:

- Carbohydrates (starches and sugars) have the greatest effect, particularly low-fat and/or low-fiber and more-processed foods.
- Fat has a glycemic effect of zero. Think of it as neutral.
- Protein generally balances the effects of carbohydrates as it causes the release of glucagon and insulin, which help keep blood sugar stable.

■ Fiber also lowers a food's glycemic index because the fiber itself isn't digested and it slows the rise of blood sugar.

Unfortunately, it's impossible to know a full meal's overall glycemic index because you rarely eat one food in isolation, nor do you usually eat 50 grams of a particular food. Sure, you might eat 50 grams of potato, but not 50 grams of carrots (that would be 1½ pounds of carrots!).

## The Glycemic Index vs. Glycemic Load

There is a more thoughtful approach that mitigates the limitations of the glycemic index. It's known as the glycemic load. The glycemic load looks at the actual amount of specific foods you eat in any given meal and calculates the overall effect of that meal's carbohydrates on your blood sugar. You can determine glycemic load by multiplying the glycemic index of a food by the amount of carbs in it and dividing by 100. Let's walk through it.

Let's say a carrot has a glycemic index of 92 and 4 grams of carbohydrates. Its glycemic load, then, is .92 x 4, or 3.68. Mashed potatoes, on the other hand, have a glycemic index of 98 with 37 grams of carbohydrates, so the GL is .98 x 37, or 36.26. Just as with the glycemic index, the lower the glycemic load, the better.

That part seems pretty straightforward, right? But here's the salient point: When you eat according to the Virgin Diet Plate, you're mixing the right kinds (and amounts) of carbohydrates, protein, and fats. And that's important because the hormonal impact of protein can offset some of the insulin impact of carbohydrates. So while the glycemic index can be important, the glycemic load, as well as the balance of the calories consumed, is much more important.

Now that you've got a handle on all that, I'm going to throw you a curveball. There's one type of sugar that registers low on the glycemic index but—counterintuitively—is the most detrimental of all. And that sugar is fructose. I do a deep dive on fructose in *The Virgin Diet*, but let me serve up the Cliffs Notes for you here. Fructose is metabolized differently than other sugars. It makes a beeline straight for your liver, which almost single-handedly bears the burden of dealing with it. And the liver does that by metabolizing the fructose and storing it as fat.

That's horror enough, but fructose also fails to raise leptin, a hormone that functions to tell you that because you just ate, you're full and you should stop eating. So what you can deduce is that when you ingest fructose, which is *low* on the glycemic index, you are consuming a sugar that makes you fat and hungry. It's also the most atherogenic of all sugars, meaning it contributes to plaque buildup in your arteries, and it can trigger insulin resistance and metabolic syndrome. But wait, there's more! Fructose goes through a process called glycation (when protein binds to sugar without the need of enzymes) seven to ten times more than other sugars. The result is substances called advanced glycation end products (AGEs!), which lead to accelerated aging. Eek!

So while the glycemic load can provide some guidance, ideally, I'd like you to focus on the *impact* the sugar is having on you. That makes intuitive sense, right? If you stick with foods low in fructose with a low glycemic load, you'll be fine. Foods and sweeteners with a high glycemic load (i.e., 20 and above) and those high in fructose (high-fructose corn syrup, agave, fruit juice concentrate, and juice) should be avoided.

All of that aside, here's the bottom line on the glycemic index, glycemic load, and fructose: Eat whole, unprocessed foods. If you simply stick with lean protein, plenty of non-starchy veggies, fibrous carbs like lentils and beans, and good fats such as coconut oil and olive oil, you'll be eating in a way that helps you lose weight fast, keeps your energy high, and keeps your blood sugar stable. And a very easy way to do that is to just follow the recipes in this book!

## VIRGIN DIET SUCCESS

### *Tamara George—Brentwood, TN*

The Virgin Diet experience was life-changing for me. I was overweight and struggling with health issues. After the Virgin Diet I feel and look 100 percent better. I was going around in circles before I tried the Virgin Diet; now I'm headed toward the straight and narrow and loving it!

My weight loss on the diet has impacted the lives of my family so much that my husband, who is an avid health and fitness guy, now turns to me for his daily Virgin Shake. My friends all want to try the Virgin Diet. They can't believe that I simply changed my eating habits, include a 1-hour workout five days a week, and try to get at least 8 hours of sleep. Granted, with my schedule, it's not always easy, but the good part is that I get to start over every day and get it right.

Tamara "Taj" Johnson-George is a member of the Grammy-nominated R&B trio Sisters With Voices, which is currently featured on the reality show *SWV: Sisters With Voices* on WE TV.

## *My Original Virgin Diet Recipe*

## TAJ'S CHICKEN TENDERS

*Serves 4*

My husband and son love to eat fried chicken. I couldn't expect them to give up on their favorites without a fight. Instead, I changed their unhealthy favorites into healthier options. That's when I came up with my Chicken Tenders—they love it and it has half the calories of regular fried chicken.

4 (6-ounce) organic free-range chicken breasts
1 to 2 tablespoons Dijon mustard
1 cup brown rice flour
½ teaspoon ground cumin
½ teaspoon cayenne pepper (or more if you'd like!)
1 teaspoon sea salt, or to taste
3 to 4 tablespoons organic coconut oil or olive oil

Cut each breast into 4 "tenders." Put the chicken into a bowl, add the mustard, and toss until all pieces are lightly coated.

In a plastic bag, combine the flour, cumin, cayenne, and salt. Add half the tenders. Shake until all are coated, and remove from the flour. Shake the other half of the tenders.

Preheat your skillet with half of the oil, and add half of the tenders. (You do not want to crowd the pan, so you will have to do it in two batches.) Cook over medium heat. Turning to cook on all sides, cook until the tenders are golden brown and the chicken is cooked through. Add the rest of the oil (or as necessary) and cook the second batch.

JJ's note: You can spice these up for variety by using Italian seasoning instead of cumin and cayenne. For a tasty dipping sauce, see my Finger-Lickin'-Good Barbecue Sauce (page 210).

To see Tamara's interview, visit thevirgindietcookbook.com/bonus.

## HEAL THYSELF

I know many of you are here because you've learned that the Virgin Diet will get you off the merry-go-round of traditional, ineffective deprivation diets and finally help you lose weight, fast. Yes! For that, you've come to the right place. But one of the surprising bonuses of the Virgin Diet is that you'll also be eating foods that *heal* you. Just as Hippocrates said, food can be your medicine. That's right—the idea that food has healing properties has been around for a *very* long time, and it's embraced by cultures throughout the world. And today we have more research to support it than ever before.

Food can restore your energy, balance your hormones, reduce inflammation, relieve your achy joints, pull you out of the doldrums, reduce your cholesterol, and fight cancer. Just a little motivation to choose wisely, huh? Yes, you'll love having the weight pour off your body and the fact that you can slip into smaller-size clothes, but I guarantee the *wow!* of how you feel will make you want to eat this way for the rest of your life.

So here are my top food choices for healing and feeling fantastic. You'll notice some crossover with my top swaps, and some are also foods I recommend for fast fat loss, so if a food appears on more than one list, it's safe to say I hope you get it on your plate immediately!

**Coconut milk**—Coconut milk is dairy-free and is easy to digest even if you have digestive problems. It's anti-bacterial, anti-fungal (because it's rich in yeast-killing caprylic acid) and anti-viral, so it's a powerful immune system booster. It stabilizes blood sugar and is anti-inflammatory. It also helps dry skin and hair and nourishes the thyroid gland.

**Aloe juice**—Aloe juice can act as a laxative, lower blood sugar, soothe skin disorders, and raise the secretory immunoglobulin A (IgA), meaning it protects your gut and mucosal surfaces (your skin on the inside). And yes, it is a juice, but it is a vegetable juice and very low in sugar, so the benefits are worth it!

**Apples**—Apples have long been a part of our healing lexicon; we all know one a day "keeps the doctor away." Why? Apples contain pectins that heal the gut; they also contain compounds that both help ward off arterial plaque and contribute to keeping your brain healthy.

**Fresh garlic**—Garlic kills off bad bacteria and has been shown to reduce inflammation, which is widely acknowledged as a precursor to diseases from diabetes to cancer.

**Red onions**—These powerful vegetables are a rich source of quercetin, an antioxidant that fights damage caused by free radicals. They also contain high amounts of sulfur, which helps rebuild collagen and purify the liver.

**Oregano leaves**—Oregano leaves are anti-fungal and anti-bacterial. Plus, they're dense with antioxidants and pack a vitamin K punch.

**Grass-fed beef**—The most specific benefit of grass-fed beef over commercially raised, hormone- and antibiotic-laced meat is that it is high in omega-3 fatty acids, which help prevent heart disease and bolster the immune system. It's also lower in both total and saturated fat than its feedlot brethren, and it contains a fatty acid called CLA (conjugated linoleic acid) that has been shown to be an effective fat burner!

**Free-range poultry**—Pastured hens have been shown to have higher levels of omega-3 fatty acids, higher levels of vitamins A and E, and less fat and cholesterol than caged birds.

**Wild cold-water fish**—Salmon is one of the most popular fish in this category, though all are rich sources of protein and omega-3 fatty acids. The omega-3s' anti-inflammatory properties are beneficial for heart health and may serve to prevent diabetes and Alzheimer's.

**Cruciferous vegetables**—This category of veggies includes broccoli, cauliflower, and Brussels sprouts. They're all packed with vitamins, including A, C, folic acid, and K, and the minerals calcium and potassium. Eat up—they may help reduce your risk of cancer!

**Leafy green vegetables**—You'll find kale, spinach, arugula, and collard greens in this power-healing category of water-rich vegetables. They're filled with fiber, amino acids, phytochemicals, and antioxidants—all of which serve to nourish and reenergize your body and slow the aging process. Wait till you see how they make your skin and hair glow, too!

**Berries**—Berries are the deal! Strawberries, blueberries, blackberries, raspberries, cranberries…if it's a berry, it gets a high healing grade. They're high in vitamin C, minerals, and phytochemicals and are chock-full of powerful antioxidants and anti-inflammatories. That means berries should be a go-to source for cleansing toxins, reducing the aging effects of free radicals, lowering your cholesterol, reducing your risk of diabetes, slowing aging, and improving cognitive function. Need I say more?

**Slow-roasted or dehydrated nuts and seeds**—Like many of the other healing foods on my list, nuts like almonds, walnuts, and Brazil nuts, and seeds like pumpkin and hemp, are rich sources of protein, fiber, healthy fats, antioxidants, and vitamins and minerals. They're also effective soldiers against free radicals, inflammation, and aging. Soaking and then slow-roasting or dehydrating makes them easier to digest and lowers the anti-nutrient lectins and phytates.

**Extra-virgin olive oil**—The anecdotal evidence of the ancient power of olive oil is now supported by loads of research, most of which shows that the monounsaturated, heart-healthy fats in olive oil reduce inflammation. Olive oil is also loaded with vitamins A and E and amino acids, so it aids in the repair of connective tissue and contributes to healthy, glowing skin.

**Green tea**—Research indicates that green tea reduces inflammation and the risk of cancer, stroke, and heart disease. It's rich in quercetin, nature's antihistamine. And as if that's not enough, it also boosts metabolism and supports fat burning. Recent studies show that green tea may help prevent type 2 diabetes and osteoporosis.

**Flaxseeds**—Flaxseeds are a prize source of omega-3 fatty acids, especially for vegetarians. They're also high in fiber, which aids digestion and keeps you full longer, and they're a great source of antioxidants. They're recommended for everything from soothing and healing the gut to preventing heart disease. Be sure to grind them so that you can reap all of their benefits.

**Chia seeds**—Like flaxseeds, chia seeds are one of the best plant-based sources of omega-3 fatty acids. That means they're effective in reducing inflammation, enhancing brain function, and lowering cholesterol. They're high in minerals that contribute to energy metabolism and weight control. As a rich source of antioxidants, they also fight free radicals in the body, and the fiber in chia seeds helps regulate digestion and bowel function.

**Quinoa**—Quinoa is an ancient power food and, to many people's surprise, is a seed, not a grain. It's a highly regarded source of protein that is loaded with amino acids. It's packed with fiber, contains enough riboflavin (vitamin $B_2$) to have a positive impact on brain and muscle cell metabolism, and is a notable source of iron.

**Legumes**—Beans, peas, and lentils are strong choices for getting soluble (cholesterol-lowering) and insoluble (digestion-supporting) fiber into your diet. They're also high in protein and rich in folic acid, copper, iron, and magnesium; and they contain pre-biotics, which encourage beneficial bacteria growth in your gut. Best of all, they help even out your blood sugar.

**Sweet potatoes**—Sweet potatoes have twice as much fiber as other potatoes and a ton of vitamin $B_6$ (which keeps arteries flexible and healthy). They're a valuable source of vitamins C and D, and they have enough potassium to lower your blood pressure. Sweet!

## FOOD CATEGORIES

Even when you're eating whole, unprocessed foods, some choices are better than others, especially when viewed through the lens of accelerating your fat loss and reviving your health. So take the extra step of familiarizing yourself with my top choices for protein, fats, non-starchy vegetables, high-fiber starchy carbohydrates, and fruit. Or at least keep this crib sheet close by for quick reference; it's an easy way to make sure you're optimizing your efforts and getting the best possible results!

**Optimal Protein Choices★**
Cold-water fish and shellfish—wild salmon, Alaskan halibut, sole, sardines, wild
    scallops
Game—venison
Lamb
Lean chicken
Lean red meats—beef, bison
Lean turkey
Pork
Vegan proteins, including pea, hemp, rice, potato, cranberry, and chlorella

★Choose free-range, cage-free, grass-fed, and no-hormone-added sources of protein whenever possible, and avoid farm-raised fish. Avoid fish at risk for medium or high levels of the toxic heavy metal mercury.

## Optimal Fat Choices

Avocados

Chia seeds

Coconut milk or oil

Cold-water, wild fish

Freshly ground flaxseeds

Grass-fed ghee*

Macadamia nut oil

Malaysian red palm fruit oil

Olives and olive oil

Soaked and low-roasted or dehydrated nuts and seeds (not peanuts), and nut butters

## Optimal Non-Starchy Vegetable Choices

Arugula

Asparagus

Bamboo shoots

Bean sprouts

Beet greens

Bell peppers (red, yellow, green)

Broccoli

Brussels sprouts

Cabbage

Cassava

Cauliflower

Celery

Chicory

Chives

Collard greens

Coriander

Cucumbers

Dandelion greens

Eggplants

Endive

Fennel

Garlic

Green beans

Jalapeño peppers

Kale

Kohlrabi

Leeks

Lettuce

Mushrooms

Mustard greens

Onions

Parsley

Radicchio

Radishes

Shallots

Shirataki noodles

Spaghetti squash

Spinach

Summer squash

Swiss chard

Turnip greens

Watercress

Zucchini

## Allowable High-Fiber Starchy Carbohydrate Choices**

Adzuki beans

Amaranth

Artichokes

Black beans

Brown and wild rice (be sure they're not GMO)

Brown rice pasta

Brown rice wraps

Buckwheat

*Ghee is also known as clarified butter. It doesn't contain any milk solids (where the potentially reactive protein molecules of regular butter live), so it's safe to consume even in Cycle 1.

**Ideally, buy beans dry, then rinse and soak them. Otherwise, be sure they are organic and packed in BPA-free cans.

Carrots
Chickpeas (garbanzo
    beans)
Cowpeas
French beans
Great Northern beans
Jicama (raw)
Kidney beans
Leeks

Legumes
Lentils
Lima beans
Millet
Mung beans
Navy beans
Okra
Pinto beans
Pumpkin

Quinoa pasta
Split peas
Squash—acorn,
    butternut, other
    winter varieties
Sweet potatoes or yams
Tomatoes
Turnips
White beans

## Optimal Fruit Choices

Fruit always raises a question mark: There's sugar in fruit, and we're cutting out sugar. But isn't fruit healthy? What's the deal?

One of the two sugars in fruit, fructose, is often simply called "fruit sugar." Earlier we touched on the harmful effects of fructose metabolism; it can be stored as fat in the liver and can wreak havoc on your metabolism. Excess amounts of fructose have also been linked to insulin resistance, diabetes, and obesity.

But the fundamental difference between fructose in fruit and the fructose you eat as high-fructose corn syrup in processed foods is that fruits are also rich in fiber, which slows down—and even reduces—the absorption of fructose. HFCS, on the other hand, without that fiber antidote, stresses out your liver, packs on pounds, and sets the metabolic stage for decay and disease.

Still, even with fruit, it's important to be selective about the kinds and amount you eat. To guide you, I've divided fruit choices into low-, medium-, and high-sugar fruits. The list reflects an update to the list in *The Virgin Diet*, with an even more finely tuned consideration of fructose content. As a general rule, though, your best bet will always be berries, as they are low in overall sugar and high in fiber and phytonutrients.

## Low-Sugar Fruit: Best Choices

Avocados

Berries—blackberries, blueberries, boysenberries, elderberries, gooseberries, loganberries, raspberries, strawberries

Cherries

Grapefruit

Guava
Lemons
Limes
Star fruit

**Medium-Sugar Fruit**

Apples

Apricots

Kiwi fruit

Melons

Nectarines

Oranges

Passion fruit

Peaches

Pears

Persimmons

Plums

Tangerines

**High-Sugar Fruit**

Think of these as "dessert," to be used sparingly in Cycle 3:

Bananas
Grapes
Mangoes
Papayas
Pineapple
Watermelon

# FIBER

You may not have noticed that each of the food categories—and all of my recipes—is designed to make sure you're getting enough fiber. Fiber, the part of plant-based foods that our bodies can't digest, is your weight loss secret weapon. It doesn't provide us with any nutrition or calories, but high-fiber, water-rich foods make us feel full on fewer calories than foods with a deficit of fiber, like meat, dairy products, and refined grains. And because it hangs out in our stomachs longer than other food, fiber slows down our digestion and makes that full feeling last longer. And here's a bonus: Fiber also helps fat zoom through our digestive systems, so less of it is absorbed. And finally, fiber feeds the good bacteria in our guts, which helps keep the bad bacteria at bay, supports a healthy immune system, and helps us absorb nutrients.

My goal is to have you eat 50 grams of fiber a day. But if you're like most people, you're probably currently eating only 5 to 14 grams a day, so be patient on this path. It may take you 2 to 3 weeks to get there. Don't try to go from 5 grams to 50 grams too quickly. The idea is for you to increase fiber over time, not overnight. If you start pounding fiber and ramp up too fast, you'll run the risk of gas, bloating, diarrhea, or constipation. And you will not be happy.

So what are some simple ways to gradually increase your fiber? Start by eating more whole foods and fewer processed foods. Nuts and seeds, beans (especially lentils), berries, and non-starchy vegetables are all fabulous sources of fiber. I also encourage you to toss a fiber blend, chia seeds, or freshly ground flaxseeds into your morning shake. When you're adding those things consistently, you'll find you're easily getting 50 grams of fiber a day.

One key component of this process is that as you increase your fiber, you must—*must*—increase your water intake. It's critical that you keep everything moving smoothly through your digestive pipes, and that you have quality poops that you can be proud of.

## MORE ABOUT WATER

I bet when I tell you I want to talk about water, you hear Charlie Brown's teacher in your head. Okay, water may not be a topic that gets your juices flowing, but for fat loss—which is the goal—and for a lot of other good metabolic reasons, it's worth knowing something about.

Your body should be about 70 percent water, but dehydration can drop that number to 50 to 60 percent. When that happens, your metabolism slows down, your stress hormones rise, and your body's inflammation increases, which can result in weight loss resistance.

I know many of you want to believe that you can meet your water quota with coffee, tea, and other similar liquids. The truth is that besides being diuretics, coffee, tea, and soft drinks are highly acidic and actually dehydrate you. You need to drink even more water to overcome their dehydrating effects. Sodas, especially diet ones, shouldn't even be in the picture.

You may know that by the time you realize you're thirsty, it's too late—you're already dehydrated. So to avoid having it go that far, sip water throughout the day. And find ways to make it second nature; always have water within arm's reach. Ditch the expensive designer water in plastic bottles, and instead carry a reusable bottle and keep it full. No matter where you are or how you're spending your time, you're not going to have any trouble finding places to fill up.

If regular filtered water doesn't thrill you, try sparkling water in glass bottles with a little lime (sassy!). I love spa water with cucumbers, oranges, lemon, lime, and maybe a little mint or basil. You might also consider putting a water filter on every tap in your home and tracking your water intake in your food journal. Remember that what you monitor, you can improve.

Water does an awesome job of curbing hunger, too, and tossing 5 to 10 grams of fiber into a glass of water 30 to 60 minutes before you eat will make you much less likely to reach for seconds.

Believe it or not, as simple as water seems, there's a method to making it work for you. Here's the water schedule I recommend you adhere to for the best results:

- Within 30 minutes of waking up: 8 to 16 ounces
- 30 to 60 minutes before each meal (reduces appetite): 8 ounces
- During a meal: limit to 4 to 8 ounces
- Start drinking water again 60 minutes after each meal.
- Between meals: 16 ounces or more
- Before bed: 8 ounces (shuts down midnight hunger pangs)

Notice that the only time I really want you to limit how much water you drink is during meals, when too much water can dilute stomach enzymes that break down protein. Otherwise, drink up!

If you're wondering how much water is right for you, there are no hard-and-fast rules. The standard rule of thumb is to drink the amount of water equal to half of your weight in ounces, so if you weigh 150 pounds, the reasoning goes that your target water intake would be 75 ounces a day. Of course, this equation doesn't work so well once you get outside of the normal weight range.

An easier, more common recommendation is to drink eight 8-ounce glasses a day. Even though I've gotten push-back on this more times than I can count, with people quick to say there's no science to support it, here's the deal. We don't need double-blind, placebo-based studies to verify that water is essential for good health. We know how important it is. So ignore the naysayers and drink *at least* 64 ounces a day. If you're heavier, live in a hot climate, or exercise rigorously, you need to increase that amount. Simple, easy, and important.

I'm not alone in saying this. The Institute of Medicine (IOM) released a report that made some general recommendations of 91 ounces (that's 11-plus cups a day) for women and 125 ounces (15-plus cups a day) for men. Their guidelines reference *total* fluid intake, including fluid from all food and beverages. And that usually breaks down this way: Approximately 80 percent of our water comes from specifically drinking water and other beverages, and the other 20 percent comes from food such as fruits and veggies, which are mostly water.

Assuming these percentages are accurate for most of us, the IOM report recommended that women take in approximately 9 cups of water daily and that men get 12½ cups. Exercise, pregnancy and breast-feeding, and high altitude can all increase our need for fluids by 1 to 3 cups a day.

## HEADING CHALLENGES OFF AT THE PASS

I'm thrilled you're setting yourself up for success by reading and cooking from this book! But sometimes just following the plan isn't enough; there are times when you have to give a little thought as to how you'll stay the course if your schedule changes, or you don't have access to your own fridge, or your kids are lobbying hard for mac and cheese. As with most challenges, these are totally manageable opportunities to be creative and have some fun.

### 10 Strategies to Make the Virgin Diet Work Anywhere

Convenience and availability often trump food quality and healthiness on the road. But that doesn't mean you shouldn't even try to fight the urge to dive into the chili-cheese fries during your two-hour flight delay. There are ways to eat smart when you travel so you not only stay on track with your weight loss, but you also won't have to deal with the physical and emotional crash that follows an empty carb binge. Here are 10 simple rules for averting dietary disaster when you dine out.

1. **Mix and match.** Give the entire menu a once-over when you sit down. Let's say you'd like to choose the salmon but it comes with garlic-cheddar risotto. The

Parmesan-encrusted fillet, on the other hand, comes with spinach sautéed in olive oil and garlic. Politely ask your server to switch the sides. Solved!

2. **Start your meal with a salad.** Keep it simple and dress it with olive oil and vinegar or fresh lemon juice. It's a healthy starter worth adding to any meal, especially since it might prevent you from overindulging on the main course. One study showed that people who started with a salad ate less of the meal that followed.

3. **Bypass the gargantuan salad "desserts."** Candied walnuts, taco strips, dried fruit, rice noodles, and wontons that top off entrée salads are sugar and fat bombs. Likewise, skip the sugary vinaigrettes and creamy dressings. Customize your salad with avocado or guacamole, salsa, chicken, and black beans. Ask for a low-sugar vinaigrette, or simply oil and vinegar, on the side.

4. **Beware of red flags.** Any entrée described as breaded, fried, crunchy, crispy, glazed, or creamy translates into a fast-fat-loss brick wall. Order your lean protein and non-starchy veggies grilled, baked, steamed, poached, or broiled.

5. **You know what assuming does.** Restaurants are notorious for slipping egg into that innocuous chicken dish, or gluten into, well, just about everything. Ask your server questions before you order so you're confident that your meal is compliant with the Virgin Diet. Check to see if they have a gluten-free menu; lots of restaurants are jumping on the bandwagon. Trust me, ignorance will not feel like bliss when your fish comes drowning in a syrupy soy glaze even though the menu didn't say so. And if you eat it, don't think you'll be able to blame your server!

6. **Don't invite the enemy to the table.** Banish the bread basket before your server even sets it down. If you need something to munch on before your salad, ask for a small bowl of olives, or crudités with hummus or guacamole. Yum.

7. **Double up.** Two appetizers as your main course provide better portion control than a gigantic entrée, and they'll fill you up just fine. Here's a chance to be creative and introduce some variety—think hummus with veggies alongside grilled chicken kabobs with salsa, or maybe grilled scallops and an organic greens salad...you get the idea. There are nutritional home runs on the starter side of the menu; look no further!

**8. Share or cut it in half.** Split that monster broccoli-garlic-stuffed chicken breast in half and share it with your dining partner, or get half of it to go before you even dive in. You'll save money and calories.

**9. Three bites and fork down.** Your business date insists you must try the pistachio chocolate upside-down cake, and who are you to argue since you're trying to score his six-figure account? Instead of demurely declining, go ahead and have three polite bites (we're talking bites you would eat on *Oprah*, not during an 11 p.m. fridge raid), and ask your server to remove the fork. Trust me, your date will have no problem finishing that cake.

**10. Get ideas, not absolutes, from the menu.** Why let the menu dictate what you'll eat? Use it as a guide, not an ultimatum, for how you should enjoy your dinner. Even if they charge a few bucks extra, many restaurants happily accommodate substitutions if you're polite about asking.

Once these rules become second nature, eating on the go not only becomes easier, it can be a chance to have delicious, nutritious food you might not be inclined to make at home, or to explore culinary treats unique to wherever you are in the world. Go forth and conquer!

## VIRGIN DIET SUCCESS

### Cindy Russo—Brooklyn, CT

It was early December 2012 and I was awake with heartburn (which was not unusual) late one night. I turned on the TV and saw JJ talking about the the Virgin Diet and her book. I am 49 years old and have suffered with heartburn for most of my life. I have had skin issues; environmental allergies (including sinus surgery at 35); digestive issues (bloating and gas); and ADHD symptoms since I was a child. I have always had a lean frame but a big belly. I'm 5'5" and weighed 152 pounds—and looked pregnant at 48!

My typical breakfast was some kind of "gluteny carby" junk. I ate healthy for the most part, counting calories and eating lots of salads, but I had a serious love affair with pasta and Italian bread. I munched on whole-grain crackers and low-fat cheese for snacks, and low-fat Ice cream or frozen yogurt was always in my freezer. I exercised regularly, doing yoga, walking, and weight machines, but I could not lose weight unless I "cleansed," which basically was starving myself for two days and only drinking liquids.

I knew after listening to JJ that night that I needed the Virgin Diet. I did Cycle 1 of the diet over the holidays—yeah, poor planning some might say, but I was ready and I used to gain 5 pounds over the holidays. My family thought I was nuts, but I did not even eat one cookie. I was so motivated!

Now I weigh 135 pounds. My heartburn is nonexistent (whereas before I was told I needed surgery to correct it); my energy is limitless; I never need allergy meds; my skin is glowing; my mood is steady, as is my focus (no more ADHD symptoms); and most satisfying to me, my belly is flatter! I no longer look like the pregnant grandma. My boyfriend also now eats what I make and takes leftovers for lunch. He gave up beer and pizza! Most dramatic for me: My 5-year-old granddaughter suffered from yeast infections, joint pain, and sinus headaches. My daughter took her for allergy testing and was told she was not allergic to anything. Upon my suggestion, she switched from cow's milk to almond or coconut, eliminated all the other dairy and gluten, and her symptoms have improved dramatically. I'm so happy that she will not suffer a lifetime of genetically inherited maladies like her "grandmuhmuh." Thank you, JJ . . . I wish we'd met sooner!

### *My Original Virgin Diet Recipe*

## SEXY CINDY'S SIMPLE AND SATISFYING SLOW-COOKER DAIRY- AND GLUTEN-FREE BEEF STROGANOFF WITH SOUR CREAM

Serve this with a small side salad if desired. I served it to my boyfriend, who has a hearty dude-like appetite and used to live for pasta and dairy. He could not tell the difference. He even grabbed the leftovers for lunch and made all his mechanic buddies at work very jealous!

And yes, it's complete with "sour cream"—my dairy-free version (you need that creamy, tangy taste to finish it or it's just not stroganoff).

*Serves 8—freeze some for leftovers!*

2 pounds stew beef (I use a lean, grass-fed beef free of hormones and antibiotics; you can substitute grass-fed beef sirloin tips to shorten the cooking time)

1 cup gluten-free flour (I prefer Bob's Red Mill Gluten-Free All-Purpose Flour), tossed in a large bowl with generous seasonings of salt, pepper, garlic powder, and onion powder (remove 2 tablespoons of the flour mixture and set aside)

*continued*

A few tablespoons of coconut oil or ghee, to brown the beef

1 (32-ounce) box organic beef broth (I prefer Emeril's organic; you won't use it all)

1 (6-ounce) can organic tomato paste

½ cup coconut aminos

1 medium onion (I use organic Vidalias), sliced in half lengthwise, then into ½-inch-wide slices

1 (8-ounce) package mushrooms (organic baby bellas are my first choice)

1 (16-ounce) package gluten-free pasta (I used a brown rice linguine), or you can also serve this over rice

Start by cutting the beef into big bite-sized pieces (not JJ's "polite bite" size, as you want to be able to find them later), and toss the pieces in the seasoned flour mixture. Use tongs to pick out the floured meat pieces and transfer them to a plate. Heat your oil of choice in a skillet over medium-high heat and quickly sear the meat pieces, turning on all sides. You don't need to cook it through here—you just want to seal in the juices and brown it a little. Dump the seared meat into a slow cooker or a large heavy-bottom pot with a lid.

In a large bowl or measuring cup, whisk about two-thirds of the beef broth with the tomato paste and coconut aminos until smooth. Pour this over the beef in the pot so it reaches ½ to 1 inch above the meat. I cooked this meal in the slow cooker on high for 5 hours because I started it late in the day, but if you have time, cooking for 8 hours on low is better for the tenderness and juiciness of the meat. Leave the lid on the slow cooker and try to resist opening and stirring, as this greatly affects temperature and cooking time. If you are using a pot on the stove, bring it to a boil, reduce to very low, cover the pot, and cook for 2 to 3 hours, stirring occasionally to prevent the meat from sticking to the pan.

After about 4 hours on high or 6 hours on low in the slow cooker, dump in your onion and mushrooms, stir, re-cover, and cook to the desired tenderness (about 1 hour on high or 2 hours on low). If you cook too long, the onions will become mushy, so use your best judgment here based on taste. When it's done the meat will be very tender and you won't need a knife to cut it.

Start the water boiling to cook your pasta or rice and cook according to the package directions.

Once your meat and veggies are cooked to the desired tenderness, it's time to check the consistency of your stroganoff "stock." If it is thin, you can thicken it with the 2 tablespoons of seasoned flour you initially set aside; whisk the flour with ½ cup of the broth until smooth, and then stir it into the stroganoff. Now turn off the slow cooker and remove the lid so it cools a bit, because if it's too hot, it can curdle your "sour cream."

Mix the "sour cream" into your stroganoff until it is all creamy and smooth. Spoon the stroganoff over the cooked pasta or rice.

### "Sour Cream"

1 (13.5-ounce) can unsweetened full-fat coconut milk (I prefer Native Forest non-GMO-verified, organic), refrigerated for several hours or overnight for best results
1 teaspoon fresh lemon juice
⅛ teaspoon sea salt

Take your can of coconut milk out of the refrigerator, turn it upside down, open it, and pour the thin part of the coconut milk into a container; save it for your next Virgin Diet Shake. You should be left with the thick, creamy part of the coconut milk; scoop it into a bowl.

Whisk the lemon juice and salt into the coconut cream.

To see Cindy's interview, visit thevirgindietcookbook.com/bonus.

## All in the Family

Changing the way you eat, even if it's the best choice you can make for yourself, can be daunting if you don't have support. And if you're the primary meal provider for your family, you may regard the moment you tell them that they'll all be eating healthier as their opportunity to vote you off the island.

Don't live in dread of that family meeting. Most people resist change, and if you have picky children or a husband who believes he could never be separated from his *Close Encounters* mound of spaghetti, my advice is to dive into these recipes headfirst without ever mentioning it. Simply carry on.

Just begin to cook the way I've laid out for you in this cookbook, and any anxiety you may have had will evaporate when you hear what so many of my clients hear from their families: "Why are we getting such great meals?" How is that possible? Because it's so simple to replace spaghetti with rice or quinoa pasta and to not have anyone feel like they're missing the inner hug they get from their favorite comfort food. You can replace antibiotic- and hormone-laced beef with grass-fed beef, add your normal side of broccoli (but make it organic), and swap the baked potato for a sweet potato. No one will bat an eye, and you've just made a much healthier dinner for the whole family. And if you live with a tribe of dessert eaters, serve fresh berries on some coconut milk ice cream. Done!

# TOSS AND SHOP FOR THE VIRGIN KITCHEN 3

Did you ever notice that when someone comes to you with a problem, the rest of the conversation goes much more smoothly when they also offer you a solution? Well, that's what toss and shop is all about! If any anxiety creeps in while you're tossing, rest assured it will be replaced tenfold with delight when your fridge and pantry are full to bursting with the good stuff.

## SETTING UP FOR SUCCESS

Everything about this cookbook—and my philosophy—is about setting you up for success. I want you to experience the fabulous benefits that come with the Virgin Diet—the transformation in your weight, your energy, your health, and your spirit. Those things are the return on the investment you're making in you, and if you don't get them, what's the point?

The best way to ensure it will all happen for you, as it has for thousands of people I've worked with, is to plan well so the execution is easy. When you realize the power of what food can do for you, you'll eat and shop with a reverence for it. The rich experience of eating well will bring your palate back to life, too.

So what's the first step in setting you up for success? Remove all your trigger foods from sight—you can't count on your willpower alone to save the day when your drug of choice is calling your name from the freezer. I have to do this, too—almond butter has a cracklike hold over me, and if it's in my house, I will devour the entire jar in one fell swoop. Guaranteed. (And yes, almond butter is a healthy swap, but not a whole jar at a sitting!)

So, out with the bad and in with the good.

## WHAT TO TOSS

Tossing is as important as adding for shifting the balance of your kitchen—and recipes—to the healthy side. An easy-to-remember rule of thumb is that if a "food" has a long list of nearly indecipherable ingredients, consider it toxic and pitch it.

Tossing foods that don't make the grade removes the temptation and avoids the internal battle to follow. But just because I'm recommending that you toss these foods doesn't mean you can't ever have them again; you're just reframing them as indulgences to splurge on every now and then.

Here's a starter list based on what I find most people have stocked in their kitchens:

**Toss It!**

| | |
|---|---|
| Agave, honey, maple syrups | Juices |
| Baked beans | Mayonnaise |
| Bisquick | Milk, soy milk, non-dairy creamers |
| Breads | Pasta |
| Cereals | Ranch, blue cheese, French dressings |
| Chips | Snack bars (those candy bars in disguise) |
| Corn-fed meats | Sodas—regular *or* diet |
| Crackers | Splenda or NutraSweet |
| Dried fruits | Trail mix (you know, the kind with peanuts and chocolate) |
| Frozen "diet" dinners | |
| Fruit-sweetened yogurts | Vegetable oils |

In addition to the foods listed above, you'll need to get rid of any others containing artificial sweeteners and colorings, gluten, dairy, high-fructose corn syrup, or partially hydrogenated oils. Also, get rid of frozen treats, baked goods, deep-fried foods, candy, soy-based products, and anything that came from a fast-food restaurant.

When you go through this purge, view it as liberating and throw out anything that's in doubt. *Do not* get into a wagering contest with yourself about whether something can stay. Even though you want to believe it, the "fat-free" label on the pastry or ice cream package does not make it a health food. Switching from sugar to artificial sweeteners doesn't turn the enemy into your friend. Feel the power in rejecting the hype!

One of the most important things you can do to support your own success is to educate yourself about where the 7 high-FI foods hide, especially when they're buried in otherwise seemingly healthy food. You don't need to know these by heart, but it helps to at least be familiar with them or to keep the list accessible. In chapter 1, I've included a partial list of these foods (for the complete list, refer to my earlier book, *The Virgin Diet*) and provided examples of foods in which they tend to be hidden. I've also listed how the foods are often labeled on packages—the ingredients list is not always clear! When cleaning out your pantry, and before heading to the grocery store, review the lists on pages 13 to 19.

## SIMPLIFY, SIMPLIFY, SIMPLIFY

You get the idea: The best choices are whole foods with single names and no labels. So simple! Buy as close to nature as possible. And even though eating non-organic fruits and vegetables is generally better than not eating them at all (the nutritional benefits usually outweigh the risk of pesticide exposure), I still always recommend that you buy organic whenever you can, if only for the peace of mind.

Even so, it's not necessary that all your fruits and vegetables be organic, so if you're on a budget or just need help making choices, learn which foods get the most pummeled with pesticides—visit ewg.org/foodnews/summary.php for the Environmental Working Group's complete list of both the "Dirty Dozen Plus" (a list of the most pesticide-laden fruits and veggies) and the "Clean Fifteen" (just the opposite). And whether organic or not, scrub a dub dub—always wash your fruits and veggies before you eat them! Even organic fruit can carry dirt and germs, or be the victim of "pesticide drift" from nearby farms.

I'm also going to recommend that you avoid GMOs (genetically modified organisms) whenever possible. That may take knowing just a little bit about them and where they're found, so here are the broad strokes. GMOs are plants and animals that have been genetically altered, ostensibly to increase crop yield or shelf life. They're engineered by inserting foreign genes into the DNA of the plant or animal, and the resulting crop is one that is not found in nature. The outside genes can come from bacteria, viruses, or other plants and animals. I know, that already doesn't sound good, but here's the scary part: According to the American Academy of Environmental Medicine, there are *serious health risks* associated with genetically modified food.

GMO foods are not labeled (yet!), but they're in as many as 80 percent of the processed foods available in the U.S. Above all else, avoid processed foods made with the eight genetically modified food crops—corn, soybeans, canola, cottonseed, sugar beets, Hawaiian papaya, and some zucchini and yellow squash. For more information and a complete list of where they might be slipping into your shopping cart, visit responsibletechnology.org/buy-non-gmo and download the non-GMO shopping list. Also, look for certification by the nonprofit organization the Non-GMO Project; it puts its seal on brands it verifies as GMO-free, so you can exhale.

## VIRGIN DIET SUCCESS

### Jamey Karnitz—Port Edwards, WI

I shudder at how I was living before I started the Virgin Diet. My life was a series of compromises. I had to be okay with being disappointed in myself every day or I wouldn't be able to go on. I thought I was destined to be overweight and unhappy. I had tried dieting many times, and in many unhealthy ways I had lost weight and then gained it (and more) back. So I gave up on dieting. I am on the road a lot, commuting to and from work, and I was hitting up fast-food joints at least once per day. I did not exercise. I did not stop to think how the fried processed foods were affecting every part of my life. At the same time, I was getting fed up with feeling sick all the time. I would work, come home, and immediately need to sleep. I could never stay focused on anything.

I was suffering from debilitating headaches, joint aches, depression, and symptoms of polycystic ovarian syndrome. My skin was breaking out with cystic acne (which I never had as a teen), and I was having hypoglycemic episodes nearly every day. Late last year, I saw JJ's special on PBS. The things she was saying resonated with me. I was convinced, however, that I could never eliminate all 7 food groups because I "needed" some of them. Then, at the end of December, it all came together. My friend Becky died of melanoma on December 30. She was only 33 years old. Her death forced me to take an honest look at my life.

Here I was, 35 years old and wishing for an altogether different kind of life, but carrying on the same behaviors that got me to this mediocre existence. I felt lucky to be alive, and in Becky's honor I knew I *had* to make some changes. Initially, for the first 2 months, I didn't even count calories or log my food intake—the weight fell off simply by following the Virgin Diet. I was able to lose 20 pounds in those 2 months. I also started doing some exercise DVDs 5 days per week. Then in the next 3 months, I lost another 21 pounds and was able to decrease my body fat significantly through working out and eating better. So I have lost a total of 41 pounds, more than 21 inches, and 3 dress sizes.

I realize that paying a bit more now for good food is going to mean fewer health problems and medical expenses later on. I also learned about the importance of planning and having "backup" plans for food. In the past I would go long periods of time without eating simply because I didn't have anything packed, and then when I did eat, it would be lots of food at one time. I learned about the importance of stoking the metabolic "fire," and now I carry several snack options at all times. And eliminating the problem food groups meant that for the first time in my life, I was in control of the food instead of the food controlling me. Dairy and gluten were the big culprits in my case, and if I sneak even a little bit of them back into my diet, I can tell because the cravings are insane.

So now everything has changed for me. Everything is easier. My skin is clearer, I am leaner, and I am so much more comfortable in my own skin. I find that I'm wearing less makeup and jewelry now, because it's so true that a healthy, fit body is the best accessory. I don't have to worry about hypoglycemic episodes now, and my headaches have almost disappeared. Most surprising, though, is how much more time I have now that I am awake all day! I find that I really don't need the naps I used to; maybe it's because I sleep better at night. I can pursue hobbies and work more quickly on my schoolwork now.

I think if my friend Becky was still here, she would be one of my biggest cheerleaders. Fitness was so important to her, as was living life to its fullest. I am on the path to doing that now. She inspired me, and now it's my job to keep her legacy going. I have JJ Virgin (and workout videos) to thank for this. *Thank you!*

### *My Original Virgin Diet Recipe*

## WHITE BEAN CAJUN CHICKEN WITH BLACK BEANS AND "RICE"

*Serves 4*

### *"Rice"*

1 head cauliflower
2 tablespoons olive oil
2 tablespoons dried rosemary
3 to 4 cloves garlic, chopped or minced
Sea salt and pepper to taste
1 can black beans, drained and rinsed

*continued*

Preheat the oven to 400°F. Line a 13 x 9-inch baking pan with parchment paper.

Cut the cauliflower into large pieces, place them in a blender or food processor, and process until fine. Place the cauliflower in a hand towel and squeeze to expel as much excess water as possible (really work hard on this).

Combine the cauliflower with 1 tablespoon of the olive oil, all the rosemary, and the garlic in the baking pan. Bake for 20 minutes, flipping the cauliflower over halfway through cooking.

Put the remaining 1 tablespoon olive oil in a frying pan, and transfer the cooked cauliflower to it. On medium-high heat, brown the "rice" to the desired color. Season with sea salt and pepper, then mix in the black beans and heat through. Set aside (may be made ahead of time and reheated to save on time).

### Chicken

Olive oil, for the pan

1 (15-ounce) can Great Northern beans, rinsed and drained

¼ cup flaxseeds

Juice of 1 lemon (about 3 tablespoons)

2 teaspoons (or more to taste) Tony Chachere or other Cajun seasoning

2 to 4 tablespoons Frank's Hot Sauce, plus more for serving (optional)

1 pound skinless, boneless free-range chicken breasts or tenders, trimmed of excess tissue, fat, etc.

Preheat the oven to 375°F. Line a baking pan with tin foil and rub the foil lightly with olive oil to reduce sticking.

Place the beans in a blender or food processor and blend until smooth. Scrape out and combine with the flaxseeds, 6 tablespoons water, lemon juice, and Cajun seasoning. Adjust the seasonings to taste; set aside.

Pour the Frank's Hot Sauce into a medium bowl, and dilute with water to taste. (I don't handle spicy too well, so I used a 1:2 ratio of hot sauce to water.)

Dip the chicken into the liquid briefly and then dip it into the bean mixture. Work with your hands to scoop the bean mixture around the chicken (it will mostly be on top), and place the chicken in the prepared pan.

Bake for 30 minutes, or until the chicken is done. Serve the chicken over the "rice," with more hot sauce if you're looking for excitement.

To see Jamey's interview, visit thevirgindietcookbook.com/bonus.

## ASSEMBLING YOUR TVD KITCHEN

The Virgin Diet focuses on lean protein, healthy fats, slow low carbs, and fruits and vegetables. This section will help connect you to the best places to get these nutritionally potent foods.

The first thing to know is that you don't have to rely only on grocery stores; I know they're not all created equal. Some place a premium on helping you know more about your food and where it comes from; others give more shelf space to boxes and bags of processed snacks. So I'm going to give a shout-out here to Whole Foods Markets. If you're fortunate enough to have one in your town, check out their 365 brand. You'll be pleasantly surprised to find that it's affordable—priced to compete against the major grocery store brands—while being GMO-free and organic. Thank you, Whole Foods!

People who are interested in eating well and knowing where their food comes from are often more than willing to help like-minded others expand their shopping horizons. So outside of the grocery stores, check your area to find a local CSA (Community Supported Agriculture), which is a partnership between farmers and people in the community who support the farm directly; or look for food collectives that are organized to get fresh, organic, local food to people who want it. If your town has an amazing farmer's market (and I've yet to find one that isn't a treasure chest!), get to know the people working the stands to learn more about the food and maybe even get some tips on preparation. Or go straight to the source and make an effort to meet the farmers themselves. The more you know about the source of your food, the more control you have over it and the better you'll feel about eating it.

As a general rule of thumb, whether at the farmer's market or a supermarket, buy local and in season. Local food tastes better and is more nutritious. The chemical makeup of fruits and vegetables changes as soon as they're harvested; the starches start turning to sugar and nutrients disintegrate. For the same reason, buy your produce whole or as close to its original state as possible, not already cut up: Brussels sprouts on the stalk, whole cauliflower rather than the trimmed curds, and whole heads of romaine lettuce rather than the prepackaged bags; you'll save money and get more nutrients. Food that has to travel a long way to get to your store shelf is often pumped full of preservatives to survive the trip. It also has more packaging and has a higher energy cost than food that was grown around the corner.

The same goes for the animals you eat. The health and quality of local livestock are often carefully tended to by your neighborhood farmer (can't you just see the beautiful scene?), as opposed to the neglected, stressed-out animals shuffled through an industrial facility. Support your local farmer, for your sake as well as the animals'!

## BRING HOME SOMETHING OTHER THAN THE BACON

Now, like the great hunters we are, we're going to go shopping. Let's drill down and fill up the pantry, fridge, and freezer with food that will keep you lean, happy, and healthy. Leave no room for any food or foodlike substance that does not move you toward or keep you at those goals! Keep the enemy out!

The first rule of safe grocery shopping is—make a list! The second rule of safe grocery shopping is (no, this isn't *Fight Club*)—take it with you! Never leave home without the list, and don't deviate from it. I'm protecting you from yourself here. If you'd like a downloadable copy of this list to take to the store with you, you'll find it at thevirgindietcookbook.com/bonus.

## PUT THESE IN YOUR PANTRY

When you stock up on these items for your pantry, be mindful not to buy acidic fruits and vegetables in cans unless those cans are BPA-free. BPA—bisphenol A—is an industrial chemical that can leach from plastics and cans and is thought to disrupt the endocrine system. Yikes! Buy those fruits and veggies in glass jars or BPA-free cans with as few additional ingredients on the label as possible.

Artichoke hearts
Aseptic-packed coconut milk and
    almond milk
Black beans
Brown and wild rice
Brown rice pasta
Canned wild salmon (I use Vital Choice)
Chickpeas (garbanzo beans)
Coconut oil

Diced green chiles
Dried, sprouted lentils
Extra-virgin olive oil
Gluten-free flours—coconut, almond,
    Bob's Red Mill GF Blend
Green tea
Macadamia nut oil
Nuts (choose from raw almonds,
    cashews, pecans, walnuts,

macadamia nuts, Brazil nuts,
  pistachios)
Organic chicken broth
Quinoa
Quinoa pasta

Rice noodles
Shirataki noodles
Sun-dried tomatoes in olive oil
Vinegar (red wine, balsamic, rice) for
  salad dressings

## FOR YOUR FRIDGE

Most supermarkets now have an expanded organic section with beautiful, colorful displays of fresh vegetables and fruits, so it's easier than ever to choose local, organic, and seasonal (I can't say it enough!). Do the same when you're combing through the meat and seafood shelves.

Pause, though, when you're filling your cart with fruit. You can get too much of a good thing here! Limit yourself to 2 servings a day maximum, and stick to tart, firm fruit; overripe fruit is higher in sugar. On top of that, I'd like to see you emphasize berries and cherries as your go-to fruits, and to otherwise limit your fruits to ones that are low to medium in overall sugar. Those include berries, cherries, grapefruit, cranberries, star fruit, passion fruit, guava, lemons, limes, and avocados.

And surprise—the highest sugar loads are in dried fruits (especially dates, prunes, figs, and raisins), fruit juice, agave, honey, and fruit packed in syrup. Disappointing, I know. But knowledge is power. Stay away from all of those as much as possible.

So, with all that said, here are some fridge-filling rock stars you'll want to keep on hand at all times:

Broccoli, cauliflower, and Brussels
  sprouts
Chia seeds
Coconut milk
Dijon mustard (gluten-free)
Flaxseeds (grind fresh before use)
Fresh fruit (low-sugar)
Fresh salsa
Guacamole
Hummus

Iced green tea (make fresh, no sugar
  added)
Lemons
Limes
Mushrooms
Nut butters: almond butter, pecan
  butter, walnut butter, macadamia
  nut butter, and cashew butter
Organic gluten-free turkey
  slices

Red bell peppers

Red onions

Roasted whole chicken

Salad greens (look for baby spinach and arugula)

Sparkling mineral water (I like Hint Fizz)

The vegetable bin is a hallowed space within the sanctuary of your refrigerator. It has less humidity than the greater fridge space, so vegetables keep longer. Pack it with a rainbow of colorful vegetables and fruits and keep it full. It will help you make better choices and quietly call to you to start meals with a salad—always a good thing! Make it your mission to try a new vegetable each week.

But not all veggies should be mindlessly tossed into the vegetable bin (even though they're veggies, and there's a bin for them). There are a few that should actually be housed outside the fridge in open baskets, in a dark dry spot, so they'll ripen (if they need to) and deliver the most intense flavor. Which? These:

Avocados

Beets

Butternut squash

Garlic and onions

Kabocha squash

Sweet potatoes/yams

Tomatoes

## FOR YOUR FREEZER

A well-stocked freezer will save you when there's no fresh protein left in the fridge and you just couldn't get to the store...those days when you blink and suddenly it's dinnertime. Rather than go without (never!) or deciding it will be okay to call for pizza (don't do it!), thaw something from your stash. You may even want to consider getting an extra freezer so you can stock up on hormone- and antibiotic-free organic grass-fed beef, wild fish, and pastured chicken when there are special sales at the supermarket. After an exhausting day of work, errands, and the car pool, you'll thank me for the safety net of Operation Freezer!

My top animal protein choices are:

Grass-fed beef tenderloin

Ground turkey, grass-fed beef, or chicken breast (you may need to ask the butcher to grind this for you)

Organic chicken, turkey, and salmon sausage
Organic free-range chicken and turkey breast
Pasture-fed pork tenderloin
Seafood, including scallops, shrimp, and king crab
Wild fish*—favorites are sole, salmon, and Alaskan halibut

### Frozen Vegetables

When produce isn't in season, frozen is a great second choice. I recommend you have these staples on hand:

Chopped spinach
Stir-fry mix
Tri-colored pepper strips
Wild mushrooms

### Frozen Whole Fruits (No Sugar Added)

Frozen fruit is great for smoothies and quick desserts—just heat, add coconut milk, protein powder, and serve! Choose these:

Blackberries
Blueberries
Cherries
Raspberries
Strawberries

## LABELS

When you're doing all of this shopping on your empowering food pilgrimages, there's a big health payoff to knowing what's meant by certain labels. Companies are often rewarded by the sleight of hand that makes their processed foods appear healthy, so don't fall victim to the misdirect on their labels.

*For a detailed list of which fish have the most mercury and which have the least, refer to nrdc.org/health/effects/mercury/guide.asp.

Learn which claims are hype and which matter. They can be differentiated between certified (matter) and non-certified (hype).

## Certified Labels

**Grass-Fed**—When an animal product is labeled "grass-fed," it has met the standard of the USDA, which requires it to have been fed only grass and forage throughout its lifetime—no grains.

**Organic**—For animal meat and dairy to be labeled "organic," the animal must never have been given antibiotics, hormones, or GMO grasses.

**Naturally Grown**—The Naturally Grown certification is reserved for food produced on smallish farms that abide by the USDA Certified Organic methods of growing and sell locally.

**Non-GMO Project Verified**—The Non-GMO Project is a nonprofit dedicated to keeping our food GMO-free, and any product with this seal has gone through its verification process.

## Non-Certified Labels

**Free-Range**—For poultry to be labeled "free-range," it only needs to meet the USDA requirement of 5 minutes of open-air access a day. And open-air access is a vague prerequisite at best; it doesn't mandate grass or dirt, or even a reasonable amount of space.

**No Added Hormones, or Hormone-Free**—U.S. law forbids the use of growth hormones in poultry already. All this label means is that the producer isn't breaking the law.

**Cage-Free**—Though this label is unregulated, egg-laying hens called "cage-free" are raised without cages, as it implies. The truth is, though, that most are warehoused—packed into overcrowded barns in unsanitary conditions. Some inhumane practices like beak cutting are also overlooked under this label.

**Pasture-Fed or Pasture-Raised**—This label is usually a great choice, an indicator of the humane treatment given to the animals and their higher micronutrient load as a result. For beef, though, the label "pastured" must also be accompanied by "grass-fed," to ensure the cattle weren't fed grains; and "organic," to be sure they weren't free to graze on GMO grasses. Pastured products that are not labeled "organic" may contain levels of GMO soy and corn.

**Vegetarian-Fed**—This is an unreliable label attempting to show that the producers didn't feed livestock or poultry any animal by-products—only hay, grass, or grains. Unfortunately, this claim is hard to prove or disprove.

**Natural**—A meaningless label, often co-opted and put on less-than-healthy foods. All the "natural" label must guarantee, according to the USDA, is that there are no artificial colors, flavors, or preservatives.

## FLOURS

One of the tenets of Cycle 1 is that you eliminate the 7 high-FI foods that create food intolerance and that could be at the root of your weight loss resistance and general malaise. One of those foods is gluten. But you may be a little concerned about how you're going to make that work for 3 weeks, since you love to bake. Am I right? Fear not! This is a perfect example of how important it is to remember that this cookbook is not about deprivation, not about what you can't have, but about making better choices. And my lateral shifts make that so easy to do!

If you're craving pizza, melt a little goat cheese (if you don't react to it and are in Cycle 3 of the Virgin Diet) and tomato sauce on a portobello mushroom. Yum! To get your baking fix, substitute almond, rice, or coconut flour for wheat or rye flour in any of your recipes, and you'll get all of the indulgence without any of the punishing sugar spikes and crashes that gluten brings to the party.

Here are some other specific flour swaps:

**Bob's Red Mill Gluten-Free All-Purpose Baking Flour**—Bob's Red Mill All-Purpose is another awesome alternative if you have an allergy or sensitivity to gluten. This flour can be made into delicious homemade baked goods without any evidence they're *sans* gluten. So what's in it? Garbanzo flour, potato starch, tapioca flour, sorghum flour, and fava flour.

**Bob's Red Mill Almond Meal**—Another from Bob's. Their almond meal is ground from blanched sweet almonds. Almonds are a potent source of protein, and they're naturally low-carb and gluten-free.

**Coconut Flour**—Coconut flour is essentially ground-up coconut meat, with the fat removed to make it drier. It's a lot like wheat- and grain-based flours in its consistency, so it can be used for baking. It's also gluten-free, high in fiber and low in carbs, and a fair source of protein.

## PASTA, RICE, AND GRAINS

If you decide to stick with oats, be sure they're gluten-free. If they're not, and gluten slips by you, it may cause a serious reaction if you have (or are serving someone with) celiac disease or gluten sensitivity. I've seen clients have a "gluten-like" reaction to gluten-free oatmeal, so I recommend that you leave oats out entirely for Cycle 1 and reintroduce them in Cycle 3.

For an easy swap in the meantime, choose quinoa flakes. Quinoa flakes are similar to oatmeal; they're the result of steamrolling quinoa grains into a thin, fast-cooking flake. So they're a perfect choice when you're on the run! Have a delicious hot bowl of them for a nutritious breakfast, mix them into pancake or waffle batter, or use them to replace breaded coatings.

Quinoa also works as an alternative to corn, as do lentils and black beans. And you can get a corn-free snack fix by trading popcorn and tortilla chips for rice chips, kale chips, crudités, or homemade sweet potato chips.

Some of the toughest foods to convince people they won't miss, though, are bread and pasta. But once they give my substitutions a chance, I hear their disbelief that they don't miss them at all. Why? Because it's not about giving up what everyone enjoys about bread and pasta, it's about making better choices for your weight and health and still getting all the pleasure they bring. Try these simple switches: Instead of flour or whole-grain pasta, go with spaghetti squash, quinoa pasta, or rice pasta. See, still "pasta"!

You don't have to give up bread entirely, either. As long as you give up those store-bought loaves in favor of Paleo bread, you're fine. You can also choose rice tortillas, rice wraps, or even lettuce wraps as healthy, great-tasting ways to stay the course without feeling like you need to mourn the loss of bread.

Remember, *all* grains can raise your blood sugar and insulin. Use them sparingly, if at all. If you decide to incorporate them into some meals, the ideal choice is sprouted grains, which are germinated and are more nutritious and usually less refined than others. And when you're cooking with grains, no matter which ones, soak them first to lower their phytates (phytates are an anti-nutrient that binds with minerals to prevent their absorption).

So, after all that, if you're still gun-shy about carbs, you may feel better knowing that I eat them, too! My personal top starchy-carb faves are quinoa, hummus, spaghetti squash, black beans, and lentils. Stick with those and you'll be making nutritious choices that aren't the blood sugar equivalent of electric shock therapy. Other good choices are brown or wild rice (be certain it's non-GMO), all other legumes, sweet potatoes, buckwheat, and amaranth.

If you have the time, buy your beans dry, and rinse and soak them before boiling or baking them. They'll be more nutritious, lower in salt, and less expensive than canned beans. Soaking also ensures they'll cook evenly and cuts down on the gas they generate (plus, they'll be clean!). And you can freeze the extra as an insurance policy that you'll always have a quick meal within reach.

There are two main ways to soak beans: the long soak method and the quick soak method. To long soak, rinse the dried beans, put them in a bowl, and add enough water to cover them by about 3 inches. Just leave them overnight, and they'll be ready for you to drain and rinse in the morning.

When you're in a hurry, pour the beans into a large pot and add water until they are covered by about 3 inches. Boil for 1 minute, then cover and let stand for an hour. When the beans are tender and have doubled in size, they're done and ready to drain.

## SWEETENERS

Once upon a time, you went to the sweeteners aisle and next to the sugar you found the pastel lure of pink, blue, and yellow packets of artificial sweeteners. However, several studies found aspartame and other artificial sweeteners could, among other things, trigger sugar cravings and weight gain. Uh-oh.

If you have a sweet tooth and would like to make or eat some sweet treats without blowing your sugar budget, you'll want to brush up on how to choose the best natural sweeteners. For actual sugar, organic coconut sugar, local organic raw honey, and blackstrap molasses are better choices than straight table sugar or high-fructose corn syrup. And best of all is straight glucose, because it doesn't contain fructose.

But here's a brief look at four popular sweeteners so you can decide for yourself which ones you can safely incorporate into your diet and which ones need to go the way of those nasty pastel packets.

**Monk fruit**—Monk fruit is also marketed as "lo han guo." Monk fruit is 200 to 400 times sweeter than sugar, depending on the form you get it in. In China, monk fruit sweetener has been used for nearly a thousand years to treat obesity and diabetes. It's rich in antioxidants with anti-inflammatory benefits, and it may have some anti-cancer and anti-diabetic properties as well. So you can see why it's my go-to natural sweetener! And even though monk fruit is slightly sweeter than stevia, whenever one of my recipes calls for one or the other, you can make an even swap without impacting the outcome.

**Erythritol**—Erythritol is a sugar alcohol that was discovered in 1848. It occurs naturally in some fruits and fermented foods. Sugar alcohols are actually neither—they got their name because their biochemical structure resembles a hybrid of a sugar and alcohol. Studies show that erythritol is tooth-friendly and doesn't contribute to dental problems the way sugar does. It may even inhibit cavities from forming! Erythritol makes an ideal sweetener for people with diabetes because it has no adverse effects on blood glucose levels. I prefer xylitol over erythritol, however, as xylitol has some actual health benefits.

**Xylitol**—A naturally occurring sugar alcohol with a sweetness similar to sucrose, xylitol has 33 percent fewer calories than sugar. Xylitol is often used in dental products and chewing gums as it may help prevent cavities, and it has been shown to aid with weight loss by suppressing ghrelin, the hunger hormone. Manufacturers used to derive xylitol from birch trees, but now it more likely comes from either corn husks or as a blend of corn and birch. If you're in Cycle 1 of the Virgin Diet, be sure to find xylitol from birch (see "Healthy Sweeteners" in the Resources section).

Note: Don't let your canine companions anywhere near xylitol; it can be fatal to dogs!

**Stevia**—Stevia is an herb that grows in North and South America; it's 300 times sweeter than sugar and is available as both a liquid extract and a powder.

Some people complain that stevia has a bitter aftertaste, but it's the preferred sweetener for many people on low-carb and Paleo diets, or those with blood sugar issues. Because it has zero calories, stevia can create caloric dysregulation, a situation in which the degree of sweetness can't be connected to the caloric load, leading to cravings and overeating. If you use stevia, opt for pure, organic stevia. Many stevia "blends" contain maltodextrin (usually derived from corn) and other sweeteners.

## OILS

Oils are an essential ingredient in the delicious food you'll make, not only for the benefits they bring in flavor and texture, but also for their impact on your health. Replacing a bad oil choice with a better one can jump-start weight loss and healing in your system. Good oils provide the fatty acids your brain, nervous system, and immune system need for peak performance. Unfortunately, there's no one oil elixir to use in all kitchen activity, so here are a few of my favorites to cover all your baking, frying, dipping, and dressing dreams.

### Cook Me Oils

**Coconut oil**—This oil is pressed from the fruit of the coconut palm tree, and it's a perfect choice for baking, to use in stir-fries (it can withstand high heat without breaking down), and as a dairy-free replacement for butter. Better still, it promotes heart health and weight loss.

**Olive oil**—Olive oil is the lifeblood of the Mediterranean diet and is widely lauded for its heart-healthy monounsaturated fat content. Olive oil is a blend of refined olive oils and extra-virgin or virgin olive oil, and there's a reason to sometimes choose it over extra-virgin olive oil. It's the better choice for high-temperature cooking because of its higher smoke point (the smoke point is the temperature at which an oil starts to smoke because it's breaking down into glycerol and free fatty acids).

**Macadamia nut oil**—Macadamia nut oil, made from pressed macadamia nuts, is low in saturated fat, so it's a good alternative to butter or margarine, and you can use it in place of vegetable and other less healthful oils. Macadamia nut oil also reduces the risk of heart disease because it's high in good fat, and it has an anti-inflammatory influence in the body.

**Ghee**—Ghee is another ancient (Indian) cooking oil with medicinal benefits. It's the rich butterfat left after a process that removes the moisture and milk solids (which are mostly proteins) from butter. It's a good source of high-quality fats, and even if you have issues with dairy, you'll probably be okay with ghee.

**Malaysian red palm fruit oil**—Palm fruit oil is extracted from the fleshy fruit of the palm tree. It has been used as a healthy cooking oil for thousands of years; it's a common cooking ingredient in Southeast Asia and Africa. But—and this is key— you'll want to buy only *Malaysian palm fruit oil* (because it's sustainably raised). One of the biggest benefits of palm fruit oil is that it's a rich source of vitamins and antioxidants like vitamin E tocotrienols and carotenoids.

## Keep Me Cool Oils

**Walnut oil**—Walnut oil is made from Persian walnuts and is best uncooked or cold; when it's heated, it can become bitter. Mix it in cold sauces or drizzle it on salads, on pasta, or on grilled fish and steak. Or substitute it for olive oil for some variety in dipping. As for its health benefits, walnut oil contains omega-3 fats and is high in antioxidants.

**Cold-pressed sesame oil**—Sesame seed oil is made from the seed of the sesame plant. I specify cold-pressed because it's a process that helps retain the seed's nutrients and aroma. This oil also contains vitamins and minerals that help battle arthritis and boost bone health.

**Extra-virgin olive oil (EVOO)**—EVOO is the result of the first cold-pressing of olives, meaning the oil is extracted without heat or chemicals. It's distinguished from the other grades of olive oil by its purity and low acidity. It's best used in salad dressings, but it can be drizzled over just about anything, including grilled veggies.

**Avocado oil**—Avocado oil, with its high chlorophyll content, is pressed from the fleshy part of avocados and has all the heart-soothing monounsaturated fat of the original fruit. You can certainly cook with avocado oil because it has a very high smoke point, but I prefer to use it in salad dressings or to flavor food.

**Flaxseed oil**—Flaxseed oil is also known as linseed oil. It comes from the seeds of a blue-flowering plant found in western Canada and is a powerhouse for your health and wellness. It's one of nature's richest sources of omega-3 fatty acids, giving you more than you get from fish oil. I prefer to use freshly ground flaxseed, rather than the oil, as it has less chance of oxidizing and provides amazing lignans and fiber.

**Grapeseed oil**—Grapeseed oil is extracted from the seeds of grapes, usually as a by-product of wine-making. It's a lightly colored, flavorful oil that contains linoleic acid, an unsaturated omega-6 fatty acid. Grapeseed oil is also rich in flavonoids called oligomeric proanthocyanidins (OPCs), which are compounds that have powerful antioxidant benefits.

## NUTS AND SEEDS

If you're cooking the Virgin Diet way as a vegetarian or vegan, nuts and seeds are an essential source of protein for you and it's critical that you're mindful about getting enough. You can't keep them all to yourself, though! Everyone who wants to lose weight or maintain weight loss can benefit from the healthy fats, fiber, vitamin Bs, and other minerals, like zinc, magnesium, and potassium, squeezed into those tiny packages. When you reach for them, go for the organic, raw versions whenever possible.

And I recommend you rinse or soak your nuts and seeds to decrease the naturally occurring anti-nutrients in them and make them easier to digest. Just put them in water with a little added salt for 8 to 12 hours (cashews are an exception; soak them for only 6 hours). If you can, change the water three or four times during the soak. Once you've soaked them, you can dry them in a dehydrator or roast them in an oven (on a baking sheet) on the lowest setting for 8 hours.

## NUT BUTTERS

Nuts are ideal swaps for peanuts, so it stands to reason that their butters would be super lateral shifts for peanut butter, and they are.

Most nut butters are nutritional equals, but I generally recommend almond butter and cashew butter. Like the others, they're both rich in monounsaturated fats, which may reduce heart disease risk and help lower "bad" LDL cholesterol. The rule of thumb here is to choose the nut butters with the fewest ingredients (that may mean just nuts and salt, but gold star for you if you find ones with no added salt). All nut butters are very high in calories, though, so know when to say when.

## SAUCES

Mastering your new kitchen and all these explosively healthy recipes means that as you're twirling from counter to counter, you'll no doubt be whipping up sauces and splashing vinegar in this or that. Watch out! Sauces and salad dressings provide cover for gluten and sugar to sneak into your diet and undo your progress. Save money and reduce your risk by making your own.

If you're specifically looking for an alternative to soy sauce, though, there are worthy options you can buy. Organic coconut aminos is a soy-free sauce, made from raw low-glycemic coconut tree sap and unrefined sea salt. If you're not soy sensitive, you can add Bragg's aminos or gluten-free tamari in Cycle 3. Any of those are delicious alternative seasonings to soy sauce and can be poured on everything from salads to sushi.

## SPICES AND HERBS

The core piece of advice I give throughout this cookbook applies here, too: Seek out organic, non-GMO, non-irradiated herbs and spices. Choose the all-natural varieties and always go with fresh whenever possible. Here are the ones to have on hand because you'll use them most often in the recipes in this book:

Basil

Black peppercorns

Cinnamon

Cumin

Curcumin (turmeric)

Herbes de Provence

Italian spice blend

Mexican spice blend

Oregano

Red chiles

Red pepper (cayenne)

Rosemary

Sea salt

## BEVERAGES

Hydrate, hydrate, hydrate! You'll support your weight loss efforts by reducing your risk of overeating, and you'll keep your system humming and your skin glowing. That means you should seriously limit liquids that do the opposite to you—diuretics like coffees (flavored and otherwise) and teas. You *can* have them, and I often recommend green tea for its fat-burning properties, but the balance of your liquids should come from still and sparkling water. For your Sunday morning frothy-drink jones, make your own lattes, frappuccinos, and cappuccinos with coconut milk or coconut creamer so you don't trigger a dairy intolerance or get more sugar than you bargained for.

Unsweetened coconut milk is my favorite you'll-never-miss-dairy swap because it's rich in fat-burning medium-chain triglycerides (MCTs). But unsweetened almond milk is also a delicious lateral shift. There are a lot of these milks on the market and many are camouflaged in "healthy" packaging, so buyer beware. When in doubt, always pick the one labeled "unsweetened." Hopefully coconut or almond milk will make you happy, because rice milk just doesn't provide the benefits the others do and is higher in carbohydrates.

And what about alcohol? Once you've gone through Cycles 1 and 2 of the Virgin Diet, you'll have plenty to celebrate. And you can do that with an adult beverage in Cycle 3! An occasional glass of red wine is not only okay, it can be good for your heart and slow down the aging process, something attributed to the powerful polyphenol resveratrol (pinot noir is highest in resveratrol). Tequila is another permissible choice; unlike most alcohols it's not grain-, rye-, barley-, or corn-based. Just make sure that you're not making this an everyday celebration.... Think of alcohol as sugar, because it's metabolized similarly.

## KITCHEN TOOLS

An artist is nothing without the right brush! So to prepare for all the gorgeous, delicious kitchen masterpieces you're going to whip up, you'll need the right tools at your fingertips. You're likely to have many of these already, but take a quick inventory and add to your cupboards where you see the need.

| | |
|---|---|
| Can opener | Electric hand mixer |
| Coffee grinder for herbs and spices | Food processor |
| Colander | Graters: 1 box and 1 Microplane grater |
| Cutting boards: 2, wood or plastic | Heat-resistant spatulas |
| Dry and liquid measuring cups | Ice cream maker |

Instant-read meat thermometer

Kitchen scale

Kitchen shears

Kitchen timer

Knives: a chef's knife, a paring knife, and serrated knives

Ladle

Magic Bullet or NutriBullet blender for traveling

Mason jars

Measuring spoons

Mixing bowls

Parchment paper

Pots and pans: cast-iron, enamel, and/or hard anodized nonstick skillets; stainless steel pots and saucepans

Salad spinner

Shallow roasting pan (baking pan)

Slow cooker

Steamer basket or insert

Storage containers

Tongs

Vegetable peeler

Vitamix or blender

Whisk

Wooden spoons

## VIRGIN DIET SUCCESS

### *Melody Copelan—Toccoa, GA*

"Fast foods, fried foods, and constantly eating out" describes the way I used to eat. Being too tired to cook and in too much pain to do much else paints a picture of how I have felt for years. Having been diagnosed with gastroesophageal reflux disease 6 years ago, I couldn't go one day without my medicine. I struggled with fatigue, gas, bloating, brain fog, digestive issues, trouble sleeping, and dark circles under my eyes, and then there was the unmanageable joint pain and stiffness. In October 2011, I was diagnosed with psoriatic arthritis. The medicines that my rheumatologist put me on had awful side effects, and they either didn't work or lowered my immune system so much that I was sick all the time. My life was so incomplete when I should have been on top of the world.

One of my four daughters was a senior in high school, and in December of 2011 my 3-month-old grandson came to live with us. Instead of being able to live fully, my body was crumbling in on itself. I had trouble doing simple tasks, such as holding an infant for extended periods of time and simple household chores. Fortunately, I have three wonderful daughters and an awesome husband who picked up the slack and took care of me. However, keeping up with my sweet girls and a fast-growing little one was becoming increasingly difficult. A weekend beach trip in May 2012 was spent in the room in pain, and my condition was worsening. By December, I was on my fourth medicine for the arthritis and still nothing was working; I was sick and tired of being sick and tired. I began searching the Internet, looking for answers. Somewhere, there had to be an answer that didn't include medicine.

Finally, I found *The Virgin Diet*. I read the first few pages on my tablet's preview, decided to buy it, began reading it immediately, and thought JJ wrote this book just for me. Making a decision to follow the plan exactly, I began my journey. Within 2 weeks I came off my medication for GERD and never took another dose of medicine for arthritis. By the end of my 21 days, I felt like a different person. Joint pain, gas and bloating, brain fog, and digestive issues were gone. Even the dark circles under my eyes were visibly better. You get the picture, and these are just a few of the symptoms that following the Virgin Diet has relieved. My energy level was through the roof. I felt so much better that I was scared to test for intolerances.

It was day 45 before I decided that I had to know what would happen if I added some of these foods back into my diet. Gluten immediately caused my joint pain to return, and dairy and soy caused stomach and digestive issues as well as gas and bloating. This realization made it much easier for me to stay away from those foods! In March 2013, I went for a follow-up with my rheumatologist and she could not find any inflammation in any of my joints (except the wrist that I broke 7 years ago). On top of that, she couldn't believe how much better I looked.

It has been 6 months and I have lost 40 pounds. I no longer come home from work and collapse. I have begun walking and am adding a toning routine. My family has been so supportive, and they make sure I have the things I need to continue feeling great. It has made them more aware of the foods they consume. My husband is finally on board, and although not yet following the plan, he has made some big changes in his diet and after only a week is seeing results. My sister was able to bust her yearlong weight plateau and at the same time has moved to a healthier lifestyle. Several of my friends are following the plan and have seen big changes in their lives. That is probably the most rewarding for me— helping others get healthy.

Because my health is better, I am able to do more. Being able to keep up with my grandson and three teenage daughters has made my life full again. My family is excited to have their wife and mother healthy, and when I see *my* mom, she tells me how proud she is of me. I'm excited to feel and look younger than I have in years. Thank you, JJ, for showing me that food relates directly to how my body works and feels, and for helping me take my life back.

*My Original Virgin Diet Recipe*

## PICO DE GALLO AVOCADO

*Serves 4 to 6*

1 pound Roma tomatoes, diced
1 red onion, diced
1 jalapeño, diced
¼ cup fresh cilantro, chopped
1½ teaspoons olive oil
1 avocado, diced
½ lime, juiced

Combine the tomatoes, onion, jalapeño, cilantro, and olive oil in a bowl. In a separate bowl combine the avocado and lime juice (this will keep the avocado from turning brown). Stir the avocado and lime juice into the Pico mixture. Enjoy with grilled chicken, shrimp, or fish.

To see Melody's interview, visit thevirgindietcookbook.com/bonus.

## TIME-EFFICIENT MEAL PREP

If there's one thing we all have in common, it's that time is at a premium and we can't afford to spend more of it in the kitchen than we have to. No one is wearing a red cape and making every meal of every day from scratch, so don't feel like you have to, either. To stay the course with meals that will help you lose weight and make you feel fabulous from the inside out, be smart about how you approach meal preparation. All it takes is some planning and knowing a few shortcuts.

First, keep your pantry, fridge, and freezer as well stocked as possible, so you always have the building blocks of a healthy, energizing, weight loss–promoting meal. It's the safety net for your goals—always be able to quickly put your hands on the ingredients of a Virgin Shake or a colorful, crisp salad. Soups and stir-fries can also be fast go-to's in a well-stocked kitchen. Just a little bit of up-front effort pays big dividends when you're crunched at mealtime.

I've recommended that you have at least one big grocery excursion day a week to reduce the time gobbled up by a hundred short shopping runs. Another way to get time back and relieve the stress that a daily preoccupation with meal planning can bring is to use the weekend to architect and build some meals for the entire week. If you can take a couple of hours on Sunday to prepare and freeze meals, you've given yourself a running start, and the week ahead will suddenly seem a lot less daunting.

For the times you do decide to put on your chef's apron and stir things up, double or triple the recipe and freeze the additional portions. Or stick the extra in the fridge for lunches the next day. If you have a slow cooker, you know that it can also save you on busy days. But there are times when you won't even have time to get that started, so freezing and leftovers become emergency stopgaps. Repurposing is a stress-busting godsend! You'll get the rhythm of this in no time.

So there you have it! You know the best foods to buy, you've got all the right tools, and you cannot be stopped! Go forth and conquer the amazing recipes in this cookbook, and seize the weight loss, high energy, and healthy long life that are waiting for you!

# PART II

# THE VIRGIN DIET RECIPES

Yes, I know you understand that breakfast is the most important meal of the day. But that doesn't mean a sugar-loaded grab-and-go will cut it.

Research shows that people who eat a protein-packed breakfast lose weight more easily and keep it off longer than those who eat a sugary breakfast or skip it all together. I can't even bear the thought that you might be a skipper! If you skip, you're slowing your metabolic rate, and you're likely to gorge at lunch. Or before. And probably straight through the rest of the day until you pass out. So, no, skipping isn't helping you lose weight.

Eat within an hour of waking up, and make sure your breakfast (whether it's one of my addictive, filling, fat-burning shakes or something that requires a fork) has clean, lean protein; healthy fats; and high-fiber, slow-releasing carbohydrates. A substantial, balanced breakfast is the key to kicking you into your day energized, with your blood sugar stable and the urge to snack kept at bay.

## BLUEBERRY POWER MUFFINS

Power muffins! It's about time! Your cup of coffee is so happy. And since they're gluten-free and naturally sweet, you can indulge without worrying about digestive upset or the muffin becoming a muffin top.

Serve these with a side of nitrate-free chicken breakfast sausage or uncured bacon, or 2 to 4 ounces of last night's leftover protein.

*Makes 12 muffins*

1⅓ cups Bob's Red Mill Gluten-Free All-Purpose Biscuit and Baking Mix
¾ cup (3 ounces) ground raw almonds

¼ cup chia seeds

¼ cup freshly ground flaxseeds

2 teaspoons monk fruit extract

2 teaspoons aluminum-free baking powder

1 teaspoon ground cinnamon

¼ teaspoon sea salt

1⅓ cups unsweetened coconut milk (such as So Delicious)

¼ cup macadamia nut oil

1 tablespoon vanilla extract

⅔ cup fresh or frozen organic blueberries, thawed if frozen

Preheat the oven to 350°F. Line a 12-cup muffin pan with paper liners.

Combine the baking mix, almonds, chia seeds, flax meal, monk fruit extract, baking powder, cinnamon, and salt in a large bowl; whisk well.

Combine the coconut milk, oil, and vanilla extract in a separate bowl. Add the wet ingredients to the dry, and stir with a rubber spatula or wooden spoon until just moistened. Gently fold in the blueberries.

Spoon the batter into the lined muffin cups. Bake until the tops are lightly browned and a toothpick inserted into the center comes out clean, 27 to 29 minutes. Remove from the oven and cool completely in the muffin pan.

## Nutrient Content per Serving

| | | | | | |
|---|---|---|---|---|---|
| **Calories:** | 175 | **Fat:** | 11 grams | **Protein:** | 4 grams |
| **Fiber:** | 4 grams | **Saturated Fat:** | 1 gram | **Carbs:** | 16 grams |
| **Sodium:** | 330 mg | | | | |

## COCONUT-ALLSPICE STEEL-CUT OATS WITH PROTEIN BOOST

There might not be a better way to start the morning than with this protein-rich breakfast, full of tropical island flavors. In less than 10 minutes you'll be enjoying this warm and satisfying meal. Bring on the day!

*Makes 1 serving*

¾ cup water

¼ cup quick-cooking gluten-free steel-cut oats

½ teaspoon monk fruit extract

½ teaspoon coconut extract

⅛ teaspoon ground allspice

⅓ cup unsweetened coconut milk (such as So Delicious)

1 scoop vanilla vegan protein powder

1 tablespoon unsweetened shredded coconut

Bring the water to a boil in a small saucepan over medium-high heat. Stir in the oats, monk fruit extract, coconut extract, and allspice. Cover, reduce the heat to medium-low, and simmer, stirring often, until tender and the liquid has been absorbed, 5 to 7 minutes.

Meanwhile, combine the coconut milk and protein powder in a small bowl, and stir until the powder has dissolved.

Stir the coconut milk mixture into the oats, add the shredded coconut, and serve immediately.

### Nutrient Content per Serving

| | | | | | |
|---|---|---|---|---|---|
| Calories: | 306 | Fat: | 11 grams | Protein: | 18 grams |
| Fiber: | 9 grams | Saturated Fat: | 6 grams | Carbs: | 40 grams |
| Sodium: | 117 mg | | | | |

## SWEDISH-STYLE PECAN PANCAKES WITH ORANGE AND STRAWBERRIES

To add an elegant touch to a weekend morning, try these Swedish-style pancakes. They're thin and crepe-like, and traditionally served rolled up on a plate with jam. I dropped the jam sugar bomb and swapped in a delicious strawberry-orange topping. Pecans add a little protein crunch and slow sugar absorption. But you'll need more protein than that; I serve mine with a side of chicken breakfast sausage.

*Makes 2 servings*

### *Fruit Topping*

1 cup strawberries, sliced

1 small orange, peeled, sectioned, and coarsely chopped

¼ teaspoon stevia extract

### *Pancakes*

⅓ cup Bob's Red Mill Gluten-Free All-Purpose Baking Flour

1½ scoops vanilla vegan protein powder

2 tablespoons arrowroot

½ teaspoon aluminum-free baking powder

¼ teaspoon baking soda

½ teaspoon stevia extract

2 tablespoons finely chopped pecans

¾ cup unsweetened coconut milk (such as So Delicious)

½ teaspoon vanilla extract

2 teaspoons coconut oil

Combine the strawberries, orange, and stevia extract in a bowl; let stand for at least 15 minutes or refrigerate for up to 2 hours.

Sift the baking flour, protein powder, arrowroot, baking powder, baking soda, and stevia extract through a wire strainer into a medium bowl; add the pecans and whisk to mix.

Combine the coconut milk and vanilla extract in a separate bowl. Pour the wet ingredients into the dry, and stir with a rubber spatula until just moistened.

Heat a large nonstick skillet over medium heat. Add 1 teaspoon of the coconut oil and swirl to coat. Cook 4 pancakes at a time; for each, spoon 2 slightly rounded tablespoons into the pan and spread into a thin 3-inch-diameter pancake. Cook until the tops of the pancakes have some bubbles and the bottoms are golden, about 3 minutes. Turn and cook 3 minutes longer, or until golden brown and cooked through. Repeat with the remaining oil and batter. Serve topped with the fruit mixture.

## Nutrient Content per Serving

| | | | | | | |
|---|---|---|---|---|---|---|
| Calories: | 297 | Fat: | 12 grams | Protein: | 12 grams |
| Fiber: | 8 grams | Saturated Fat: | 3 grams | Carbs: | 40 grams |
| Sodium: | 356 mg | | | | |

## HOT QUINOA FLAKE CEREAL WITH WARM BERRY COMPOTE

Breakfast should always make you feel good, and how can you resist one with warm berries? This hearty, highly satisfying breakfast will warm your belly and give you a protein kick to start your day. I like to use So Delicious unsweetened coconut milk, which tastes great and is also rich in minerals and good fats.

*Makes 1 serving*

1 cup fresh strawberries, hulled and sliced

½ cup fresh blueberries

¾ teaspoon vanilla extract

¼ teaspoon monk fruit extract

⅓ cup unsweetened coconut milk (such as So Delicious)

1 scoop vanilla vegan protein power

1 cup water

⅛ teaspoon ground cinnamon

⅓ cup quinoa flakes cereal

2 tablespoons chopped slow-roasted pecans (see page 128)

1 tablespoon chia seeds (optional)

Combine the strawberries, blueberries, ¼ teaspoon of the vanilla extract, and the monk fruit extract in a small saucepan. Cook over low heat, stirring occasionally, until the fruit is warm and tender, about 4 minutes.

Meanwhile, combine the coconut milk and protein powder in a small bowl and stir until the powder has dissolved; set aside.

Combine the water, the remaining ½ teaspoon vanilla, and the cinnamon in a small saucepan and bring to a boil over medium-high heat. Add the cereal, reduce to medium, and cook, stirring often, until thickened, about 1½ minutes. Remove from the heat and stir in the coconut milk mixture, pecans, and chia seeds (if using).

## Nutrient Content per Serving

| | | | | | | |
|---|---|---|---|---|---|---|
| **Calories:** | 433 | **Fat:** | 19 grams | **Protein:** | 14 grams |
| **Fiber:** | 14 grams | **Saturated Fat:** | 3 grams | **Carbs:** | 57 grams |
| **Sodium:** | 76 mg | | | | |

## BACON-AND-MUSHROOM SWEET POTATO HASH

Hash often flies under the radar as a humble breakfast dish, but this recipe may make you rethink that. It's a stick-to-your-ribs blend of bacon, mushrooms, and the vitamin A–rich sweet potato. Think about making double—it's simple to reheat as a side dish for your next meal.

*Makes 1 serving*

1 small sweet potato (about 5 ounces), peeled, halved lengthwise, and sliced into thin half-moons

4 slices nitrate-free bacon

1 medium red onion, thinly sliced

2 garlic cloves, sliced

¼ teaspoon dried basil

¼ teaspoon ground cumin

4 ounces white mushrooms, sliced

¼ teaspoon sea salt

⅛ teaspoon freshly ground black pepper

Place the sweet potato in a small saucepan and add enough cold water to cover by 2 inches. Bring to a boil and cook until the potato is crisp-tender, about 2 minutes; drain and set aside.

Cook the bacon in a large nonstick skillet over medium heat until crisp, 6 to 7 minutes. Drain on a plate lined with a paper towel, and then cut into 1-inch pieces.

Pour off all but 1 tablespoon fat from the skillet and heat the skillet over medium-high heat. Add the onion, garlic, basil, and cumin and cook for 1 minute. Stir in the mushrooms and cook, stirring occasionally, until they are starting to brown, 5 to 6 minutes. Add the sweet potatoes and continue cooking until they are tender, 4 to 5 minutes longer. Remove from the heat and stir in the bacon, salt, and pepper.

### Nutrient Content per Serving

| | | | | | |
|---|---|---|---|---|---|
| Calories: | 326 | Fat: | 10 grams | Protein: | 15 grams |
| Fiber: | 6 grams | Saturated Fat: | 3 grams | Carbs: | 43 grams |
| Sodium: | 1292 mg | | | | |

## BASIC VIRGIN DIET SHAKE

I often hear from my clients that a shake for breakfast is the cornerstone for them in fast fat loss. This one is the original. It's naturally sweet and loaded with fiber. You'll never believe something so tasty could be so good for you!

*Makes 1 serving*

2 scoops vegan protein powder
1 to 2 scoops fiber blend
1 to 2 scoops chia seeds or freshly ground flaxseeds
8 to 10 ounces unsweetened coconut milk or almond milk (such as So Delicious)
½ to 1 cup low-sugar fruit (such as blueberries, raspberries, blackberries)
5 to 10 ice cubes

Combine the protein powder, fiber blend, chia seeds, coconut milk, fruit, and ice cubes in a blender. Mix on high speed until smooth. Thin with cold water if desired.

### Nutrient Content per Serving

| | | | | | |
|---|---|---|---|---|---|
| Calories: | 331 | Fat: | 13 grams | Protein: | 24 grams |
| Fiber: | 17 grams | Saturated Fat: | 5 grams | Carbs: | 36 grams |
| Sodium: | 371 mg | | | | |

# WHAT TO LOOK FOR IN A SHAKE

Replace a meal a day with a healthy shake to support fat loss, optimal nutrition, and ideal body composition.

**Choose a high-quality protein base:** I recommend vegan rice, pea, chlorella, or chia protein, or blends of these. If you suspect a dairy allergy after you reintroduce dairy into your diet, do not choose a whey protein product.

**Avoid:** Soy, egg, and milk protein powders; and artificial colors and sweeteners such as aspartame and sucralose.

**Look for:** GMO-free and hormone (rBGH)–free. Make sure your protein powder is low in sugar—stick with a very small amount of natural sweetener or sugar alcohol (e.g., stevia or xylitol), 5 grams per serving max. Look for shakes made with 10 grams or less of net carbs per serving—the less the better so you can add fruit and veggies without raising the carb count excessively.

## MIXED BERRY AND AVOCADO PROTEIN SHAKE

When you sneak avocado into this delicious shake, you're upping the healthy fat content and turning your fat-burning machinery to 11.

*Makes 1 serving*

2 scoops vanilla vegan protein powder
1 cup unsweetened coconut milk (such as So Delicious)
1 cup frozen organic mixed berries
½ small ripe avocado
1 to 2 tablespoons freshly ground flaxseeds
¼ to ½ cup cold water

Combine the protein powder, coconut milk, mixed berries, avocado, flax meal, and ¼ cup water in a blender. Mix on high speed until smooth. Thin with additional cold water if desired.

### Nutrient Content per Serving

| | | | | | |
|---|---|---|---|---|---|
| **Calories:** | 402 | **Fat:** | 22 grams | **Protein:** | 26 grams |
| **Fiber:** | 17 grams | **Saturated Fat:** | 6 grams | **Carbs:** | 40 grams |
| **Sodium:** | 244 mg | | | | |

## CHOCOLATE-CHERRY-CHIA PROTEIN SHAKE

Enjoy this decadent shake anytime, for any meal. In fact, sub it for two meals to step up fat burning and get double its protein boost. So good!

*Makes 1 serving*

2 scoops chocolate vegan protein powder

1 cup frozen organic unsweetened pitted dark cherries

1 cup unsweetened almond milk (such as So Delicious)

1 tablespoon raw or homemade almond butter (see page 128)

1 to 2 tablespoons chia seeds

¼ to ½ cup cold water

Combine the protein powder, cherries, almond milk, almond butter, chia seeds, and ¼ cup water in a blender. Mix on high speed until smooth. Thin with additional cold water if desired.

### Nutrient Content per Serving

| | | | | | |
|---|---|---|---|---|---|
| Calories: | 431 | Fat: | 21 grams | Protein: | 30 grams |
| Fiber: | 15 grams | Saturated Fat: | 3 grams | Carbs: | 41 grams |
| Sodium: | 574 mg | | | | |

## GREEN COCONUT PROTEIN SHAKE

Don't let the color throw you! This nutrient-rich meal is delicious, can be made in minutes, and will power you for hours. Substitute ice for the cold water for a thicker, chillier treat.

*Makes 1 serving*

2 scoops vanilla vegan protein powder

1 cup unsweetened coconut milk (such as So Delicious)

1 cup organic baby kale or baby spinach

¼ small ripe avocado

¼ medium apple, peeled and cut into chunks

2 teaspoons chia seeds

¼ teaspoon coconut extract

¼ to ½ cup cold water

Combine the protein powder, coconut milk, kale, avocado, apple, chia seeds, coconut extract, and ¼ cup water in a blender. Mix on high speed until smooth. Thin with additional cold water if desired.

## Nutrient Content per Serving

| | | | | | |
|---|---|---|---|---|---|
| Calories: | 333 | Fat: | 18 grams | Protein: | 25 grams |
| Fiber: | 14 grams | Saturated Fat: | 6 grams | Carbs: | 29 grams |
| Sodium: | 280 mg | | | | |

## PEACH-BERRY-ALMOND PROTEIN SHAKE

We don't think of peaches enough, do we? But they're so deliciously juicy, not to mention a super source of detoxifying fiber and minerals. Throw in blueberries and almonds, and this shake is nothing short of a nutrient powerhouse.

*Makes 1 serving*

2 scoops vanilla vegan protein powder

1 cup unsweetened almond milk (such as So Delicious)

½ cup frozen organic sliced peaches

½ cup frozen organic blueberries

1 tablespoon raw or homemade almond butter (see page 128)

1 to 2 tablespoons freshly ground flaxseeds

¼ teaspoon almond extract

¼ to ½ cup cold water

Combine the protein powder, almond milk, peaches, blueberries, almond butter, flax meal, almond extract, and ¼ cup water in a blender. Mix on high speed until smooth. Thin with additional cold water if desired.

## Nutrient Content per Serving

| | | | | | |
|---|---|---|---|---|---|
| Calories: | 392 | Fat: | 19 grams | Protein: | 28 grams |
| Fiber: | 15 grams | Saturated Fat: | 2 grams | Carbs: | 37 grams |
| Sodium: | 442 mg | | | | |

## STRAWBERRY "MILKSHAKE" PROTEIN SHAKE

This thick and creamy shake tastes like a treat from childhood but delivers the very adult benefits that come from all the phytonutrients in strawberries. The polyphenols give you a powerful antioxidant boost while fiber helps regulate blood sugar and blood pressure. Yum!

*Makes 1 serving*

2 scoops vanilla vegan protein powder

1½ cups unsweetened coconut milk (such as So Delicious)

1 cup frozen organic unsweetened strawberries

1 to 2 tablespoons chia seeds

½ teaspoon vanilla extract

Combine the protein powder, coconut milk, strawberries, chia seeds, and vanilla extract in a blender. Mix on high speed until smooth. Thin with cold water if desired.

## Nutrient Content per Serving

| | | | | | |
|---|---|---|---|---|---|
| **Calories:** | 337 | **Fat:** | 15 grams | **Protein:** | 24 grams |
| **Fiber:** | 14 grams | **Saturated Fat:** | 7 grams | **Carbs:** | 34 grams |
| **Sodium:** | 247 mg | | | | |

## RISE AND SHINE MOCHA ESPRESSO PROTEIN SHAKE

If you're not one to pop out of bed ready to greet the day, this will help ease you into it. The soothing chocolate is a mood enhancer, and the espresso will help dilate your blood vessels and bring you back to life. In the meantime, it will have quietly slipped you an invigorating protein-and-good-fat boost. You're welcome!

Add a few ice cubes before blending to make a thicker shake. And if you don't have instant espresso or coffee powder on hand, substitute ¼ cup strong brewed coffee.

*Makes 1 serving*

2 scoops chocolate vegan protein powder

1 cup unsweetened almond milk (such as So Delicious)

1 tablespoon raw or homemade almond butter (see page 128)

1 to 2 tablespoons freshly ground flaxseeds

1 teaspoon instant espresso powder or coffee powder

⅛ teaspoon ground cinnamon

¼ teaspoon vanilla extract

¼ to ½ cup cold water

Combine the protein powder, almond milk, almond butter, flax meal, espresso powder, cinnamon, vanilla extract, and ¼ cup water in a blender. Mix on high speed until smooth. Thin with additional cold water if desired.

## Nutrient Content per Serving

| Calories: | 346 | Fat: | 19 grams | Protein: | 28 grams |
|---|---|---|---|---|---|
| Fiber: | 11 grams | Saturated Fat: | 2 grams | Carbs: | 22 grams |
| Sodium: | 569 mg | | | | |

## NUTTY CHAI BREAKFAST BLAST SHAKE

The spicy lushness of chai makes this shake slightly sweet, creamy, and rich—a taste so decadent you'll almost forget it's good for you! For a more intense chai flavor, add ¼ teaspoon ground cinnamon.

*Makes 1 serving*

2 scoops chai vegan protein powder

1 cup unsweetened coconut milk (such as So Delicious)

1 cup fresh baby spinach

½ medium apple, peeled and cut into chunks

1 tablespoon raw cashew butter

1 to 2 tablespoons freshly ground flaxseeds

¼ to ½ cup cold water

Combine the protein powder, coconut milk, spinach, apple, cashew butter, flax meal, and ¼ cup water in a blender. Mix on high speed until smooth. Thin with additional water if desired.

## Nutrient Content per Serving

| Calories: | 382 | Fat: | 19 grams | Protein: | 27 grams |
|---|---|---|---|---|---|
| Fiber: | 12 grams | Saturated Fat: | 7 grams | Carbs: | 37 grams |
| Sodium: | 277 mg | | | | |

# WRAPS, SALADS, AND SANDWICHES 5

Don't you just love a wrap? They just seem to tenderly caress our food. And when the food is this good, I get it. But of course I have just as much love for salads—which are a lot like wraps that have been set free.

For eating healthy and losing weight, it doesn't get much better than meals designed to deliver as many heart-healthy, brain-healthy, anti-inflammatory benefits as these. The lettuce and vegetables are high in fiber, vitamins, phytochemicals, and antioxidants, and once you've added a lean protein, it's an undeniable nutritional home run.

But that health pendulum can swing the other way if you sculpt your salad into a heaping mound topped with a gooey dressing, cheese, dried fruit, glazed nuts, and crunchy noodles. Now you have dessert, and a pro-inflammatory one at that. So here are the general rules for wraps and salads:

1. Start with great greens—no iceberg for you! The deeper the green color, the better.
2. Add some non-starchy veggies—make your plate a rainbow.
3. Toss on some clean, lean protein, meaning that it shouldn't be in a mayo bath or come with crunch.
4. Add a little high-fiber starchy carb.
5. Add some healthy fat.

My wrap and salad recipes follow these rules for you, but it's worth keeping them in mind when you're eating out or traveling.

## GRILLED PESTO CHICKEN WRAP

Among the many things to love about wraps is the way they expand. And this one has room for leftovers. No doubt it's yummy and filling enough as it is, but add your raw or leftover cooked veggies for an extra nutrient, flavor, and texture kick.

*Makes 2 servings*

2 (4-ounce) organic free-range boneless, skinless chicken breast halves, pounded to ½-inch thickness
2 teaspoons olive oil
1 garlic clove, minced
¼ teaspoon ground cumin
¼ teaspoon sea salt
⅛ teaspoon freshly ground black pepper
2 brown rice tortillas
4 tablespoons Pesto Sauce (page 211)
1 cup torn baby kale
4 oil-packed sun-dried tomatoes, drained, patted dry, and sliced

Combine the chicken, oil, garlic, cumin, salt, and pepper in a medium bowl. Heat a grill pan over medium heat until hot, add the chicken, and cook for 4 to 5 minutes per side, until an instant-read meat thermometer inserted into the thickest part registers 165°F. Transfer to a cutting board and let stand for 3 minutes. Then cut across the grain into thin slices.

Heat a large nonstick skillet over medium heat until hot. Working with one at a time, place the tortillas in the skillet and cook, turning several times, until heated through, about 45 seconds.

Lay the tortillas on a work surface and spread each one with 2 tablespoons of the pesto. Top with the kale, sun-dried tomatoes, and chicken. Roll up tightly.

### Nutrient Content per Serving

| | | | | | |
|---|---|---|---|---|---|
| Calories: | 489 | Fat: | 28 grams | Protein: | 28 grams |
| Fiber: | 4 grams | Saturated Fat: | 4 grams | Carbs: | 32 grams |
| Sodium: | 644 mg | | | | |

## CHICKEN CAESAR SALAD WRAP

When you're on the go, this wrap is hard to beat. The flavorful vitamin- and mineral-rich anchovies make this portable, easy-to-eat meal a treat for your taste buds, and it's much healthier than the traditional Caesar salad with chicken. What a pleasant surprise!

*Makes 2 servings*

3 tablespoons Creamy Eggless Mayo (page 214)

½ teaspoon grated lemon zest

½ teaspoon coconut aminos

1 oil-packed anchovy, mashed to a paste with a fork

⅛ teaspoon freshly ground black pepper

6 thinly sliced romaine lettuce leaves, about 3 cups

2 (4-ounce) organic free-range boneless, skinless chicken breast halves, pounded to ½-inch thickness

1 teaspoon olive oil

¼ teaspoon sea salt

⅛ teaspoon freshly ground black pepper

2 brown rice tortillas

Combine the mayo, lemon zest, coconut aminos, anchovy, and black pepper in a medium bowl. Add the lettuce and toss to coat; set aside.

Combine the chicken, oil, salt, and pepper in a medium bowl. Heat a grill pan over medium heat until hot, add the chicken, and cook for 4 to 5 minutes per side, until an instant-read meat thermometer inserted into the thickest part registers 165°F. Transfer to a cutting board and let stand for 3 minutes. Then cut across the grain into thin slices.

Heat a large nonstick skillet over medium heat until hot. Working with one at a time, place the tortillas in the skillet and cook, turning several times, until heated through, about 45 seconds total.

Lay the tortillas on a work surface and top each one with sliced chicken and the romaine mixture. Roll up tightly.

## Nutrient Content per Serving

| | | | | | |
|---|---|---|---|---|---|
| Calories: | 468 | Fat: | 25 grams | Protein: | 28 grams |
| Fiber: | 5 grams | Saturated Fat: | 3 grams | Carbs: | 31 grams |
| Sodium: | 799 mg | | | | |

## CHICKEN SALAD WRAP

It's easy to take chicken salad for granted, but look again. This version is filled with protein, amino acids, and omega-3 fatty acids, courtesy of the walnuts and chia seeds. If you're in a hurry, don't hesitate to use that leftover chicken.

*Makes 2 servings*

1½ cups organic low-sodium chicken broth

1 tablespoon coconut aminos

2 (4-ounce) organic free-range boneless, skinless chicken breast halves

1 small unpeeled apple, cut into ¼-inch dice (about ⅔ cup)

1 celery stalk, chopped

2 green onions, finely chopped

3 tablespoons walnuts, coarsely chopped

2 tablespoons Creamy Eggless Mayo (page 214)

2 tablespoons thinly sliced fresh basil

1 tablespoon chia seeds

⅛ teaspoon sea salt

⅛ teaspoon freshly ground black pepper

2 brown rice tortillas

Combine the broth and coconut aminos in a medium saucepan and bring to a boil over medium-high heat. Add the chicken and immediately reduce to a simmer. Cook until an instant-read meat thermometer inserted into the thickest portion registers 165°F, 10 to 12 minutes. Transfer the chicken to a cutting board and let it cool, about 10 minutes. Then cut the chicken into ½-inch pieces and combine them in a bowl with the apple, celery, green onions, walnuts, mayo, basil, chia seeds, salt, and pepper; mix well.

Heat a large nonstick skillet over medium heat until hot. Working with one at a time, place the tortillas in the skillet and cook, turning several times, until heated through, about 45 seconds.

Lay the tortillas on a work surface and top each one with half the chicken salad. Roll up tightly.

## Nutrient Content per Serving

| | | | | | |
|---|---|---|---|---|---|
| Calories: | 524 | Fat: | 25 grams | Protein: | 30 grams |
| Fiber: | 8 grams | Saturated Fat: | 3 grams | Carbs: | 44 grams |
| Sodium: | 669 mg | | | | |

## BLT AND AVOCADO WRAP

You'll love this new twist on an old classic. The avocado adds some great flavor and texture, not to mention all those good fats. Be sure to have all your ingredients ready before you heat the tortillas.

*Makes 2 servings*

2 brown rice tortillas

2 tablespoons Creamy Eggless Mayo (page 214)

8 slices nitrate-free bacon, cooked

4 (¼-inch-thick) tomato slices

1 cup baby spinach or arugula

⅔ avocado, sliced

Heat a large nonstick skillet over medium heat. Working with one at a time, place the tortillas in the skillet and heat until warm and pliable, about 45 seconds.

Lay the tortillas on a work surface and spread each one with mayo. Top with the bacon, tomato, baby spinach, and avocado. Roll up tightly.

## Nutrient Content per Serving

| | | | | | |
|---|---|---|---|---|---|
| Calories: | 497 | Fat: | 33 grams | Protein: | 14 grams |
| Fiber: | 7 grams | Saturated Fat: | 6 grams | Carbs: | 35 grams |
| Sodium: | 939 mg | | | | |

## FLANK STEAK WRAP WITH CHIPOTLE MAYONNAISE AND HEIRLOOM TOMATO

There's no sacrifice in taste or quality for lunch today—steak isn't just for dinner anymore! Make this wrap with leftover cooked flank steak, pork tenderloin, or chicken and serve it at room temperature.

*Makes 2 servings*

8 ounces grass-fed flank steak, trimmed

1 teaspoon Barbecue Spice Rub (page 213)

3 tablespoons Creamy Eggless Mayo (page 214)

½ canned chipotle in adobo sauce, minced

2 brown rice tortillas

1 medium heirloom tomato, cut into 4 slices

2 romaine lettuce leaves, thinly sliced (about 1 cup)

¼ cup thinly sliced red onion

Rub the entire surface of the steak with the spice rub. Let stand at room temperature for 15 minutes.

Heat a grill pan over medium heat until hot. Add the steak and cook for 4 to 5 minutes per side for medium-rare, or to desired doneness. Transfer to a cutting board and let stand for 5 minutes. Then cut the steak diagonally across the grain into thin slices.

Combine the mayonnaise with the chipotle; set aside.

Heat a large nonstick skillet over medium heat until hot. Working with one at a time, place the tortillas in the skillet and cook, turning several times, until heated through, about 45 seconds.

Lay the tortillas on a work surface and spread each one with the mayo mixture. Top with the tomato slices, lettuce, onion, and sliced steak. Roll up tightly.

## Nutrient Content per Serving

| | | | | | | |
|---|---|---|---|---|---|---|
| Calories: | 507 | Fat: | 28 grams | Protein: | 28 grams |
| Fiber: | 5 grams | Saturated Fat: | 6 grams | Carbs: | 34 grams |
| Sodium: | 520 mg | | | | |

## TEX-MEX TURKEY WRAP WITH SALSA, AVOCADO, AND ARUGULA

Tex-Mex is like anything else that allows you to enjoy the best of two worlds. And this wrap exemplifies that by combining sensationally flavorful, nutrient-dense ingredients from both sides of the border. Make the salsa as chunky or as smooth as you'd like—for chunky, chop the tomatoes into ⅓-inch pieces; for smooth, blend the ingredients briefly in a food processor.

*Makes 2 servings*

1 medium plum tomato, seeded and chopped (about ½ cup)
2 tablespoons finely chopped red onion
1 tablespoon chopped fresh cilantro
2 teaspoons lime juice
½ small jalapeño pepper, finely chopped (optional)
⅛ teaspoon sea salt
1 small avocado
2 brown rice tortillas
2 tablespoons Creamy Eggless Mayo (page 214)
8 ounces deli-sliced nitrate-free turkey breast
1 cup baby arugula

Combine the tomato, onion, cilantro, lime juice, jalapeño, and salt in a small bowl. Slice the avocado.

Heat a large nonstick skillet over medium heat. Working with one at a time, place the tortillas in the skillet and cook, turning several times, until heated through, about 45 seconds.

Lay the tortillas on a work surface and spread each one with mayo. Top them with the turkey, avocado, arugula, and the tomato mixture. Roll up tightly.

## Nutrient Content per Serving

| | | | | | | |
|---|---|---|---|---|---|---|
| Calories: | 486 | Fat: | 26 grams | Protein: | 25 grams |
| Fiber: | 8 grams | Saturated Fat: | 3 grams | Carbs: | 9 grams |
| Sodium: | 1019 mg | | | | |

## THANKSGIVING TURKEY WRAP WITH CRANBERRY SAUCE

Turkey and cranberry is such a delicious combination, there's no way it should be relegated to a once-a-year holiday. Plus, turkey breast is a lean protein source, rich in heart-healthy nutrients. So make up a holiday of your own and dig in; I promise you won't fall asleep on the couch after this one! Brown rice tortillas are usually found in the freezer section of your grocery store.

*Makes 2 servings*

2 brown rice tortillas
2 tablespoons Creamy Eggless Mayo (page 214)
4 tablespoons Nutty Cranberry-Orange Sauce (page 212)
1 cup baby kale
8 ounces deli-sliced nitrate-free turkey breast
½ medium unpeeled apple, cut into 8 slices
2 tablespoons thinly sliced red onion

Heat a large nonstick skillet over medium heat. Working with one at a time, place the tortillas in the skillet and cook, turning several times, until heated through, about 45 seconds.

Lay the tortillas on a work surface and spread each one with mayo and cranberry-orange sauce. Top with the kale, turkey, apple slices, and onion. Roll up tightly.

### Nutrient Content per Serving

| | | | | | |
|---|---|---|---|---|---|
| Calories: | 416 | Fat: | 16 grams | Protein: | 25 grams |
| Fiber: | 4 grams | Saturated Fat: | 2 grams | Carbs: | 41 grams |
| Sodium: | 1022 mg | | | | |

## FLANK STEAK BISTRO CHOPPED SALAD

Be forewarned—this is likely to become your new favorite salad! It's not only flavorful, it also packs a serious nutrient punch. Grass-fed steak is a lean protein source that's high in omega-3 fatty acids, and the rainbow of veggies are loaded with antioxidants and support detoxification. Other vegetables, including broccoli, zucchini, and green beans, make lovely additions to this salad.

*Makes 2 servings*

8 ounces grass-fed flank steak, trimmed
1 teaspoon Dijon mustard
5 teaspoons olive oil

1 teaspoon chopped fresh rosemary

½ teaspoon sea salt

¼ teaspoon freshly ground black pepper

1 small head romaine lettuce, chopped (about 4 cups)

1 medium cucumber, peeled, seeded, and cut into ½-inch dice

1 medium red bell pepper, cut into ½-inch dice

2 celery stalks, cut into ½-inch dice

3 radishes, cut into ½-inch dice

1 small red onion, finely chopped

1 tablespoon white balsamic vinegar

Combine the steak, mustard, 1 teaspoon of the oil, and the rosemary in a medium bowl. Heat a grill pan over medium heat until hot. Season the steak with ¼ teaspoon of the salt and ⅛ teaspoon of the pepper, and add it to the pan; cook for 4 to 5 minutes per side for medium-rare, or to desired doneness. Transfer to a cutting board and let stand for 5 minutes.

While the steak rests, combine the lettuce, cucumber, bell pepper, celery, radishes, onion, vinegar, and the remaining 4 teaspoons oil, ¼ teaspoon salt, and ⅛ teaspoon pepper in a separate bowl.

Cut the steak diagonally across the grain into thin slices. Divide the salad between two plates, and top it with the steak.

## Nutrient Content per Serving

| | | | | | |
|---|---|---|---|---|---|
| Calories: | 387 | Fat: | 21 grams | Protein: | 29 grams |
| Fiber: | 10 grams | Saturated Fat: | 5 grams | Carbs: | 22 grams |
| Sodium: | 752 mg | | | | |

## SHEPHERD'S SALAD WITH PRAWNS

This snappy, well-dressed salad is topped with large wild prawns, which deliver a healthy dose of protein and omega-3 fatty acids. Mini, or Persian, cucumbers have thin peels that are not waxy or bitter and should be left on.

*Makes 2 servings*

4 mini or Persian cucumbers, unpeeled, cut into ½-inch dice

1 small red bell pepper, cut into ½-inch dice

3 medium plum tomatoes, seeded and chopped

½ small red onion, chopped (about ½ cup)

2 tablespoons chopped fresh parsley

1 tablespoon red wine vinegar

2 tablespoons extra-virgin olive oil

⅜ teaspoon sea salt

¼ teaspoon freshly ground black pepper

2 teaspoons olive oil

12 ounces large wild prawns, peeled and deveined

Combine the cucumbers, bell pepper, tomatoes, onion, parsley, vinegar, extra-virgin olive oil, ¼ teaspoon of the salt, and ⅛ teaspoon of the pepper in a large bowl.

Heat the olive oil in a large nonstick skillet over medium-high heat. Season the prawns with the remaining ⅛ teaspoon salt and ⅛ teaspoon pepper. Add them to the skillet and cook until pink and opaque, about 1½ minutes per side. Transfer to a plate.

Divide the salad between two plates and top each with prawns. Serve the prawns warm or at room temperature.

## Nutrient Content per Serving

| | | | | | | |
|---|---|---|---|---|---|---|
| **Calories:** | 346 | **Fat:** | 19 grams | **Protein:** | 30 grams |
| **Fiber:** | 5 grams | **Saturated Fat:** | 3 grams | **Carbs:** | 15 grams |
| **Sodium:** | 566 mg | | | | |

## SEARED AHI TUNA OVER ASIAN SLAW

*Ahi* is the Hawaiian name for yellowfin tuna. It's meaty and high in protein, omega-3 fatty acids, B vitamins, and minerals. When it's cooked—whether in your kitchen or on an outdoor grill—it should be firm but tender. Tuna is a medium-mercury fish, so if you're hooked on this dish and like to have it weekly, switch it up occasionally with salmon, shrimp, or halibut.

*Makes 2 servings*

3 cups thinly sliced napa cabbage (about ⅓ medium head)

½ medium bell pepper, thinly sliced

2 green onions, thinly sliced

2 tablespoons chopped fresh cilantro

2 ounces snow peas, thinly sliced

1 tablespoon lime juice

2 tablespoons Creamy Eggless Mayo (page 214)

¼ teaspoon sea salt

2 (6-ounce) ahi tuna steaks, about 1 inch thick

1 teaspoon Asian sesame oil

1 teaspoon coconut aminos

Combine the cabbage, bell pepper, green onions, cilantro, and snow peas in a medium bowl. In a separate bowl whisk together the lime juice, mayo, and ⅛ teaspoon of the salt; toss with the cabbage and set aside.

Combine the tuna steaks, sesame oil, and coconut aminos in a bowl and let stand for 5 minutes at room temperature.

Heat a grill pan over medium heat until hot. Season the tuna with the remaining ⅛ teaspoon salt and place it on the pan. Cook the tuna, turning it once, until well marked and cooked to medium-rare, about 3 minutes per side, or to desired doneness. Transfer the tuna to a cutting board and let it cool for 5 minutes. Then cut it across the grain into ¼-inch-thick slices.

Divide the slaw mixture between two plates and top with the tuna.

## Nutrient Content per Serving

| | | | | | |
|---|---|---|---|---|---|
| Calories: | 367 | Fat: | 15 grams | Protein: | 45 grams |
| Fiber: | 3 grams | Saturated Fat: | 2 grams | Carbs: | 10 grams |
| Sodium: | 570 mg | | | | |

## PAN-SEARED SALMON OVER TRI-COLOR SALAD WITH DIJON DRESSING

When you're buying your salmon fillets, choose wild salmon over farmed salmon, always. Wild salmon have a better fatty acid composition, naturally occurring antioxidants, and they're not exposed to antibiotics or concentrated pesticides as farmed salmon can be.

*Makes 2 servings*

### Salad

2 teaspoons lemon juice

1 tablespoon finely chopped shallots

2 teaspoons Dijon mustard

⅛ teaspoon sea salt

⅛ teaspoon freshly ground black pepper

4 teaspoons extra-virgin olive oil

½ small head radicchio, thinly sliced (about 2 cups)

1 Belgian endive, thinly sliced (about 1 cup)

3 cups baby arugula

### Salmon

1 teaspoon olive oil

2 (6-ounce) wild salmon fillets, such as king or sockeye

⅛ teaspoon sea salt

⅛ teaspoon freshly ground black pepper

Combine the lemon juice, shallots, mustard, salt, and pepper in a small bowl. Slowly whisk in the extra-virgin olive oil until well combined, and set aside. In a separate bowl combine the radicchio, endive, and arugula; set aside.

Heat the olive oil in a small nonstick skillet over medium heat. Sprinkle the salmon with the salt and pepper and place in the skillet, flesh side down; cook until the fish flakes easily with a fork, 4 to 5 minutes per side. Remove from the skillet.

Toss the dressing with the lettuces and divide the salad between two plates; top each with a salmon fillet.

### Nutrient Content per Serving

| | | | | | |
|---|---|---|---|---|---|
| Calories: | 370 | Fat: | 21 grams | Protein: | 38 grams |
| Fiber: | 2 grams | Saturated Fat: | 3 grams | Carbs: | 5 grams |
| Sodium: | 647 mg | | | | |

## VIETNAMESE CHICKEN-AND-CABBAGE SALAD

This low-carb feast is also a detoxification powerhouse. Red cabbage, which is more nutrient-dense than its green counterpart, is high in fiber and—like arugula—is full-to-bursting with antioxidants like vitamin C, which boosts the immune system and even fights cancer. For a touch of added crunch and sweetness, try stirring in some shredded apple.

### Makes 2 servings

1½ tablespoons lime juice

1 tablespoon macadamia nut oil

½ teaspoon fish sauce

1 green onion, thinly sliced

⅛ teaspoon monk fruit extract

2 cups shredded red cabbage

4 cups baby arugula

½ medium cucumber, peeled, seeded, and thinly sliced

1 carrot, shredded

2 tablespoons coarsely chopped slow-roasted cashews (see page 128)

2 tablespoons chopped fresh basil

8 ounces cooked organic free-range boneless, skinless chicken breast, shredded (about 2 cups)

Combine the lime juice, oil, fish sauce, green onion, and monk fruit extract in a small bowl.

Combine the cabbage, arugula, cucumber, carrot, cashews, basil, and chicken in a separate bowl. Pour in the dressing and toss well.

## Nutrient Content per Serving

| | | | | | |
|---|---|---|---|---|---|
| Calories: | 284 | Fat: | 14 grams | Protein: | 27 grams |
| Fiber: | 3 grams | Saturated Fat: | 2 grams | Carbs: | 14 grams |
| Sodium: | 306 mg | | | | |

## SEAFOOD SALAD WITH ITALIAN SALSA VERDE

Thanks to the seafood, this dish serves up a $B_{12}$ and selenium wallop, which makes it both heart-healthy and anti-inflammatory. Make the salsa verde and cook the seafood up to 5 hours ahead; store separately and combine just before serving.

*Makes 4 servings*

### Salsa verde

⅓ cup chopped fresh parsley

2 tablespoons chopped fresh basil

1 tablespoon chopped shallots

1 tablespoon white wine vinegar

2 teaspoons capers, drained and chopped

½ teaspoon sea salt

¼ teaspoon freshly ground black pepper

¼ cup extra-virgin olive oil

### Salad

8 ounces wild squid, cut into ½-inch-thick rings

12 ounces large wild prawns or shrimp, peeled and deveined

8 ounces wild sea scallops, quartered

½ small fennel bulb, thinly sliced

4 celery stalks, thinly sliced

1 carrot, thinly sliced

½ medium red onion, thinly sliced

Combine the parsley, basil, shallots, vinegar, capers, salt, and pepper in a small bowl. Whisk in the oil until well combined; set aside.

Bring a medium saucepan of lightly salted water to a boil over high heat. Add the squid, cook for 30 seconds, and then use a slotted spoon to transfer to a strainer; rinse under cold water, drain, and transfer to a large bowl.

Return the water to a boil and add the prawns and scallops. Cook, stirring occasionally, until the seafood is opaque, about 2 minutes. Drain, and rinse the prawns and scallops under cold water; drain again and add to the bowl with the squid. Add the fennel, celery, carrot, and red onion; stir gently to combine. Add the salsa verde and mix well.

## Nutrient Content per Serving

| | | | | | |
|---|---|---|---|---|---|
| Calories: | 302 | Fat: | 15 grams | Protein: | 30 grams |
| Fiber: | 2 grams | Saturated Fat: | 2 grams | Carbs: | 11 grams |
| Sodium: | 697 mg | | | | |

## FRISÉE AND BACON SALAD

This plate takes its inspiration from the bistro salads found all over Paris. The feathery frisée lettuce adds some nice texture and is a rich source of vitamins A and C. Make it your main dish or an ideal side salad. Vegetarians, you don't have to miss out here—just skip the bacon and enjoy!

*Makes 2 servings as a main dish or 4 as a side salad*

8 slices nitrate-free bacon

1 large head frisée lettuce, torn into bite-sized pieces

1 pint grape tomatoes, halved

3 tablespoons sliced almonds, toasted

2 tablespoons Shallot-Champagne Vinaigrette (page 215)

Cook the bacon in a medium nonstick skillet over medium heat until crisp, 6 to 7 minutes. Transfer to a plate lined with a paper towel to drain.

Combine the frisée, tomatoes, and almonds in a large bowl. Add the vinaigrette and toss well to coat. Divide the salad between two (or four) plates, crumble the bacon over the top of each salad, and serve.

Nutrient Content per Serving

| | | | | | | |
|---|---|---|---|---|---|---|
| Calories: | 262 | Fat: | 20 grams | Protein: | 10 grams |
| Fiber: | 5 grams | Saturated Fat: | 3 grams | Carbs: | 14 grams |
| Sodium: | 491 mg | | | | |

## CHICKPEA FALAFEL SALAD WITH TAHINI DRESSING

The protein-rich chickpea, which has been a much-loved staple in many of the world's cuisines for thousands of years, is the centerpiece of this tantalizing salad. The falafel is wonderfully enhanced by the flavorful, creamy tahini dressing.

*Makes 4 servings*

### *Falafel*

1 (15-ounce) can organic no-salt-added chickpeas (garbanzo beans), drained

2 green onions, chopped

1 garlic clove, minced

1 teaspoon ground cumin

¼ teaspoon curry powder

3 tablespoons olive oil

2 tablespoons chopped fresh parsley

¼ teaspoon aluminum-free baking powder

¼ teaspoon sea salt

⅛ teaspoon cayenne pepper

### *Dressing*

2 tablespoons organic tahini paste

2 tablespoons plain cultured coconut milk (such as So Delicious)

1 tablespoon lemon juice

1 teaspoon grated lemon zest

1 teaspoon extra-virgin olive oil

¼ teaspoon sea salt

### *Salad*

10 cups mixed spring greens (about 5 ounces)

1 large cucumber, peeled, halved lengthwise, and sliced into half-moons

1 cup grape tomatoes, halved

Preheat the oven to 375°F. Lightly oil a large baking sheet.

Combine the chickpeas, green onions, garlic, cumin, and curry powder in the bowl of a food processor. Process until it forms a slightly coarse paste. Transfer to a bowl and stir in the oil, parsley, baking powder, sea salt, and cayenne; mix well. Form the mixture into eight 2-inch-diameter patties and place them on the prepared baking sheet. Bake until lightly browned and slightly puffed, about 20 minutes, turning once. Set aside. (The falafel patties will be very tender, but they will firm up a bit as they cool.)

Combine the tahini, coconut milk, lemon juice, lemon zest, extra-virgin olive oil, and salt in a small bowl.

Combine the mixed spring greens, cucumber, and tomatoes in a large bowl. Add the dressing and toss well to coat. Divide among four plates, and top each salad with two falafel patties.

## Nutrient Content per Serving

| | | | | | | |
|---|---|---|---|---|---|---|
| **Calories:** | 313 | **Fat:** | 18 grams | **Protein:** | 12 grams |
| **Fiber:** | 9 grams | **Saturated Fat:** | 3 grams | **Carbs:** | 32 grams |
| **Sodium:** | 435 mg | | | | |

## CUCUMBER AND RADISH SALAD WITH ARUGULA, NUTS, AND SEEDS

This dish is a vegan's dream—protein- and nutrient-rich, and flavorful. It is light and refreshing with a satisfyingly crunchy texture. Consider complementing it with a side of quinoa. If you're having it as a starter salad or adding some protein to it, reduce the seeds and nuts by half. It can also be made ahead; just store the dressing separately.

*Makes 2 servings*

4 mini or Persian cucumbers, unpeeled, ends trimmed, cut into ¼-inch-thick slices

4 radishes, sliced

2 cups baby arugula

⅓ cup thinly sliced red onion

2 tablespoons coarsely chopped raw walnuts

2 tablespoons coarsely chopped raw pecans

1½ teaspoons sesame seeds

1½ teaspoons chia seeds

2 tablespoons Toasted Macadamia Nut Dressing (page 216)

Combine the cucumbers, radishes, arugula, onion, walnuts, pecans, sesame seeds, and chia seeds in a bowl. Add the dressing and toss well to coat. Divide between two plates and serve.

### Nutrient Content per Serving

| | | | | | |
|---|---|---|---|---|---|
| Calories: | 272 | Fat: | 24 grams | Protein: | 6 grams |
| Fiber: | 5 grams | Saturated Fat: | 2 grams | Carbs: | 11 grams |
| Sodium: | 169 mg | | | | |

## JICAMA, APPLE, AND PEAR SLAW

This is one of those fresh, snappy, flavorful salads that instantly drop you into a summer scene. It has a nice balance of sweet and tart flavors with a crisp, refreshing texture, and it keeps well—so save some for tomorrow, if you can!

*Makes 4 servings*

1 cup shredded red cabbage
1 cup shredded green cabbage
1 medium apple, unpeeled, cored, and cut into thin matchsticks
1 medium ripe pear, cored and cut into thin matchsticks
½ small jicama, peeled and cut into thin matchsticks (about 1 cup)
3 green onions, chopped
4 teaspoons cider vinegar
1 tablespoon macadamia nut oil
1 tablespoon chopped fresh cilantro
¼ teaspoon sea salt

Toss the cabbages, apple, pear, jicama, green onions, vinegar, oil, cilantro, and salt together in a large bowl. Let stand for 30 minutes, tossing occasionally to allow the flavors to bloom.

### Nutrient Content per Serving

| | | | | | |
|---|---|---|---|---|---|
| Calories: | 122 | Fat: | 4 grams | Protein: | 1 gram |
| Fiber: | 7 grams | Saturated Fat: | 0 grams | Carbs: | 22 grams |
| Sodium: | 161 mg | | | | |

## ROASTED SWEET POTATO SALAD

The orange color of sweet potatoes comes from beta-carotene, which we convert to vitamin A. Like all antioxidants, beta-carotene helps fight heart disease, cancer, and inflammation. Tossing the potatoes with the dressing when they're warm allows them to absorb more of the flavor. And by all means, add other vegetables, depending on what's in season. Cauliflower also works especially well in place of the sweet potatoes.

*Makes 4 servings*

2 medium sweet potatoes (about 1 pound), peeled and cut into ¾-inch cubes

1 medium red bell pepper, cut into ¾-inch dice

1 medium red onion, cut into ¾-inch dice

6 teaspoons macadamia nut oil

2 celery stalks, sliced

¼ cup slow-roasted cashews (see page 128)

1 tablespoon white wine vinegar

2 tablespoons chopped fresh parsley

1 teaspoon Dijon mustard

¼ teaspoon sea salt

¼ teaspoon freshly ground black pepper

Preheat the oven to 425°F. Lightly oil a large baking sheet.

Combine the potatoes, bell pepper, and onion in a bowl; toss with 2 teaspoons of the oil. Transfer to the baking sheet and roast, stirring occasionally, until the vegetables are tender and browned, 28 to 30 minutes. Transfer to a bowl and stir in the celery and cashews.

In a small bowl, whisk together the vinegar, parsley, mustard, salt, and pepper. Slowly whisk in the remaining 4 teaspoons oil, and then toss with the vegetables. Serve warm or at room temperature.

## Nutrient Content per Serving

| | | | | | | |
|---|---|---|---|---|---|---|
| Calories: | 208 | Fat: | 11 grams | Protein: | 3 grams |
| Fiber: | 4 grams | Saturated Fat: | 2 grams | Carbs: | 25 grams |
| Sodium: | 241 mg | | | | |

## SHRIMP SUMMER ROLLS WITH TAMARI-GINGER DIPPING SAUCE

These light, refreshing rolls not only taste good, they do good—the shrimp and ginger both soothe inflammation. Be sure to have all your ingredients prepared and laid out before you dampen the spring roll wrappers. Because of the tamari, this is a Cycle 3 recipe only.

*Makes 2 servings*

3 tablespoons reduced-sodium wheat-free tamari

1 tablespoon rice vinegar

2 teaspoons grated fresh ginger

4 (8-inch) rice spring roll wrappers

8 shrimp (about 8 ounces), cooked and halved lengthwise

16 medium fresh basil leaves

4 medium romaine lettuce leaves, fibrous rib trimmed to flatten

3 tablespoons thinly sliced fresh mint

1 medium beet, cooked and sliced into very thin matchsticks

1 medium red bell pepper, cut into very thin strips

1 cucumber, peeled, seeded, and sliced lengthwise into very thin strips

Combine the tamari, vinegar, and ginger in a small bowl and set aside.

Fill a large bowl with warm water. Soak one spring roll wrapper in the water until it becomes pliable, about 30 seconds. Pat excess water from the wrapper with a paper towel. Place 4 shrimp halves in a row across the middle of the wrapper. Top each with a basil leaf. Arrange a lettuce leaf on the bottom third of the wrapper, trimming it if necessary to leave a 1-inch border along the edges. Top the lettuce with one-fourth of the mint, beet, bell pepper, and cucumber. Fold about 1 inch on the right and left sides of the wrapper in toward the center; then roll the wrapper from the bottom toward the top, jelly roll–style, to enclose the filling. Transfer the roll to a plate and cover it with a dampened paper towel. Repeat with the remaining ingredients.

To serve, cut each roll in half crosswise and serve with the tamari dipping sauce.

## Nutrient Content per Serving

| | | | | | |
|---|---|---|---|---|---|
| Calories: | 235 | Fat: | 1 gram | Protein: | 26 grams |
| Fiber: | 5 grams | Saturated Fat: | 0 grams | Carbs: | 30 grams |
| Sodium: | 1194 mg | | | | |

# SNACKS 6

First, I'm going to just put this out there: I'm anti-snacking for fat loss and fast metabolism. Why? Generally speaking, snacking raises insulin levels and racks up calories like the numbers on a gas pump. And late-night snackers (come on, if you're a snacker, is there any better time?) store more calories than those who stick to three squares a day.

So my hope is to have you avoid snacking as much as possible, and if you're following my Golden Rules of Meal Timing—(1) Eat within an hour of waking up; (2) Eat every 4 to 6 hours; and (3) Stop eating at least 3 hours before bed—you should be able to without much angst.

But I do know there are times when you need a snack. You might already know to avoid the butter-soaked popcorn at the movie, but when you're genuinely hungry (which is really the only time I want you to snack), what should you do? Snack well! These recipes are all about turning you into the world's smartest snacker. That means you don't make it a three-times-a-day habit and do choose the best fat-burning foods you can. Some of my favorites include:

- Apple slices with almond butter
- Kale chips
- Raw nuts and seeds
- Half a serving of a protein shake with berries, kale, and unsweetened coconut or almond milk
- Celery sticks with cashew butter
- Sliced natural turkey with avocado
- Hummus and crudités
- My Virgin Diet Bar, if you're on the go

And, of course, there are many more to follow.

## BABAGANOUSH

This traditional Middle Eastern dip is made with all nutritious ingredients and makes a wonderful afternoon snack with cut-up raw vegetables. When you buy the eggplants, look for ones with unblemished skin that don't yield easily to pressure when squeezed. Like you.

*Makes 6 to 8 servings (2 cups)*

2 (1-pound) eggplants, pricked all over with the tip of a sharp knife
2 tablespoons organic tahini paste
2 tablespoons extra-virgin olive oil
1 tablespoon lemon juice
1 garlic clove
½ teaspoon sea salt
¼ teaspoon freshly ground black pepper

Preheat the oven to 375°F.

Place the eggplants on a large baking sheet and roast until they are very soft, 45 to 50 minutes. Remove from the oven and let cool for 30 minutes or until cool enough to handle. Cut the eggplants in half and scoop out the flesh with a spoon. Place the eggplant flesh in a wire-mesh sieve or colander and drain off the excess liquid for 20 minutes.

Transfer the drained eggplant to the bowl of a food processor and add the tahini, oil, lemon juice, garlic, salt, and pepper. Process until the mixture is well combined but not a completely smooth paste. Transfer to a serving bowl. Can be stored in a covered container in the fridge for up to 1 week.

### Nutrient Content per Serving

| | | | | | |
|---|---|---|---|---|---|
| Calories: | 85 | Fat: | 6 grams | Protein: | 2 grams |
| Fiber: | 3 grams | Saturated Fat: | 1 gram | Carbs: | 7 grams |
| Sodium: | 149 mg | | | | |

## ROASTED RED PEPPER HUMMUS

Roasted red peppers bring classic protein-rich hummus to life with just a touch of sweetness—a much smarter choice than your average store-bought, bad fat–laden dip! Great to keep on hand for an afternoon snack with raw vegetables, this keeps for up to 1 week in the fridge.

*Makes 4 to 6 servings*

1 (15-ounce) can organic no-salt-added chickpeas (garbanzo beans), drained and rinsed

1 garlic clove

3 tablespoons organic tahini paste

1 bottled roasted red pepper, drained and patted dry

2 tablespoons lemon juice

2 teaspoons grated lemon zest

¼ teaspoon Tabasco sauce

2 tablespoons extra-virgin olive oil

¼ teaspoon sea salt

¼ teaspoon freshly ground black pepper

Combine the chickpeas, garlic, tahini paste, roasted red pepper, lemon juice, lemon zest, and Tabasco in the bowl of a food processor, and puree. Stir in the olive oil, salt, and pepper. Transfer to a bowl to serve.

## Nutrient Content per Serving

| | | | | | |
|---|---|---|---|---|---|
| Calories: | 159 | Fat: | 9 grams | Protein: | 5 grams |
| Fiber: | 3 grams | Saturated Fat: | 1 gram | Carbs: | 15 grams |
| Sodium: | 98 mg | | | | |

## SMOKY BLACK BEAN HUMMUS

Smoked paprika, which is available in your grocery store's spice section, lends wonderful depth of flavor to this protein-rich treat.

*Makes 4 to 6 servings*

1 (15-ounce) can organic no-salt-added black beans, drained and rinsed

1 garlic clove

2 tablespoons organic tahini paste

2 tablespoons lime juice

1 teaspoon grated lime zest

1 teaspoon ground cumin

¾ teaspoon smoked paprika

½ teaspoon ground chipotle pepper

3 tablespoons extra-virgin olive oil

2 tablespoons chopped fresh cilantro

¼ teaspoon salt

Combine the beans, garlic, tahini paste, lime juice, lime zest, cumin, paprika, and chipotle pepper in the bowl of a food processor, and puree. Stir in the oil, cilantro, and salt. Transfer to a bowl to serve. Can be stored in a covered container in the fridge for up to a week.

### Nutrient Content per Serving

| | | | | | |
|---|---|---|---|---|---|
| Calories: | 146 | Fat: | 10 grams | Protein: | 4 grams |
| Fiber: | 3 grams | Saturated Fat: | 1 gram | Carbs: | 11 grams |
| Sodium: | 59 mg | | | | |

## AVOCADO-LIME BLACK BEAN SALSA

*Salsa* is the Spanish word for sauce, which says little about how much this zesty version can bring food to life. When you control the ingredients and make your own, salsa can be a healthy choice to spoon over fish or chicken or to accompany cut-up raw vegetables.

*Makes 4 servings*

1 (15-ounce) can organic no-salt-added black beans, drained and rinsed
1 avocado, cut into ½-inch dice
1 medium plum tomato, seeded and chopped (about ½ cup)
1 tablespoon lime juice
1 teaspoon grated lime zest
2 tablespoons chopped fresh cilantro
½ teaspoon sea salt
1 small jalapeño pepper, finely chopped

Combine the beans, avocado, tomato, lime juice, lime zest, cilantro, salt, and jalapeño in a bowl.

### Nutrient Content per Serving

| | | | | | |
|---|---|---|---|---|---|
| Calories: | 161 | Fat: | 7 grams | Protein: | 6 grams |
| Fiber: | 8 grams | Saturated Fat: | 1 gram | Carbs: | 19 grams |
| Sodium: | 248 mg | | | | |

## KALE CHIPS WITH CUMIN AND SEA SALT

It feels like cheating to reap all the nutritious benefits of kale by snacking on these savory chips. You can store them in a covered container for a day or two, but kale chips are at their best the day they are made.

*Makes 2 to 4 servings*

1 bunch kale (about 1 pound), washed and thoroughly dried

1 tablespoon olive oil

½ teaspoon ground cumin

¼ teaspoon sea salt

⅛ teaspoon ground chipotle pepper

Preheat the oven to 325°F.

Tear the kale into 1½-inch pieces. Toss them in a large bowl with the oil, gently rubbing the leaves with your fingers to help spread the oil evenly. Add the cumin, salt, and chipotle pepper and toss well.

Arrange the kale in a single layer on two large baking sheets. Bake, one batch at a time, turning the leaves once, until crisp, 16 to 18 minutes. Allow the kale chips to cool on the baking sheet. Serve immediately or store in a covered container.

## Nutrient Content per Serving

| | | | | | |
|---|---|---|---|---|---|
| Calories: | 66 | Fat: | 4 grams | Protein: | 3 grams |
| Fiber: | 1 gram | Saturated Fat: | 1 gram | Carbs: | 6 grams |
| Sodium: | 172 mg | | | | |

## ROASTED JALAPEÑO GUACAMOLE WITH TOASTED PUMPKIN SEEDS

The amount of heat in this slightly smoky guacamole depends entirely on how hot your jalapeños are. Taste them first to determine how much you want to use—only you know how much fire you can handle!

*Makes 4 servings*

6 tablespoons raw pumpkin seeds

2 medium jalapeño peppers

1 avocado, coarsely mashed with a fork

3 tablespoons finely chopped red onion

1 small plum tomato, seeded and chopped

3 tablespoons chopped fresh cilantro

1 teaspoon lime juice

¼ teaspoon sea salt

Preheat the oven to 300°F.

Spread the pumpkin seeds on a medium baking sheet. Bake, stirring occasionally, until lightly toasted, 10 to 12 minutes. Spread them out on a plate and cool for 5 minutes.

Preheat the broiler.

Place the jalapeños on the baking sheet. Broil 4 inches from the heat, turning them occasionally, until the skin is blistered, 4 to 5 minutes. Remove from the oven and allow to cool for 5 minutes. Then peel off and discard the charred skins, remove the seeds and stems, and finely chop the peppers.

Combine the pumpkin seeds, jalapeños, avocado, onion, tomato, cilantro, lime juice, and salt in a bowl; mix well.

### Nutrient Content per Serving

| | | | | | |
|---|---|---|---|---|---|
| Calories: | 184 | Fat: | 15 grams | Protein: | 5 grams |
| Fiber: | 4 grams | Saturated Fat: | 2 grams | Carbs: | 8 grams |
| Sodium: | 153 mg | | | | |

## CLASSIC TAPENADE ON ENDIVE

Tapenade, the traditional olive paste or spread, is intensely flavored, so a little goes a long way. But it will be enough to give you the heart-healthy and anti-inflammatory polyphenol goodness in all those olives.

*Makes 8 servings*

1 cup pitted Kalamata olives
¾ cup pitted Picholine olives
1 oil-packed anchovy fillet
1 garlic clove
2 tablespoons chopped fresh basil
2 tablespoons chopped fresh parsley
2 tablespoons extra-virgin olive oil
Fresh Belgian endive leaves, for serving

Combine the olives, anchovy, garlic, basil, and parsley in the bowl of a food processor. Pulse until the mixture is finely chopped. Transfer to a bowl and stir in the oil.

Spoon a small amount of the tapenade onto the wide or cut end of each endive leaf. The tapenade can be made up to 1 week ahead and kept in a covered container in the refrigerator.

### Nutrient Content per Serving

| | | | | | |
|---|---|---|---|---|---|
| Calories: | 156 | Fat: | 13 grams | Protein: | 2 grams |
| Fiber: | 4 grams | Saturated Fat: | 1 gram | Carbs: | 9 grams |
| Sodium: | 975 mg | | | | |

## ROASTED ARTICHOKE DIP

Antioxidant-rich artichokes help digestion and are loaded with disease-fighting polyphenols. Be sure to read the label and buy frozen artichokes with no added ingredients. This dip can be stored in a covered container in the refrigerator for up to 5 days.

*Makes 6 to 8 servings*

2 (9-ounce) packages frozen artichoke hearts, thawed
6 garlic cloves
2 tablespoons olive oil
1 medium Vidalia or other sweet onion, chopped
½ avocado
3 tablespoons Creamy Eggless Mayo (page 214)
1 tablespoon lemon juice
½ teaspoon sea salt
2 tablespoons chopped fresh parsley or basil (optional)

Preheat the oven to 450°F. Lightly oil a large baking sheet.

Combine the artichoke hearts, garlic, and 1 tablespoon of the oil in a medium bowl. Spread the artichokes and garlic out in a single layer on the prepared baking sheet. Roast, stirring occasionally, until the artichokes are lightly browned and the garlic is tender, 20 to 22 minutes. Remove from the oven and let cool for 5 minutes.

Meanwhile, heat the remaining 1 tablespoon oil in a medium nonstick skillet over medium heat. Add the onion and cook, stirring occasionally, until golden, 12 to 15 minutes; let cool for 5 minutes.

Combine the artichoke hearts, garlic, onion, avocado, mayonnaise, lemon juice, and salt in the bowl of a food processor. Process until smooth, and transfer to a bowl. Top with the parsley or basil, if using.

### Nutrient Content per Serving

| | | | | | | |
|---|---|---|---|---|---|---|
| Calories: | 142 | Fat: | 10 grams | Protein: | 3 grams |
| Fiber: | 5 grams | Saturated Fat: | 1 gram | Carbs: | 11 grams |
| Sodium: | 240 mg | | | | |

## CINNAMON ROASTED PECANS

Pecans are a nutrient powerhouse in and of themselves, and just a handful a day can increase the amount of age-defying antioxidants in your body, which may help prevent cancer and chronic disease. Pack these addictive nuts away in bags of 10 pecans each to ensure you don't overdo it!

*Makes 1½ cups*

1½ cups slow-roasted pecans (see page 128)

½ teaspoon macadamia nut oil

½ teaspoon ground cinnamon

¾ teaspoon monk fruit extract

¼ teaspoon sea salt

Preheat the oven to 200°F.

Combine the pecans and oil in a medium bowl, and toss well. Combine the cinnamon, monk fruit extract, and salt in a separate bowl. Add the spice mixture to the nuts and stir well to coat.

Place the nuts in a single layer on a large baking sheet and bake for 10 minutes. Remove from the oven and let cool for at least 10 minutes before serving. Store in a covered container at room temperature.

### Nutrient Content per Serving (1 Ounce)

| | | | | | |
|---|---|---|---|---|---|
| Calories: | 104 | Fat: | 11 grams | Protein: | 1 gram |
| Fiber: | 1 gram | Saturated Fat: | 1 gram | Carbs: | 2 grams |
| Sodium: | 73 mg | | | | |

## SMOKED PAPRIKA AND CAYENNE ROASTED ALMONDS

Almonds are a source of healthy fats and protein, and they help reduce bad cholesterol. But that doesn't mean you can go crazy—a few a day will do the trick. This is a zingy snack to keep on hand and will keep well for several weeks in the refrigerator.

*Makes 1½ cups*

1½ cups slow-roasted almonds (see page 128)

½ teaspoon olive oil

½ teaspoon smoked paprika

¼ teaspoon ground cumin

¼ teaspoon monk fruit extract

½ teaspoon sea salt

⅛ teaspoon cayenne pepper

Preheat the oven to 200°F.

Combine the almonds and oil in a medium bowl and toss well. Combine the paprika, cumin, monk fruit extract, salt, and cayenne in a small bowl; add to the nuts and stir well to coat.

Place the nuts in a single layer on a large baking sheet and bake for 10 minutes. Remove from the oven and let cool for at least 10 minutes before serving. Store in a covered container in the fridge.

### Nutrient Content per Serving

| | | | | | |
|---|---|---|---|---|---|
| Calories: | 157 | Fat: | 14 grams | Protein: | 5 grams |
| Fiber: | 3 grams | Saturated Fat: | 1 gram | Carbs: | 6 grams |
| Sodium: | 146 mg | | | | |

## SEA SALT AND BLACK PEPPER CASHEW CHEESE

Cashews have the same heart-healthy fat found in olive oil. You can crumble this "cheese" into a salad, use it to snack on with vegetables, or add it to a wrap. It stores well for up to 10 days in the refrigerator.

*Makes 1 cup*

1½ cups raw cashews
1 tablespoon lemon juice
1 tablespoon extra-virgin olive oil
½ teaspoon ground coriander
½ teaspoon sea salt
¼ teaspoon freshly ground black pepper
⅛ teaspoon cayenne pepper

Place the cashews in a bowl and add enough cold water to cover them by 3 inches. Let the cashews soak for at least 5 hours or overnight.

Drain the cashews, place them in the bowl of a food processor, and add the lemon juice, oil, coriander, salt, black pepper, and cayenne. Process, stopping to scrape down the sides of the bowl occasionally, until the mixture is smooth and begins to hold together. Transfer to a bowl and serve.

### Nutrient Content per Serving

| | | | | | |
|---|---|---|---|---|---|
| Calories: | 137 | Fat: | 11 grams | Protein: | 4 grams |
| Fiber: | 1 gram | Saturated Fat: | 2 grams | Carbs: | 6 grams |
| Sodium: | 149 mg | | | | |

## ROMESCO DIP

Drizzle this classic Catalan sauce—rich in disease-fighting antioxidants and omega-3 fatty acids—over asparagus or green beans, serve it as a dip with a crudités platter, or serve it with baked or grilled fish, chicken, or meat. It can be kept in a covered container in the refrigerator for up to 5 days.

*Makes 8 servings*

1 tablespoon chia seeds
¼ cup water
3 medium red bell peppers
2 tablespoons olive oil
¼ cup sliced raw almonds
2 garlic cloves, cracked
1 medium plum tomato
1 tablespoon sherry vinegar
1 teaspoon smoked paprika
½ teaspoon sea salt
¼ teaspoon freshly ground black pepper
1 tablespoon extra-virgin olive oil

Preheat the broiler. Lightly oil a large baking sheet.

Soak the chia seeds in the water for 20 minutes.

Place the bell peppers on the baking sheet and broil them, about 4 inches from the heat, turning every 2 to 3 minutes, until the skins are blistered and charred, 10 to 12 minutes. Transfer the peppers to a bowl, cover with plastic wrap, and let steam for 10 minutes. Then peel off the charred black skins and discard the stems, seeds, and ribs.

Combine the oil, almonds, and garlic in a small skillet over medium heat. Cook, stirring often, until the almonds and garlic are lightly golden, 3 to 4 minutes. Remove from the heat.

Combine the peppers and tomato in a blender; puree. Add the almond mixture and the chia seeds; puree. Add the vinegar, paprika, salt, and pepper; puree. Transfer to a bowl and stir in the extra-virgin olive oil. Chill until ready to serve.

### Nutrient Content per Serving

| | | | | | |
|---|---|---|---|---|---|
| Calories: | 94 | Fat: | 8 grams | Protein: | 2 grams |
| Fiber: | 2 grams | Saturated Fat: | 1 gram | Carbs: | 5 grams |
| Sodium: | 148 mg | | | | |

## FREEZE-DRIED FRUIT, NUT, AND SEED MIX

Freeze-dried fruits are available at many major health food stores. Don't confuse them with dried fruit, which is much higher in calories and sugar, and often also has *added* sugar.

*Makes 8 servings*

1 cup organic freeze-dried raspberries
1 cup organic freeze-dried strawberries
1 cup organic freeze-dried blueberries
¼ cup raw pumpkin seeds
¼ cup raw sunflower seeds
½ cup slow-roasted cashews (see page 128)

Combine the raspberries, strawberries, blueberries, pumpkin seeds, sunflower seeds, and cashews in a bowl. Store in an airtight container at room temperature.

### Nutrient Content per Serving (1 Ounce)

| | | | | | | |
|---|---|---|---|---|---|---|
| Calories: | 138 | Fat: | 8 grams | Protein: | 4 grams |
| Fiber: | 3 grams | Saturated Fat: | 1 gram | Carbs: | 14 grams |
| Sodium: | 40 mg | | | | |

## CACAO-NUT BUTTER SPREAD

You'll love me for this—it's a healthy take on the very unhealthy Nutella. So, enjoy your guilty pleasure without any of the guilt! Experiment with using nuts in different combinations to find the mix you like best. And add a touch of cinnamon and/or nutmeg if you'd like!

*Makes ¾ cup*

½ cup slow-roasted almonds (see page 128)
½ cup slow-roasted pecans (see page 128)
2 tablespoons raw cacao nibs
1¼ teaspoons monk fruit extract
4 teaspoons coconut butter

Combine the almonds, pecans, cacao nibs, monk fruit extract, and coconut butter in a food processor and process to form a smooth paste, stopping occasionally to scrape down the sides of the bowl with a rubber spatula.

Transfer to a covered container and store in the refrigerator for up to 3 weeks. Allow to soften slightly at room temperature before serving.

### Nutrient Content per Serving (1 Tablespoon)

| | | | | | |
|---|---|---|---|---|---|
| Calories: | 184 | Fat: | 18 grams | Protein: | 4 grams |
| Fiber: | 4 grams | Saturated Fat: | 5 grams | Carbs: | 6 grams |
| Sodium: | 25 mg | | | | |

## HOMEMADE ALMOND BUTTER

You may know by now that almond butter is my weakness … and like me, you'll want to eat this whole batch! But let there be restraint! Stick with 1 to 2 tablespoons (put it away before you start, trust me here). Even too much of a healthy food can be unhealthy.

*Makes ⅔ cup*

1 cup slow-roasted almonds (see below)
1 teaspoon monk fruit extract
4 teaspoons coconut butter
Pinch of ground cinnamon

Combine the almonds, monk fruit extract, coconut butter, and cinnamon in the bowl of a food processer and process to form a smooth paste, stopping occasionally to scrape down the sides of the bowl with a rubber spatula.

Transfer the mixture to a covered container and store in the refrigerator for up to 3 weeks. Allow to soften slightly at room temperature before serving.

### Nutrient Content per Serving (1 Tablespoon)

| | | | | | |
|---|---|---|---|---|---|
| Calories: | 164 | Fat: | 15 grams | Protein: | 5 grams |
| Fiber: | 3 grams | Saturated Fat: | 4 grams | Carbs: | 6 grams |
| Sodium: | 117 mg | | | | |

## SLOW-ROASTED NUTS

Slow roasting brings out the flavor in nuts, helps lower the anti-nutrients in them (the lectins and phytates), and improves their digestibility. And when you roast your own, you can be sure they're not being exposed to high heat, which may damage the fats. One note, though: If your oven doesn't go as low as 140°F, you'll need a dehydrator.

*Makes 1½ cups*

1½ cups raw nuts (cashews, walnuts, almonds, pecans, macadamias)
½ teaspoon sea salt

Place the nuts in a bowl and add enough water to cover by 3 inches; then stir in the salt. Let the nuts soak overnight.

Preheat the oven to 140°F.

Drain the nuts and spread them out on a baking sheet, or place them in a dehydrator. Bake or dehydrate the nuts for 8 hours. Remove from the oven or dehydrator and let cool completely (the nuts will crisp up as they cool).

For best results, store the nuts in a resealable plastic bag in the refrigerator.

## Nutrient Content per Serving (1 Ounce)

| | | | | | | |
|---|---|---|---|---|---|---|
| **Calories:** | 157 | **Fat:** | 12 grams | **Protein:** | 5 grams |
| **Fiber:** | 1 gram | **Saturated Fat:** | 2 grams | **Carbs:** | 9 grams |
| **Sodium:** | 148 mg | | | | |

No doubt you've heard the life-coaching advice "Keep the main thing the main thing." Well, I can't think of a more important reason to stay focused than your goals on the Virgin Diet. Build your meals around these centerpieces; they'll fuel your weight loss, keep you feeling full and happy, kick-start your energy, and contribute to the overall effervescence that is you.

## BEEF, PORK, AND LAMB

I'm a big fan of clean, lean protein—emphasis on lean. It can help stave off hunger and keep blood sugar levels stable. And in addition to being good sources of protein, beef, pork, and lamb contain other important nutrients, including iron, zinc, and the B vitamins.

But to get the biggest bang for your buck, choose wisely when picking your meat. All beef, pork, and lamb are high in protein, but they're not all created equal. If you get yours from a factory-farmed source, it can be high in saturated fat and pumped full of antibiotics and hormones. Make sure you support your own health—and humane, sustainable farming—by voting with your dollars for grass-fed and antibiotic-free and hormone-free lean cuts.

### GRASS-FED BEEF TENDERLOIN STEAKS WITH SAUTÉED SHIITAKES

Beef tenderloin is lean and tender, but it's a somewhat less flavorful cut of meat. The mushrooms enhance the meaty flavor, and also provide immune and cardiovascular support (and bioavailable iron) in the bargain. I'm feeling better already....

Make the mushrooms without wine until Cycle 3; use an additional ¼ cup of broth in its place.

*Makes 4 servings*

1 tablespoon plus 2 teaspoons macadamia nut oil

1 large shallot, chopped

12 ounces shiitake mushrooms, stems removed, caps quartered

1 tablespoon chopped fresh tarragon

½ cup dry red wine

¾ cup organic low-sodium beef broth

2 teaspoons coconut aminos

½ teaspoon sea salt

¼ teaspoon freshly ground black pepper

4 (4-ounce) grass-fed beef tenderloin steaks, about 1 inch thick, trimmed

Heat 1 tablespoon of the oil in a large nonstick skillet over medium-high heat. Add the shallot and cook until starting to soften, 1 to 2 minutes. Add the mushrooms and tarragon and cook until the mushrooms have softened and started to brown, 6 to 7 minutes. Stir in the wine, bring to a boil, and cook for 1 minute. Add the broth and coconut aminos, return to a boil, and cook until slightly reduced, about 4 minutes. Stir in ¼ teaspoon of the salt and ⅛ teaspoon of the pepper; transfer to a bowl and cover to keep warm.

Wipe out the skillet with a paper towel; add the remaining 2 teaspoons oil and heat over medium heat. Season the steaks with the remaining ¼ teaspoon salt and ⅛ teaspoon pepper, and add them to the skillet. Cook the steaks, turning once, until medium-rare, 3 to 4 minutes per side, or until desired doneness. Transfer the steaks to serving plates.

Return the skillet to medium-high heat and add the mushrooms. Cook until hot, about 1 minute. Spoon the mushrooms over the steaks to serve.

### Nutrient Content per Serving

| | | | | | | |
|---|---|---|---|---|---|---|
| Calories: | 262 | Fat: | 13 grams | Protein: | 20 grams |
| Fiber: | 3 grams | Saturated Fat: | 3 grams | Carbs: | 9 grams |
| Sodium: | 618 mg | | | | |

## SHALLOT-THYME MARINATED FLANK STEAK

The flank is a flavorful cut, so even though it's not one of the tenderest, you won't want to miss out on having this dish. Marinating helps soften the meat, as does cutting it into thin strips.

*Makes 4 servings*

1 medium shallot, chopped

1 tablespoon chopped fresh thyme

2 tablespoons balsamic vinegar

1 tablespoon coconut aminos

1 tablespoon Dijon mustard

2 tablespoons olive oil

1½ pounds grass-fed flank steak, trimmed

¾ teaspoon sea salt

¼ teaspoon freshly ground black pepper

Combine the shallot, thyme, vinegar, coconut aminos, mustard, and olive oil in a large bowl. Add the flank steak and turn to coat. Refrigerate for at least 30 minutes and up to 2 hours, turning the steak occasionally.

Prepare a grill for direct high heat.

Season steak with salt and pepper. Place the steak on the grill, directly over the heat, and close the lid. Cook for 4 to 5 minutes per side for medium-rare (or until desired doneness). Transfer the steak to a cutting board and let stand for 5 minutes before cutting it diagonally across the grain into thin slices.

## Nutrient Content per Serving

| | | | | | |
|---|---|---|---|---|---|
| Calories: | 342 | Fat: | 19 grams | Protein: | 35 grams |
| Fiber: | 1 gram | Saturated Fat: | 6 grams | Carbs: | 5 grams |
| Sodium: | 620 mg | | | | |

## MEATBALLS IN TOMATO SAUCE

I consulted my friend Dr. Ed Bauman, founder and president of Bauman College: Holistic Nutrition and Culinary Arts, about using flax in recipes. This is what he had to say:

*Flax can be used in baking recipes as a binder and fiber. The oils are better protected when the flax is whole vs. ground, but in a pancake, cookie, or muffin, the heat is not so extreme or direct as to damage the omega-3 fatty acids that are embedded in the whole flax seed. Flax oil, on the other hand, is highly perishable and not to be used in baking.*

So the flaxseeds in these meatballs not only maintain their high omega-3 fatty acid content (as does the grass-fed ground beef), they also lend a sassy texture you can't wait to sink your teeth into.

*Makes 4 servings*

1 pound grass-fed lean ground beef

2 garlic cloves, minced

¼ cup chopped fresh parsley

2 tablespoons ground flaxseeds

1 teaspoon dried basil

½ teaspoon dried oregano

¾ teaspoon sea salt

¼ teaspoon freshly ground black pepper

1 tablespoon olive oil

1½ cups Go-To Marinara Sauce (page 209)

Combine the beef, garlic, parsley, flax meal, basil, oregano, salt, and pepper in a medium bowl and mix well. Form the mixture into twenty 1-inch balls.

Heat the oil in a large nonstick skillet over medium heat. Add the meatballs and cook, turning occasionally, until browned on all sides, 6 minutes. Transfer the meatballs to a medium saucepan and add the marinara sauce. Bring the mixture to a simmer over medium heat. Cover, reduce the heat to medium-low, and simmer until the meatballs are cooked through, about 10 minutes. Serve the meatballs with the sauce.

### Nutrient Content per Serving

| | | | | | |
|---|---|---|---|---|---|
| Calories: | 267 | Fat: | 14 grams | Protein: | 24 grams |
| Fiber: | 3 grams | Saturated Fat: | 3 grams | Carbs: | 11 grams |
| Sodium: | 816 mg | | | | |

## TEX-MEX BURGERS WITH AVOCADO SALSA

This succulent burger will give you all the satisfaction you get when you sink your teeth into a burger without any of the anxiety that comes when you haven't handpicked the meat. Make the salsa first to allow the flavors to combine and bloom. The burgers puff up on the grill; the indentation in the patties helps them cook more evenly.

*Makes 4 servings; makes 1½ cups salsa*

### *Salsa*

1 avocado, cut into ¼-inch dice

1 plum tomato, seeded and cut into ¼-inch dice

½ medium red bell pepper, cut into ¼-inch dice

1 small jalapeño pepper, finely chopped

3 tablespoons finely chopped red onion

2 tablespoons chopped fresh basil

1 tablespoon lime juice

¼ teaspoon sea salt

### Burgers

1 pound grass-fed lean ground beef

2 slices nitrate-free bacon, cooked and coarsely chopped

1 teaspoon ground cumin

½ teaspoon onion powder

¼ teaspoon smoked paprika

½ teaspoon sea salt

¼ teaspoon freshly ground black pepper

4 organic Boston or romaine lettuce leaves

Combine the avocado, tomato, bell pepper, jalapeño, onion, basil, lime juice, and salt in a medium bowl. Set aside.

Prepare a grill for direct high heat.

Gently combine the beef, bacon, cumin, onion powder, paprika, salt, and pepper in a medium bowl. Working the mixture as little as possible, form it into four ½-inch-thick patties. Make a small indentation in the center of each patty with your thumb.

Place the burgers on the grill, close the lid, and cook for 4 minutes per side for medium, or to desired doneness. Remove from the grill; place each burger on a lettuce leaf and top with the salsa.

### Nutrient Content per Serving

| | | | | | | |
|---|---|---|---|---|---|---|
| Calories: | 259 | Fat: | 14 grams | Protein: | 25 grams |
| Fiber: | 5 grams | Saturated Fat: | 4 grams | Carbs: | 9 grams |
| Sodium: | 576 mg | | | | |

## EASY PASTA BOLOGNESE

This Italian staple is *delizioso*! You'll never believe it's diet food! The combination of lean ground beef and protein-rich quinoa pasta is so flavorful, you'll want to serve it to a crowd (yes, you will be showered with compliments!).

Make the sauce without wine until Cycle 3; use ¼ cup beef broth in its place.

### Makes 4 servings

12 ounces grass-fed lean ground beef

½ medium onion, chopped

2 celery stalks, finely chopped

1 carrot, finely chopped

4 garlic cloves, minced

1 teaspoon dried basil

½ teaspoon dried oregano

½ cup dry red wine

1 (28-ounce) can organic diced tomatoes

3 tablespoons organic tomato paste

8 ounces quinoa linguine pasta

½ teaspoon sea salt

¼ teaspoon freshly ground black pepper

Heat a large nonstick skillet over medium-high heat and add the beef. Cook, stirring and breaking the beef into crumbles with a wooden spoon, until it is no longer pink, 4 to 5 minutes. Add the onion, celery, carrot, garlic, basil, and oregano and cook, stirring occasionally, until the vegetables start to soften, 3 to 4 minutes. Pour in the wine, bring to a boil, and cook until it has nearly evaporated, about 1 minute. Add the diced tomatoes and tomato paste and bring to a boil. Then reduce the heat to medium and simmer until slightly thickened, 15 to 18 minutes.

Meanwhile, bring a large saucepan of water to a boil. Add the pasta and cook according to the package directions; drain.

Remove the skillet from the heat and season the meat sauce with the salt and pepper.

Divide the pasta among four bowls and top each with the sauce.

## Nutrient Content per Serving

| | | | | | |
|---|---|---|---|---|---|
| Calories: | 447 | Fat: | 7 grams | Protein: | 29 grams |
| Fiber: | 6 grams | Saturated Fat: | 2 grams | Carbs: | 64 grams |
| Sodium: | 736 mg | | | | |

## PORK TENDERLOIN FAJITAS

The pork tenderloin is a cut from the tenderest part of the pig, and from the second it first sizzles in your skillet, it will fill your kitchen with fantastic aromas. Wrap the fajitas up in gluten-free brown rice wraps.

*Makes 4 servings*

4 teaspoons Malaysian red palm fruit oil

1 pound natural lean pork tenderloin, trimmed and cut into 2-inch-long, ¼-inch-wide strips

1 medium onion, thinly sliced

1 medium red bell pepper, thinly sliced

1 medium green bell pepper, thinly sliced

3 garlic cloves, minced

1 teaspoon dried oregano

1 teaspoon ground cumin

2 plum tomatoes, quartered lengthwise

2 teaspoons coconut aminos

4 brown rice tortillas

Sliced avocado (optional)

Tomato salsa (optional)

Plain cultured coconut milk (such as So Delicious; optional)

Heat 2 teaspoons of the oil in a large nonstick skillet over medium-high heat. Add half of the pork and cook, turning occasionally, until browned and nearly cooked through, about 4 minutes; transfer to a plate. Add the remaining pork to the skillet and repeat.

Heat the remaining 2 teaspoons oil in the skillet. Add the onion, bell peppers, garlic, oregano, and cumin; cook, stirring occasionally, until the vegetables are slightly softened, 4 to 5 minutes. Add the tomatoes and cook until slightly wilted, 2 to 3 minutes. Stir in the pork and the coconut aminos, and cook until the pork is hot and cooked through, 1 to 2 minutes.

Heat a large nonstick skillet over medium heat until hot. Working with one at a time, place the tortillas in the skillet and cook, turning several times, until heated through, about 45 seconds.

Lay the tortillas on a work surface and top each one with one-fourth of the pork mixture. Then top with the avocado slices, tomato salsa, and/or cultured coconut milk, if desired, and fold to enclose the filling.

## Nutrient Content per Serving

| | | | | | |
|---|---|---|---|---|---|
| **Calories:** | 327 | **Fat:** | 10 grams | **Protein:** | 25 grams |
| **Fiber:** | 4 grams | **Saturated Fat:** | 3 grams | **Carbs:** | 33 grams |
| **Sodium:** | 269 mg | | | | |

## SPICE-RUBBED PULLED PORK

Spice up your game-day tailgate with this instant pigskin classic and score big points with your team (I couldn't resist)! And to be sure you can enjoy yourself, too, make this in advance and reheat it on game day.

*Makes 4 servings*

1 pound natural lean pork loin, trimmed, cut into 2-inch pieces

1 tablespoon Barbecue Spice Rub (page 213)

6 tablespoons Homemade Ketchup (page 211)

2 tablespoons cider vinegar

2 tablespoons water

¼ teaspoon monk fruit extract

Combine the pork and the rub in a saucepan; toss thoroughly to completely coat the pork. Stir in the ketchup, vinegar, water, and monk fruit extract.

Bring the mixture to a simmer over medium heat. Reduce the heat to medium-low, cover, and simmer, stirring occasionally, until the pork is very tender, 50 to 55 minutes. Remove from the heat and transfer the mixture to a bowl. Shred the pork with two forks. Return the pork to the saucepan and heat over medium heat until hot, about 1 minute.

## Nutrient Content per Serving

| | | | | | |
|---|---|---|---|---|---|
| Calories: | 142 | Fat: | 3 grams | Protein: | 22 grams |
| Fiber: | 1 gram | Saturated Fat: | 1 gram | Carbs: | 5 grams |
| Sodium: | 284 mg | | | | |

## HERB-MARINATED PORK CHOPS WITH BALSAMIC DRIZZLE

These pork chops are a great choice for a family on the go because you can double the balsamic sauce, keep it for a week in the refrigerator, and use it on hot or cold chicken. Use the time you save for you!

*Makes 4 servings*

1 tablespoon chopped fresh parsley
2 teaspoons chopped fresh thyme
2 teaspoons chopped fresh sage
1 teaspoon Dijon mustard
1 tablespoon olive oil
1 garlic clove, minced
4 (4-ounce) natural lean boneless center-cut pork chops, ½ inch thick, trimmed
½ cup balsamic vinegar
¼ teaspoon monk fruit extract
¼ teaspoon sea salt
¼ teaspoon freshly ground black pepper

Combine the parsley, thyme, sage, mustard, oil, and garlic in a medium bowl. Add the pork chops and turn to coat. Refrigerate, covered, for 1 hour.

Meanwhile, combine the vinegar and monk fruit extract in a small saucepan and bring to a boil over medium-high heat. Reduce the heat to medium and simmer until the mixture is syrupy, 6 to 7 minutes; remove from the heat.

Heat a grill pan over medium heat until hot. Season the pork chops with the salt and pepper, and place on the grill pan. Cook the pork, turning once, until it is cooked through and well marked, 4 to 5 minutes per side. To serve, drizzle with the balsamic sauce.

## Nutrient Content per Serving

| | | | | | |
|---|---|---|---|---|---|
| Calories: | 157 | Fat: | 8 grams | Protein: | 13 grams |
| Fiber: | 0 grams | Saturated Fat: | 2 grams | Carbs: | 6 grams |
| Sodium: | 212 mg | | | | |

## PORK SOUVLAKI KABOBS WITH TZATZIKI

These zesty kabobs burst with Greek flavor, which is delicately offset by the tangy lemon juice in the marinade. The pork is all lean protein, and you'll never miss the dairy in this wonderfully flavorful version of tzatziki, so indulge guilt-free!

If you are using bamboo skewers, soak them in warm salted water for 30 minutes before using.

*Makes 4 servings*

1 pound natural lean pork loin, trimmed, cut into 24 cubes

1 small red bell pepper, cut into 12 pieces

1 small green bell pepper, cut into 12 pieces

1 tablespoon olive oil

1 tablespoon chopped fresh parsley

1 tablespoon plus 1 teaspoon lemon juice

1 teaspoon dried oregano

½ cup plain cultured coconut milk (such as So Delicious)

½ small cucumber, grated and then squeezed to remove excess liquid

½ garlic clove, minced

¾ teaspoon sea salt

¼ teaspoon freshly ground black pepper

Preheat the broiler. Lightly oil a broiler pan.

Combine the pork, bell peppers, oil, parsley, 1 tablespoon of the lemon juice, and the oregano in a bowl; let stand at room temperature for 15 minutes.

Thread the pork and bell peppers, alternating, onto four 12-inch skewers.

Combine the cultured coconut milk, cucumber, garlic, remaining 1 teaspoon lemon juice, and ¼ teaspoon of the salt in a bowl. Place the skewers on the prepared pan and season with the remaining ½ teaspoon salt and the pepper. Broil 4 inches from the heat, turning every 2 minutes, until cooked through, a total of about 8 minutes. Serve the skewers with the tzatziki.

## Nutrient Content per Serving

| | | | | | |
|---|---|---|---|---|---|
| Calories: | 198 | Fat: | 8 grams | Protein: | 22 grams |
| Fiber: | 2 grams | Saturated Fat: | 3 grams | Carbs: | 8 grams |
| Sodium: | 486 mg | | | | |

## BROILED ROSEMARY-AND-FENNEL LAMB CHOPS

This satisfying dish will make you feel as though you're indulging for a special occasion. And here's something to celebrate—lamb is a lean meat that's high in protein and helps regulate blood sugar. If you don't have fresh rosemary, substitute 1 teaspoon dried.

*Makes 4 servings*

2 tablespoons olive oil

1 tablespoon chopped fresh rosemary

1 teaspoon fennel seeds, crushed

½ teaspoon garlic powder

¼ teaspoon ground coriander

8 (¾-inch-thick) grass-fed lean bone-in loin lamb chops (1¼ to 1½ pounds total)

½ teaspoon sea salt

¼ teaspoon freshly ground black pepper

Combine the oil, rosemary, fennel seeds, garlic powder, and coriander in a medium bowl. Add the lamb chops and toss well to coat; let stand at room temperature for 10 minutes.

Meanwhile, preheat the broiler and lightly oil a broiler pan.

Season the lamb with the salt and pepper, and place on the prepared broiler pan. Broil the lamb, 4 inches from the heat, turning once, for a total of 5 to 6 minutes for medium-rare.

## Nutrient Content per Serving

| | | | | | |
|---|---|---|---|---|---|
| Calories: | 305 | Fat: | 25 grams | Protein: | 19 grams |
| Fiber: | 0 grams | Saturated Fat: | 8 grams | Carbs: | 1 gram |
| Sodium: | 349 mg | | | | |

## GRILLED DIJON-LEMON LAMB KABOBS

Kabobs are always a great alternative to the standard fare of grilling season. These not only bring a little elegance to the soiree, they're also easy to prep, and the simple treatment really brings out their natural flavors.

If you are using bamboo skewers, soak them in warm salted water for 30 minutes before using.

*Makes 4 servings*

1 tablespoon Dijon mustard

1 tablespoon olive oil

2 teaspoons chopped fresh marjoram

2 garlic cloves, minced

1½ teaspoons grated lemon zest

½ teaspoon freshly ground black pepper

1½ pounds grass-fed lean boneless leg of lamb, trimmed, cut into 1-inch cubes

½ teaspoon sea salt

Combine the mustard, oil, marjoram, garlic, lemon zest, and pepper in a large bowl; stir in the lamb and toss thoroughly. Refrigerate, covered, for at least 30 minutes or up to 4 hours.

Prepare a grill for direct medium heat.

Thread the lamb onto four 12-inch skewers and season with salt. Place the kabobs on the grill, directly over the heat, and cook, turning occasionally, until cooked through, 7 to 8 minutes.

### Nutrient Content per Serving

| | | | | | | |
|---|---|---|---|---|---|---|
| Calories: | 257 | Fat: | 13 grams | Protein: | 32 grams |
| Fiber: | 0 grams | Saturated Fat: | 4 grams | Carbs: | 2 grams |
| Sodium: | 463 mg | | | | |

# POULTRY

It's essential that clean, lean protein be front and center at every one of your meals, and none quite says "go to" like poultry for weight control and the support of lean muscle mass. It easily slides across the normally impermeable lunch/dinner barrier because chicken and turkey, especially, are like a blank canvas—you can paint them with the brush of delicious sauces, marinades, or sides full of explosive flavors. They're versatile enough to be at the heart of haute cuisine or cut up for leftovers.

Poultry has even more to offer, though. It's a good source of vitamins $B_6$ (for metabolism) and $B_{12}$ (to make red blood cells, among other things) and of amino acids and selenium. So this food group alone helps fight cancer, supports heart and brain health, and encourages fast fat loss.

But remember, you have to do your homework on this one. You get the biggest health benefits from organic, pasture-raised, hormone- and antibiotic-free poultry.

Factory-farmed chicken, turkey, and duck are pumped full of antibiotics and added hormones, and the last thing I want you to eat is food full of those.

## CHICKEN TOSTADAS

Coconut milk adds a slightly sweet flavor to this Mexican treat. And more good news: It's easy to digest and contains an abundance of vitamins, minerals, and antioxidants. Cultured coconut milk is a delicious and heart-healthy stand-in for sour cream.

*Makes 4 servings*

2 brown rice tortillas

6 teaspoons macadamia nut oil

1 (16-ounce) can organic low-fat refried black beans (I like Bearitos refried beans; they make a fat-free version, and they're BPA-free)

1 medium onion, thinly sliced

2 garlic cloves, minced

½ small red bell pepper, sliced

½ small green bell pepper, sliced

1 small jalapeño pepper, finely chopped

½ teaspoon ground cumin

2 plum tomatoes, seeded and chopped

1 pound cooked chicken breast, shredded (about 4 cups)

1 tablespoon chopped fresh cilantro

1 tablespoon lime juice

½ teaspoon sea salt

1 avocado, sliced

¼ cup plain cultured coconut milk (such as So Delicious)

Preheat the oven to 400°F.

Brush the top of the tortillas with 2 teaspoons of the oil, and cut them in quarters. Place the tortilla pieces in a single layer on a large baking sheet. Bake until lightly browned and crisp, 6 to 7 minutes. Remove from the oven and spread the top of the tortilla pieces with the refried beans.

Heat the remaining 4 teaspoons oil in a large nonstick skillet over medium-high heat. Add the onion, garlic, bell peppers, jalapeño, and cumin. Cook, stirring occasionally, until slightly softened, 5 to 6 minutes. Add the tomato and cook until slightly wilted, 1 to 2 minutes. Remove from the heat and stir in the chicken, cilantro, lime juice, and salt.

Return the baking sheet to the oven and heat the refried beans for 2 minutes. Transfer to a platter and top with the chicken mixture, avocado slices, and cultured coconut milk.

## Nutrient Content per Serving

| | | | | | | | |
|---|---|---|---|---|---|---|---|
| Calories: | 500 | Fat: | 18 grams | Protein: | 44 grams |
| Fiber: | 11 grams | Saturated Fat: | 3 grams | Carbs: | 39 grams |
| Sodium: | 782 mg | | | | |

## BBQ GLAZED CHICKEN

No need to wait for summertime—whether it's an outdoor occasion or you just want something light and simple for dinner, this BBQ Glazed Chicken should come to mind. But you're not skimping on nutrition; in addition to the lean protein in the chicken, the palm fruit oil adds antioxidants in the form of carotenes and tocotrienols. With a simple rub, a little sauce, and a grill, you'll have this meal on your table in less than 30 minutes. One note, though—don't rely on color when determining if chicken is cooked through. Use an instant-read meat thermometer to ensure it is done but not overcooked.

*Makes 4 servings*

2 organic free-range bone-in, skinless chicken breast halves (about 1½ pounds)
1 tablespoon Malaysian red palm fruit oil
1 tablespoon Barbecue Spice Rub (page 213)
¼ cup All-Purpose Finger-Lickin'-Good Barbecue Sauce (page 210), plus more for serving (optional)

Preheat a grill for indirect medium heat.

Brush the chicken with the oil, and then pat the spice rub evenly over the chicken to coat.

Place chicken on the grill, away from the heat source, and cook, flesh side up, for 15 minutes. Turn the chicken over and grill for an additional 10 minutes. Turn the chicken again, brush with half the barbecue sauce, and cook for 5 minutes. Turn and brush with the remaining sauce. Grill until an instant-read meat thermometer inserted into the thickest portion of the breast registers 165°F, 5 to 6 minutes longer.

Remove the chicken from the grill and place on a work surface. Cut each breast in half crosswise, and serve with additional sauce if desired.

## Nutrient Content per Serving

| | | | | | | |
|---|---|---|---|---|---|---|
| Calories: | 222 | Fat: | 7 grams | Protein: | 35 grams |
| Fiber: | 0 grams | Saturated Fat: | 3 grams | Carbs: | 2 grams |
| Sodium: | 248 mg | | | | |

## COCONUT RED CURRY CHICKEN

Thai red curry paste packs spice as well as Thai curry flavor. It's made with dried red chiles, so if you prefer milder dishes, cut the paste back to 1 teaspoon.

*Makes 4 servings*

3 teaspoons coconut oil

1 pound organic free-range boneless, skinless chicken breast halves, cut into ¼-inch-thick strips

1 medium onion, sliced

1 medium red bell pepper, sliced

1 tablespoon minced fresh ginger

3 garlic cloves, minced

1½ teaspoons red curry paste (such as Thai Kitchen)

1 cup unsweetened coconut milk (such as So Delicious)

2 teaspoons fish sauce

½ teaspoon monk fruit extract

2 tablespoons chopped fresh cilantro

Heat 2 teaspoons of the oil in a large nonstick skillet over medium-high heat. Add the chicken and cook, stirring occasionally, until no longer pink, 3 to 4 minutes. Transfer the chicken to a plate and reserve.

Return the skillet to the stove and heat the remaining 1 teaspoon oil. Add the onion, bell pepper, ginger, and garlic and cook, stirring occasionally, until slightly softened, 3 to 4 minutes. Stir in the red curry paste and cook, stirring, for 1 minute. Reduce the heat to medium-low, add the chicken and the coconut milk, and gently simmer until the chicken is cooked through, about 2 minutes. Remove from the heat and stir in the fish sauce, monk fruit extract, and cilantro.

### Nutrient Content per Serving

| | | | | | |
|---|---|---|---|---|---|
| Calories: | 190 | Fat: | 7 grams | Protein: | 24 grams |
| Fiber: | 1 gram | Saturated Fat: | 5 grams | Carbs: | 7 grams |
| Sodium: | 346 mg | | | | |

## CHICKEN SLOPPY JOES OVER BROWN RICE

Sloppy Joes scream "summer," but you can whip up this picnic fave any time of the year. Make this version with lean ground chicken—it has a little more fat than ground chicken breast, but less than "ground chicken," which may include any and all parts of the bird (yep, as scary as it sounds).

*Makes 4 servings*

1 tablespoon coconut oil or Malaysian red palm fruit oil

1 medium onion, chopped

1 medium green bell pepper, chopped

3 garlic cloves, minced

1 teaspoon chili powder

½ teaspoon dried oregano

½ teaspoon dried cumin

1 pound organic free-range lean ground chicken

½ cup Homemade Ketchup (page 211)

¼ teaspoon sea salt

¼ teaspoon freshly ground black pepper

2 cups warm cooked brown rice

Heat the oil in a large nonstick skillet over medium-high heat. Add the onion, bell pepper, and garlic and cook, stirring occasionally, until slightly softened, 4 to 5 minutes. Add the chili powder, oregano, and cumin and cook, stirring, for 30 seconds. Stir in the chicken, breaking it into crumbles with a wooden spoon, and cook until it begins to brown, about 6 to 7 minutes. Stir in the ketchup and cook, stirring, until very hot, about 2 minutes. Remove from the heat and season with the salt and pepper. Serve over the rice.

## Nutrient Content per Serving

| | | | | | |
|---|---|---|---|---|---|
| Calories: | 358 | Fat: | 18 grams | Protein: | 25 grams |
| Fiber: | 4 grams | Saturated Fat: | 6 grams | Carbs: | 33 grams |
| Sodium: | 403 mg | | | | |

## CHICKEN WITH 40 CLOVES OF GARLIC

Yes, 40! Don't worry, your breath will be fine. So will your heart, thanks to all of garlic's antioxidant properties. It also enhances the immune system, reduces inflammation, and helps the liver release toxins. So now you want to make it 80, right?

This dish, in various iterations, has been around forever. Surprisingly, the garlic is sweet and not pungent or overwhelming. By placing the paste under the skin, you flavor the meat and can remove the skin after cooking.

*Makes 6 servings*

2 tablespoons olive oil

2 tablespoons chopped fresh rosemary

¾ teaspoon sea salt

½ teaspoon freshly ground black pepper

1 (3½- to 4-pound) organic free-range chicken

40 garlic cloves, unpeeled

1 medium onion, chopped

2 celery stalks, chopped

1½ cups organic low-sodium chicken broth

Preheat the oven to 400°F.

Stir the oil, rosemary, salt, and pepper together in a small bowl to form a paste. Use your fingertips to gently loosen the skin on the chicken breast, legs, and thighs. Rub the paste over the meat under the skin. Tuck the wings under the bird and tie the legs with kitchen twine. Transfer the chicken to a shallow roasting pan and add the garlic, onion, celery, and broth.

Roast the chicken until an instant-read meat thermometer inserted into the thickest part of the thigh registers 170°F, 65 to 70 minutes. Remove from the oven and let the chicken cool for 5 minutes. Discard the onion and celery. Then remove the skin and carve the chicken. Serve it with the garlic cloves and pan juices.

## Nutrient Content per Serving

| | | | | | |
|---|---|---|---|---|---|
| **Calories:** | 387 | **Fat:** | 22 grams | **Protein:** | 36 grams |
| **Fiber:** | 1 gram | **Saturated Fat:** | 5 grams | **Carbs:** | 9 grams |
| **Sodium:** | 426 mg | | | | |

## ASIAN CHICKEN IN LETTUCE CUPS

There's beauty in a meal that doesn't require utensils, am I right? These wraps are low in carbs and high in flavor. Just use the lettuce leaves as wraps, roll them around the chicken, and dig in.

*Makes 4 servings*

1 tablespoon Malaysian red palm fruit oil

1 pound organic free-range lean ground chicken

1½ tablespoons grated fresh ginger

4 garlic cloves, minced

3 green onions, thinly sliced

½ medium red bell pepper, cut into ¼-inch dice

2 celery stalks, finely chopped

1 carrot, finely chopped

¼ cup chopped fresh cilantro

¼ cup slow-roasted cashews, coarsely chopped (see page 128)

2 tablespoons lime juice

2 teaspoons fish sauce

8 Boston lettuce leaves

Heat the oil in a large nonstick skillet over medium-high heat until very hot. Add the chicken, ginger, garlic, and green onions and cook, breaking the chicken into smaller pieces with a wooden spoon, until it is starting to brown and is cooked through, 7 to 8 minutes. Transfer to a bowl and stir in the bell pepper, celery, carrot, cilantro, cashews, lime juice, and fish sauce.

Place two lettuce leaves on each of four plates, and top each with one-half cup of the chicken mixture.

## Nutrient Content per Serving

| Calories: | 278 | Fat: | 17 grams | Protein: | 23 grams |
|---|---|---|---|---|---|
| Fiber: | 2 grams | Saturated Fat: | 5 grams | Carbs: | 9 grams |
| Sodium: | 336 mg | | | | |

## POUNDED CHICKEN PAILLARDS TOPPED WITH TOMATO AND FRESH BASIL SALAD

Even though the chicken has never done anything to you, pound it anyway (but be gentle—you shouldn't be using force). It's a great way to release a little stress, and, better yet, it will ensure quick, even cooking so the meat retains its tenderness and natural juices. Pounding the chicken between two pieces of plastic wrap makes it easier to evenly flatten the breast without tearing the meat and makes for easier cleanup.

*Makes 4 servings*

### Chicken

1 tablespoon olive oil

1 tablespoon lemon juice

¾ teaspoon dried oregano

¼ teaspoon sea salt

⅛ teaspoon freshly ground black pepper

4 (4-ounce) organic free-range boneless, skinless chicken breast halves

### Salad

1 pound Campari tomatoes or large vine-ripened cherry tomatoes, quartered

1 cup loosely packed fresh basil, thinly sliced

4 cups baby spinach or baby arugula

½ small red onion, thinly sliced

1 tablespoon balsamic vinegar

2 tablespoons extra-virgin olive oil

1 tablespoon capers, drained and chopped

¼ teaspoon sea salt

⅛ teaspoon freshly ground black pepper

Combine the oil, lemon juice, oregano, salt, and pepper in a large bowl and set aside. Sandwich one chicken breast half between two pieces of plastic wrap and use a meat mallet with a smooth surface or a rolling pin to gently pound the chicken to an even ⅛-inch thickness. Repeat with the remaining breast halves. Add the chicken to the bowl and turn once to coat with the mixture. Allow to stand at room temperature for 10 minutes.

Prepare a grill for direct grilling over medium heat, or preheat the broiler and lightly oil a broiler pan.

Meanwhile, combine the tomatoes, basil, baby spinach, onion, vinegar, extra-virgin olive oil, capers, salt, and pepper in a bowl and toss well.

Place the chicken on the grill or under the broiler and cook (with the grill lid closed) for 2 to 3 minutes per side, or until the chicken is cooked through. Serve the chicken topped with the salad.

### Nutrient Content per Serving

| | | | | | |
|---|---|---|---|---|---|
| Calories: | 259 | Fat: | 13 grams | Protein: | 25 grams |
| Fiber: | 3 grams | Saturated Fat: | 2 grams | Carbs: | 10 grams |
| Sodium: | 450 mg | | | | |

## TURKEY MEAT LOAF WITH KALE

Use "lean ground turkey" to get the best taste and nutrition in this dish. It's a perfect compromise between ultra-lean ground turkey breast, which results in meat loaf that's too dry, and "ground turkey," which includes all parts and can be quite high in saturated fat.

*Makes 6 servings*

1 tablespoon Malaysian red palm fruit oil

1 small onion, chopped

3 garlic cloves, minced

1 teaspoon dried oregano

6 ounces kale, stems removed, leaves finely chopped (about 3 cups)

1½ pounds natural lean ground turkey

½ cup gluten-free oats

½ cup Homemade Ketchup (page 211)

¾ teaspoon sea salt

¼ teaspoon cayenne pepper

Preheat the oven to 350°F. Line a baking sheet pan with parchment paper.

Heat the oil in a large nonstick skillet over medium-high heat. Add the onion, garlic, and oregano and cook, stirring occasionally, until starting to soften, 1 to 2 minutes. Add the kale and cook, stirring often, until tender, about 4 minutes. Transfer to a large bowl and let cool for 5 minutes.

Add the turkey, oats, ¼ cup of the ketchup, the salt, and the cayenne to the bowl and mix well. Transfer to the prepared baking sheet and form into an 8 x 4 x 2-inch loaf. Spread the top with the remaining ¼ cup ketchup.

Bake until an instant-read meat thermometer registers 175°F when inserted into the thickest part of the loaf, 48 to 50 minutes. Remove from the oven and let cool for at least 10 minutes before slicing.

## Nutrient Content per Serving

| | | | | | | |
|---|---|---|---|---|---|---|
| Calories: | 214 | Fat: | 5 grams | Protein: | 30 grams |
| Fiber: | 2 grams | Saturated Fat: | 2 grams | Carbs: | 13 grams |
| Sodium: | 479 mg | | | | |

## MEDITERRANEAN TURKEY-AND-PEPPERS SKILLET

The delicate balance of Mediterranean flavorings adds flair to this dish, and the texture of the lean turkey is complemented by the crunchy, nutrient-rich red bell peppers. Serve this over quinoa or brown rice for a complete, fast, and easy meal.

*Makes 4 servings*

2 tablespoons olive oil

1 pound natural turkey breast cutlets, cut into ½-inch-wide strips

½ teaspoon sea salt

¼ teaspoon freshly ground black pepper

1 medium onion, sliced

1 medium red bell pepper, sliced

1 medium green bell pepper, sliced

½ medium fennel bulb, sliced

6 garlic cloves, sliced

1 teaspoon dried basil

1 tablespoon white balsamic vinegar

¼ cup fresh basil, sliced

Heat 1 tablespoon of the oil in a large nonstick skillet over medium-high heat. Combine the turkey, ¼ teaspoon of the salt, and ⅛ teaspoon of the pepper in a bowl. Add half of the turkey to the skillet and cook, turning occasionally, until very lightly browned, about 3 minutes. Transfer the turkey to a plate. Add the remaining turkey to the skillet and repeat.

Heat the remaining 1 tablespoon oil in the skillet over medium-high heat. Add the onion, bell peppers, fennel, garlic, and dried basil. Cook, stirring occasionally, until the vegetables are tender and starting to brown, 7 to 8 minutes. Stir in the turkey, vinegar, remaining ¼ teaspoon salt, and remaining ⅛ teaspoon pepper and cook, stirring often, until the turkey is completely cooked through and hot, 1 to 2 minutes. Remove from the heat and stir in the fresh basil.

## Nutrient Content per Serving

| | | | | | |
|---|---|---|---|---|---|
| Calories: | 237 | Fat: | 8 grams | Protein: | 29 grams |
| Fiber: | 4 grams | Saturated Fat: | 1 gram | Carbs: | 12 grams |
| Sodium: | 372 mg | | | | |

## CILANTRO TURKEY BURGERS WITH CHIPOTLE KETCHUP

Clearly, there's something about a burger we just can't ignore! But it's hard to eat them guilt-free these days, knowing what we know about grain-fed beef. That's why I made this one. Combine lean turkey with cilantro, which is high in potassium, and you've got a high-nutrient patty right there. Once you pile on spinach and avocado, you'll not only be full, you'll be energized for hours.

### Makes 4 servings

½ cup Homemade Ketchup (page 211)
½ to 1 canned chipotle pepper in adobo sauce, minced
1 pound natural lean ground turkey
3 tablespoons chopped fresh cilantro
¼ cup gluten-free oats
½ teaspoon chili powder
½ teaspoon garlic powder
½ teaspoon sea salt
¼ teaspoon freshly ground black pepper
4 brown rice tortillas
1 cup baby spinach
8 tomato slices
1 avocado, sliced

Combine the ketchup and chipotle pepper in a bowl, and set aside.

Combine the turkey, cilantro, oats, chili powder, garlic powder, salt, and pepper in a medium bowl, taking care not to overwork the mixture. Form into four ½-inch-thick patties.

Heat a grill pan over medium heat. Add the patties and cook for 5 to 6 minutes per side, until an instant-read meat thermometer registers 175°F in the thickest part.

Heat a large nonstick skillet over medium heat until hot. Working with one at a time, place the tortillas in the skillet and cook, turning several times, until heated through, about 45 seconds.

Lay the tortillas on a work surface and top each one with one-fourth of the spinach, 2 tomato slices, one-fourth of the avocado slices, 2 tablespoons of the ketchup mixture, and a patty. Fold the wraps around the burgers and serve immediately.

## Nutrient Content per Serving

| | | | | | |
|---|---|---|---|---|---|
| Calories: | 469 | Fat: | 21 grams | Protein: | 30 grams |
| Fiber: | 8 grams | Saturated Fat: | 4 grams | Carbs: | 41 grams |
| Sodium: | 784 mg | | | | |

## GRILLED TURKEY CUTLETS WITH CHIMICHURRI

Add an international flair to these grilled turkey cutlets with chimichurri, the Argentinian sauce used as a marinade for grilled meat. It can also be added to chicken or fish.

*Makes 4 servings*

### Chimichurri
3 tablespoons chopped fresh cilantro
3 tablespoons chopped fresh basil
4 teaspoons lime juice
1 tablespoon finely chopped onion
4 teaspoons extra-virgin olive oil
¼ teaspoon sea salt

### Turkey
1 tablespoon olive oil
1 garlic clove, minced
1 tablespoon lime juice
¼ teaspoon ground cumin
¼ teaspoon smoked paprika

4 (5-ounce) natural turkey breast cutlets

¼ teaspoon sea salt

⅛ teaspoon freshly ground black pepper

Combine the cilantro, basil, lime juice, onion, oil, and salt in a small bowl; set aside.

Combine the oil, garlic, lime juice, cumin, and paprika in a large bowl; add the turkey and turn to coat. Let the turkey stand at room temperature for 15 minutes.

Heat a grill pan over medium heat. Season the turkey with the salt and pepper, and place on the grill pan. Cook the turkey, turning once, until well marked and cooked through, 4 to 5 minutes per side. Serve with the chimichurri sauce.

### Nutrient Content per Serving

| | | | | | |
|---|---|---|---|---|---|
| Calories: | 230 | Fat: | 9 grams | Protein: | 34 grams |
| Fiber: | 0 grams | Saturated Fat: | 1 gram | Carbs: | 1 gram |
| Sodium: | 350 mg | | | | |

## CHICKEN MARSALA

The herbs and spices in this much-loved dish always fill the kitchen with delicious scents, and now you can enjoy it knowing it's the same classic flavor in a good-for-you version! But remember—only in Cycle 3, due to the wine, and make sure to use dry Marsala, not the sweet dessert wine version.

*Makes 4 servings*

4 (4-ounce) organic free-range boneless, skinless chicken breast halves

¼ teaspoon plus ⅛ teaspoon sea salt

¼ teaspoon freshly ground black pepper

2 tablespoons arrowroot

2 tablespoons olive oil

8 ounces cremini mushrooms, thinly sliced

1 small shallot, finely chopped

3 garlic cloves, minced

1 tablespoon chopped fresh sage

¾ cup organic low-sodium chicken broth

½ cup dry Marsala wine

Sprinkle the chicken with ¼ teaspoon of the salt and ⅛ teaspoon of the pepper. Spread the arrowroot on a plate and lightly dredge both sides of the chicken.

Heat 1 tablespoon of the oil in a large nonstick skillet over medium-high heat. Add the chicken and cook until lightly browned, about 3 minutes per side. Transfer the chicken to a plate and reserve.

Heat the remaining 1 tablespoon oil in the skillet over medium-high heat. Add the mushrooms and cook, stirring occasionally, until lightly browned around the edges, about 5 minutes. Stir in the shallot, garlic, and sage and cook until slightly softened, 1 to 2 minutes. Pour in the broth and wine; bring to a boil and cook until the mixture begins to thicken, about 2 minutes. Reduce the heat to medium and add the reserved chicken. Cook, turning occasionally, until an instant-read meat thermometer inserted horizontally into the thickest part of the chicken registers 165°F, 4 to 5 minutes.

Remove from the heat and stir in the remaining ⅛ teaspoon salt and ⅛ teaspoon pepper.

### Nutrient Content per Serving

| | | | | | |
|---|---|---|---|---|---|
| Calories: | 269 | Fat: | 10 grams | Protein: | 25 grams |
| Fiber: | 1 gram | Saturated Fat: | 2 grams | Carbs: | 12 grams |
| Sodium: | 480 mg | | | | |

## GRILLED MARINATED DUCK BREASTS

Duck may not be the first lean meat that comes to your mind, but don't give it short shrift. It's a delicious, moist, dark meat that "eats" like red meat. And it's a high-quality protein (and vitamin and mineral) source when you're looking for a change from chicken.

*Makes 4 servings*

4 (6-ounce) boneless duck breasts
1 tablespoon grated orange zest
1 tablespoon grated fresh ginger
2 teaspoons grated lemon zest
2 garlic cloves, minced
1 tablespoon coconut aminos
1 tablespoon dry sherry (optional)
2 teaspoons Asian sesame oil

Using a sharp knife, carefully remove the duck skin and discard it.

Combine the orange zest, ginger, lemon zest, garlic, coconut aminos, sherry (if using), and sesame oil in a medium bowl. Add the duck breasts and turn to coat. Cover and refrigerate for at least 2 and up to 6 hours.

Remove the duck from the refrigerator and let it stand at room temperature for 10 minutes. Meanwhile, heat a grill pan over medium heat until hot.

Wipe off the excess marinade and place the duck on the hot pan. Cook, turning once, until an instant-read meat thermometer inserted into the thickest part of the breast registers 140°F, about 5 minutes per side. Transfer to a cutting board and let stand for 3 minutes before slicing.

### Nutrient Content per Serving

| | | | | | |
|---|---|---|---|---|---|
| Calories: | 231 | Fat: | 6 grams | Protein: | 39 grams |
| Fiber: | 0 grams | Saturated Fat: | 1 gram | Carbs: | 3 grams |
| Sodium: | 279 mg | | | | |

## FISH AND SHELLFISH

Seafood could well be considered one of Earth's perfect foods. It's low in saturated fat, is plentiful in protein, iron, and B vitamins, and is the richest provider of omega-3 fatty acids of any food on the planet. And that one healthy fat alone helps prevent heart disease and reduce high blood pressure and inflammation. It also boosts brain power, improves immune function, and eases joint pain.

You'll get the biggest nutritional benefit from cold-water wild fish, starting with those lowest on the food chain (like sardines and anchovies). But those are not universally loved, and it's hard to ignore the nutrient density and taste sensation that is wild salmon.

All my mouthwatering fish and shellfish recipes make the best seafood choices for you and deliver exquisite meals from which to reap its nutritional benefits.

### SCALLION SHRIMP STIR-FRY WITH SNOW PEAS

No matter how exotic this dinner sounds, know this: You can have it on the table in less than 15 minutes. Now everyone is smiling! Put a healthy twist on the traditional dish by serving it over steamed brown rice, and use the tamari in Cycle 3.

*Makes 4 servings*

1 tablespoon coconut oil
1 tablespoon grated fresh ginger
3 garlic cloves, minced
8 ounces snow peas
1½ pounds wild shrimp, peeled and deveined
2 tablespoons coconut aminos or reduced-sodium wheat-free tamari

½ teaspoon chili garlic sauce

4 green onions, thinly sliced

Heat the oil in a large nonstick skillet over medium-high heat. Add the ginger and garlic and cook, stirring, for 30 seconds. Add the snow peas and cook, stirring, until they are bright green, 1 to 2 minutes. Stir in the shrimp and cook until pink, about 1 minute. Add the coconut aminos (or tamari) and chili garlic sauce and cook for 15 seconds. Stir in the green onions and cook, stirring, until the shrimp is cooked through, 1 to 1½ minutes longer.

## Nutrient Content per Serving

| | | | | | |
|---|---|---|---|---|---|
| Calories: | 170 | Fat: | 4 grams | Protein: | 27 grams |
| Fiber: | 2 grams | Saturated Fat: | 3 grams | Carbs: | 7 grams |
| Sodium: | 353 mg | | | | |

## PAN-SEARED SCALLOPS WITH BACON AND SPINACH

This dish brings the elegance of dining out into your own home. You'll savor the mildly sweet flavor of the scallops, and because they're a rich source of vitamin $B_{12}$ and omega-3 fatty acids, you'll be giving your cardiovascular system a treat, too.

For moist, tender scallops, cook until they just turn opaque in the center.

*Makes 4 servings*

3 slices nitrate-free bacon

1 medium onion, thinly sliced

1 large shallot, sliced

4 garlic cloves, sliced

2 (10-ounce) packages frozen organic spinach, thawed and squeezed dry

½ teaspoon sea salt

¼ teaspoon freshly ground black pepper

1 pound wild sea scallops (16 to 20 per pound)

Heat a large nonstick skillet over medium heat. Add the bacon and cook, turning occasionally, until crisp, 6 to 7 minutes. Drain on a plate lined with a paper towel; chop and set aside.

Pour off all but 1 tablespoon bacon fat from skillet, setting aside 2 teaspoons for cooking the scallops. Heat the fat in the skillet over medium-high heat. Add the onion, shallot, and garlic; cook, stirring occasionally, until softened and lightly browned, 6 to 7 minutes. Add the spinach and cook, stirring, until hot, about 2 minutes. Stir in the bacon, ¼ teaspoon of the salt, and ⅛ teaspoon of the pepper. Transfer to a bowl and keep warm.

Wipe out the skillet and heat the reserved 2 teaspoons bacon fat over medium-high heat. Season the scallops with the remaining ¼ teaspoon salt and ⅛ teaspoon pepper. Place the scallops in the skillet and cook, turning once, until nicely browned and just opaque in the center, 5 to 6 minutes.

Divide the spinach among four plates and top with the scallops.

## Nutrient Content per Serving

| | | | | | |
|---|---|---|---|---|---|
| Calories: | 283 | Fat: | 6 grams | Protein: | 35 grams |
| Fiber: | 3 grams | Saturated Fat: | 2 grams | Carbs: | 17 grams |
| Sodium: | 710 mg | | | | |

## DIJON-AND-ALMOND-CRUSTED HALIBUT WITH LEMON AND PARSLEY

Go fish! This Alaskan fish has firm white meat and a delicately sweet flavor. For a richer, more luxurious version, use macadamia nuts in place of the almonds.

*Makes 4 servings*

⅓ cup raw almonds
4 (6-ounce) wild halibut fillets
½ teaspoon sea salt
¼ teaspoon freshly ground black pepper
4 teaspoons Dijon mustard
3 tablespoons chopped fresh parsley
1 tablespoon lemon juice
1 teaspoon grated lemon zest
5 teaspoons extra-virgin olive oil

Preheat the oven to 400°F. Lightly brush a baking sheet with olive oil.

Place the almonds in the bowl of a food processor and pulse until coarsely chopped. Transfer to a plate.

Season the halibut with the salt and pepper; brush the flesh side of each fillet with 1 teaspoon of the mustard. Dip the mustard side of each fillet into the almonds, pressing firmly to help the nuts adhere. Place the fillets, nut-crusted side facing up, on the prepared baking sheet.

Bake the halibut until the fish flakes easily with a fork and the nuts are browned, about 10 minutes. Remove from the oven.

Combine the parsley, lemon juice, lemon zest, and olive oil in a small bowl. Spoon over the fish and serve immediately.

## Nutrient Content per Serving

| | | | | | |
|---|---|---|---|---|---|
| **Calories:** | 470 | **Fat:** | 37 grams | **Protein:** | 29 grams |
| **Fiber:** | 2 grams | **Saturated Fat:** | 6 grams | **Carbs:** | 4 grams |
| **Sodium:** | 559 mg | | | | |

## STIR-FRIED SHRIMP WITH GINGER, BLACK BEANS, AND CASHEWS

Between the shrimp and the black beans, there's no shortage of protein here. Shrimp are also a highly concentrated source of omega-3 fatty acids and antioxidants, and they have anti-inflammatory properties, so eat up! But because fermented black beans are made with black soybeans, save this recipe for Cycle 3.

You can find authentic fermented black beans, without added ingredients like sugar, at Asian food stores. Also, take care that your fish sauce doesn't contain gluten.

*Makes 4 servings*

1½ tablespoons fermented black beans
2 tablespoons water
1½ pounds wild shrimp, peeled and deveined
1 tablespoon grated fresh ginger
1½ teaspoons Asian sesame oil
4 teaspoons coconut oil
3 garlic cloves, minced
8 ounces asparagus, trimmed, cut into 1½-inch pieces
2 cups shredded napa cabbage
⅓ cup slow-roasted cashews (see page 128)
1½ teaspoons coconut aminos
2 cups cooked brown rice, for serving (optional)

Combine the black beans with the water in a small bowl; set aside. In a separate bowl, toss the shrimp, ginger, and sesame oil.

Heat 2 teaspoons of the coconut oil in a large nonstick skillet over medium-high heat until very hot. Add the shrimp and cook, turning once, until they are opaque and almost cooked through, about 2 minutes. Transfer to a plate.

Return the skillet to the stove and heat the remaining 2 teaspoons oil until very hot. Add the garlic and cook, stirring, for 10 seconds. Add the asparagus and cook, stirring, until bright green, 1 minute. Stir in the cabbage and cashews and cook, stirring often, until the cabbage is wilted, about 2 minutes. Add the black beans, shrimp, and coconut aminos; cook, stirring often, until hot, 1 to 1½ minutes. Serve immediately, over the rice, if using.

## Nutrient Content per Serving

| | | | | | |
|---|---|---|---|---|---|
| Calories: | 280 | Fat: | 13 grams | Protein: | 32 grams |
| Fiber: | 2 grams | Saturated Fat: | 5 grams | Carbs: | 11 grams |
| Sodium: | 170 mg | | | | |

## LEMON AND HERB BROILED SOLE

Like most fish, sole delivers the goods when it comes to omega-3 fatty acids, but it's also an underappreciated source of B vitamins. And it's low in mercury. So this is a perfect, healthy meal for a busy weeknight—it's ready in less than 10 minutes!

*Makes 4 servings*

2 tablespoons olive oil

1 tablespoon grated lemon zest

1 tablespoon chopped fresh parsley

1 garlic clove, minced

2 teaspoons lemon juice

½ teaspoon sea salt

½ teaspoon coarsely ground black pepper

4 (6-ounce) wild sole fillets

Preheat the broiler. Lightly oil a large baking sheet.

Combine the oil, lemon zest, parsley, garlic, lemon juice, salt, and pepper in a small bowl. Place the fish on the prepared baking sheet and spread the lemon-herb mixture over the top of the fillets.

Broil until the fish flakes easily with a fork, 3 to 4 minutes.

## Nutrient Content per Serving

| | | | | | |
|---|---|---|---|---|---|
| Calories: | 167 | Fat: | 10 grams | Protein: | 18 grams |
| Fiber: | 0 grams | Saturated Fat: | 2 grams | Carbs: | 1 gram |
| Sodium: | 717 mg | | | | |

## HALIBUT EN PAPILLOTE

I know you don't need a reason other than "It's delicious!" to make this simple, elegant meal in a packet . . . but here it is, anyway: There are no pots and pans to wash! All you have to do is enjoy it.

*Makes 4 servings*

1 medium red onion, thinly sliced

1 pint grape tomatoes, halved

6 teaspoons olive oil

4 (6-ounce) wild halibut fillets

12 ounces asparagus, trimmed

6 teaspoons balsamic vinegar

½ teaspoon sea salt

⅛ teaspoon freshly ground black pepper

Preheat the oven to 450°F. Tear four 12 x 18-inch sheets of aluminum foil. Lightly brush one side of each sheet with oil.

Combine the onion, tomatoes, and 2 teaspoons of the oil in a bowl.

Arrange one sheet of foil so that the long side is closest to you. Fold it in half, matching short end to short end; then open it like a book. Place one fourth of the tomato mixture in the center of the right half of the foil sheet. Place a halibut fillet next to the tomato mixture and one-fourth of the asparagus next to the halibut. Drizzle with 1 teaspoon of oil and 1½ teaspoons of vinegar. Season evenly with salt and pepper. Fold the foil over the filling, then tightly crimp the edges to form a packet. Repeat with the remaining ingredients.

Place the packets on a large baking sheet and bake in the center of the oven until the packets are puffed, 11 to 12 minutes. Remove from the oven and transfer each packet to a plate. With the tip of a sharp knife, carefully cut an X into the top of each packet to allow the steam to escape. Then fold back the foil and serve immediately.

## Nutrient Content per Serving

| | | | | | | |
|---|---|---|---|---|---|---|
| **Calories:** | 453 | **Fat:** | 33 grams | **Protein:** | 29 grams |
| **Fiber:** | 3 grams | **Saturated Fat:** | 5 grams | **Carbs:** | 10 grams |
| **Sodium:** | 446 mg | | | | |

## BLACKENED SALMON

No swimming upstream necessary (I couldn't resist). This meal is easy to prepare and loaded with essential omega-3 fatty acids. Add a dollop of cultured coconut milk mixed with a squeeze of lemon to give your palate even more pleasure.

*Makes 4 servings*

½ teaspoon smoked paprika

½ teaspoon sweet paprika

½ teaspoon ground cumin

½ teaspoon ground coriander

¼ teaspoon dried thyme

¾ teaspoon sea salt

¼ teaspoon cayenne pepper

4 (6-ounce) wild salmon fillets, such as king or sockeye

1 tablespoon olive oil

Lemon wedges, for serving

Combine the smoked and sweet paprikas, cumin, coriander, thyme, salt, and cayenne in a small bowl. Rub the mixture over the salmon fillets.

Heat the oil in a large nonstick skillet over medium-high heat. Add the salmon and cook for 4 to 5 minutes per side, until the fish flakes easily with a fork. Serve with the lemon wedges.

## Nutrient Content per Serving

| | | | | | |
|---|---|---|---|---|---|
| Calories: | 275 | Fat: | 13 grams | Protein: | 36 grams |
| Fiber: | 0 grams | Saturated Fat: | 2 grams | Carbs: | 1 gram |
| Sodium: | 625 mg | | | | |

## POACHED SALMON WITH RÉMOULADE SAUCE

I'm recommending wild salmon here and (always!) evangelizing for its high omega-3 fatty acid content, but you can use this rémoulade sauce on any grilled or pan-seared fish.

*Makes 4 servings*

½ cup Creamy Eggless Mayo (page 214)

2 tablespoons finely chopped shallots

1 teaspoon capers, drained and chopped

2 teaspoons chopped fresh parsley

1 teaspoon lemon juice

¼ teaspoon Tabasco sauce

1 (8-ounce) bottle clam juice

½ cup dry white wine

½ cup water

1 medium onion, thinly sliced

2 celery stalks, thinly sliced

1 carrot, thinly sliced

4 (6-ounce) wild salmon fillets, such as king or sockeye

Combine the mayo, shallots, capers, parsley, lemon juice, and Tabasco in a small bowl. Refrigerate until ready to use.

Combine the clam juice, wine, water, onion, celery, and carrot in a medium skillet over medium-high heat. Bring the mixture to a boil; then reduce the heat to medium-low, cover, and simmer for 15 minutes. Add the salmon to the skillet, cover, and return to a simmer. Cook until the fish flakes easily with a fork, 10 to 11 minutes.

Transfer the fillets to serving plates and top each with rémoulade sauce. Serve warm, at room temperature, or chilled.

## Nutrient Content per Serving

| | | | | | |
|---|---|---|---|---|---|
| Calories: | 477 | Fat: | 29 grams | Protein: | 37 grams |
| Fiber: | 2 grams | Saturated Fat: | 5 grams | Carbs: | 10 grams |
| Sodium: | 511 mg | | | | |

## SALMON PUTTANESCA

You might be more familiar with puttanesca sauce on pasta, but its robust flavor is a perfect counterpoint to flavorful wild salmon. Savor the taste explosion in every bite!

*Makes 4 servings*

4 teaspoons olive oil
1 small onion, chopped
2 garlic cloves, minced
½ teaspoon dried basil
⅛ teaspoon crushed red pepper flakes
⅓ cup pitted Kalamata olives, halved lengthwise
2 teaspoons capers, drained and chopped
1 pint grape tomatoes, halved lengthwise
2 tablespoons chopped fresh parsley
½ teaspoon sea salt
4 (6-ounce) wild salmon fillets, such as king or sockeye
⅛ teaspoon freshly ground black pepper

Heat 2 teaspoons of the oil in a large nonstick skillet over medium-high heat. Add the onion, garlic, basil, and pepper flakes and cook, stirring, for 1 minute. Add the olives and capers and cook for 1 minute. Add the tomatoes and cook, stirring occasionally, until wilted, 3 to 4 minutes. Transfer to a bowl, and stir in the parsley and ¼ teaspoon of the salt.

Season the salmon with the remaining ¼ teaspoon salt and the pepper. Wipe out the skillet; add the remaining 2 teaspoons oil and heat over medium heat. Add the salmon to the skillet, flesh side down, and cook for 4 to 5 minutes per side, until the fish flakes easily with a fork. Serve topped with the tomato mixture.

### Nutrient Content per Serving

| | | | | | |
|---|---|---|---|---|---|
| Calories: | 299 | Fat: | 14 grams | Protein: | 35 grams |
| Fiber: | 1 gram | Saturated Fat: | 3 grams | Carbs: | 6 grams |
| Sodium: | 603 mg | | | | |

## GRILLED FRESH SARDINES

Sardines are so underappreciated! But that's about to change. A Mediterranean favorite served in upscale restaurants in the U.S., these bear no resemblance to the canned version. They're flavorful and can easily be considered one of the healthiest foods you can eat—they're filled with nutrients that support cardiovascular health. I hope you get hooked!

Grains of kosher coarse sea salt are smaller than most other coarse sea salt; to substitute, place regular coarse sea salt in a sealed plastic bag and crush it lightly with a rolling pin.

*Makes 4 servings*

16 fresh sardines (about 2 pounds), scaled, cleaned, and patted dry
2 tablespoons olive oil
¾ teaspoon kosher coarse sea salt
¼ teaspoon freshly ground black pepper
1 tablespoon chopped fresh parsley
Lemon wedges, for serving

Preheat a grill for direct medium heat.

Place the sardines in a large bowl and drizzle with the oil, tossing gently to coat. Season with the salt and pepper.

Place the sardines on the grill, close the lid, and cook, turning once, until they are opaque and flake easily with a fork, about 2 minutes per side. Transfer to a platter, sprinkle with the parsley, and serve accompanied by the lemon wedges.

### Nutrient Content per Serving

| | | | | | |
|---|---|---|---|---|---|
| Calories: | 363 | Fat: | 18 grams | Protein: | 46 grams |
| Fiber: | 0 grams | Saturated Fat: | 4 grams | Carbs: | 1 gram |
| Sodium: | 476 mg | | | | |

# MEATLESS MAINS

There's a fair amount of evidence that a plant-based diet is uber-healthy. But before I lend my support to that research, I have to say that I don't support it unequivocally—I've been a vegetarian, and from personal experience I recommend including animal protein in your diet. Yes, vegetarians generally consume fewer calories than omnivores do, but animal protein supports a high-functioning metabolism that burns fat fast, especially through its support of lean muscle mass.

But, and this is a big but, if you just can't go there for personal or spiritual reasons, you can still get the essential nutrition you need, lose fat fast, and maintain an active, healthy life without eating meat (provided you're not considering a donut as "vegetarian").

A plant-based diet that's high in vegetables, beans and legumes, and nuts (preferably organic) is rich in fiber. So it offers intense digestive support. It's also dense with other nutrients like vitamins and antioxidants, which ward off cancer and other chronic diseases. Simply eating *less* meat has a heart-protective effect, but all the antioxidants in vegetables also actively work on behalf of the heart.

These recipes also include protein in every meal—something that requires a bit of extra attention on a meatless diet.

## LENTIL NUT BURGERS WITH CILANTRO VINAIGRETTE

Not all vegetable burgers are created equal, and if you want to avoid the health bombs that soy and corn can set off, you're better off making your own. Lentils are a solid source of protein and lend substantial texture to a burger, so be prepared to make new friends at the barbecue.

*Makes 4 servings*

2 tablespoons chopped fresh cilantro
1 tablespoon lime juice
½ teaspoon grated lime zest
½ teaspoon sea salt
2 tablespoons plus 6 teaspoons olive oil
4 ounces white mushrooms, chopped (about 1 cup)
1 small onion, finely chopped (about ¼ cup)
3 garlic cloves, minced

1 teaspoon ground cumin

⅓ cup raw walnuts, finely chopped

1 (15-ounce) can organic black lentils, drained and rinsed (I like Westbrae Natural's canned lentils)

1 cup cooked brown rice

2 tablespoons chopped fresh parsley

¼ teaspoon freshly ground black pepper

Optional toppings: sliced cucumbers, tomatoes, and/or fennel

Combine the cilantro, lime juice, lime zest, and ¼ teaspoon of the salt in a small bowl; whisk in 2 tablespoons of the oil in a slow, steady stream. Set aside.

Heat 2 teaspoons of the remaining oil in a medium nonstick skillet over medium heat. Add the mushrooms, onion, garlic, and cumin and cook, stirring occasionally, until softened, 4 to 5 minutes. Add the walnuts and cook until the nuts are lightly toasted, 2 to 3 minutes. Transfer to a bowl.

Combine the lentils and rice in the bowl of a food processor and pulse until coarsely chopped; add to the mushrooms. Stir in the parsley, remaining ¼ teaspoon salt, and the pepper. Form into four ½-inch-thick patties.

Heat the remaining 4 teaspoons oil in a large nonstick skillet over medium heat. Add the patties and cook, turning once, until browned and heated through, 9 to 10 minutes. Transfer to serving plates and top with any of the optional toppings and the cilantro vinaigrette.

## Nutrient Content per Serving

| | | | | | |
|---|---|---|---|---|---|
| Calories: | 356 | Fat: | 21 grams | Protein: | 12 grams |
| Fiber: | 9 grams | Saturated Fat: | 2 grams | Carbs: | 33 grams |
| Sodium: | 301 mg | | | | |

## MUSHROOM LENTIL LOAF WITH BARBECUE GLAZE

Meat loaf always brings back memories of growing up, and now you can share this comforting meal with your own family. It's a meatless loaf for both vegetarians and carnivores alike. Sprouted lentils are easier to digest and can even bring out additional vitamins and enzymes. Want more good news? No need to take the time to sprout your own (you're hungry, after all!)—just buy a bag of dry, sprouted lentils and get busy making delicious food!

### Makes 4 servings

3 tablespoons chia seeds

⅓ cup water

2 cups organic dry, sprouted green lentils (such as TruRoots)

2 tablespoons olive oil

8 ounces cremini mushrooms, coarsely chopped

1 small onion, finely chopped

2 celery stalks, finely chopped

1 small red bell pepper, finely chopped

3 garlic cloves, minced

2 teaspoons chopped fresh thyme

1 teaspoon ground coriander

¾ cup gluten-free oats

2 teaspoons coconut aminos

½ teaspoon sea salt

¼ teaspoon freshly ground black pepper

¼ cup All-Purpose Finger-Lickin'-Good Barbecue Sauce (page 210) or Homemade Ketchup (page 211), plus more for serving (optional)

Preheat the oven to 350°F. Line an 8 x 4-inch loaf pan with aluminum foil, leaving a 3-inch overhang on each side.

Combine the chia seeds with the water in a small bowl and set aside.

Cook the lentils according to the package directions for a tender texture. (You should end up with about 4 cups.)

Heat the oil in a large nonstick skillet over medium-high heat, and add the mushrooms. Cook, stirring occasionally, until slightly softened, about 3 minutes. Stir in the onion, celery, bell pepper, garlic, thyme, and coriander and cook, stirring occasionally, until the vegetables are slightly softened, about 4 minutes. Transfer to a large bowl.

Place 3 cups of the lentils in the bowl of a food processor, and puree. Add the pureed and whole lentils to the bowl containing the mushrooms. Stir in the oats, chia seed mixture, coconut aminos, salt, and pepper; mix well. Firmly press the mixture into the prepared loaf pan. Spread the top with the barbecue sauce or ketchup.

Bake until the loaf is firm and browned around the edges, 48 to 50 minutes. Remove from the oven and let cool in the pan for 5 minutes. Then lift the loaf out of the pan, using the foil overhangs as handles, and transfer it to a cutting board. Cool for an additional 20 minutes. Slice the loaf with a serrated knife and serve with additional barbecue sauce or ketchup if desired.

## Nutrient Content per Serving

| | | | | | |
|---|---|---|---|---|---|
| Calories: | 490 | Fat: | 13 grams | Protein: | 26 grams |
| Fiber: | 20 grams | Saturated Fat: | 1 gram | Carbs: | 73 grams |
| Sodium: | 444 mg | | | | |

## QUINOA FUSILLI WITH CHERRY TOMATOES, GARLIC, BASIL, AND OLIVE OIL

See, you don't have to give up pasta! This simple, elegant dish not only swaps traditional pasta's carbs for quinoa's protein, but it's just plain fun to eat—the fusilli-shaped pasta has lots of nooks to catch the sauce.

*Makes 4 servings*

8 ounces quinoa fusilli pasta
¼ cup olive oil
8 garlic cloves, thinly sliced
¼ teaspoon crushed red pepper flakes
2 pints grape tomatoes, halved
1 cup organic no-salt-added cannellini beans, drained and rinsed
½ cup thinly sliced fresh basil
½ teaspoon sea salt

Bring a large pot of lightly salted water to a boil. Add the pasta and cook according to the package directions.

While the pasta is cooking, heat the oil in a large nonstick skillet over medium-high heat. Add the garlic and pepper flakes and cook, stirring, until fragrant, about 30 seconds. Add the grape tomatoes and cook, stirring occasionally, until softened, 6 to 7 minutes. Stir in the beans and cook for 1 minute.

Drain the pasta and add it to the tomato mixture. Cook, tossing, until hot, 1 minute. Remove from the heat and stir in the basil and salt.

### Nutrient Content per Serving

| | | | | | |
|---|---|---|---|---|---|
| Calories: | 416 | Fat: | 16 grams | Protein: | 10 grams |
| Fiber: | 8 grams | Saturated Fat: | 2 grams | Carbs: | 63 grams |
| Sodium: | 222 mg | | | | |

## VEGETARIAN CHILI

You'll never miss the meat! Bring this protein-packed chili to your next potluck and all you'll hear is how incredibly tasty and filling it is. Chocolate is an ingredient in classic chilis, where it adds depth of flavor. Here the chocolate shake powder not only adds that flavor, it also adds valuable protein. And the beans just pile it on (if you can, buy them dry and soak them first). This chili can always be made ahead of time and frozen.

Ground ancho chile pepper can be found in the spice section of the supermarket.

*Makes 4 servings*

4 teaspoons coconut oil or Malaysian red palm fruit oil

1 medium onion, chopped

4 garlic cloves, minced

1 medium green bell pepper, chopped

1 medium red bell pepper, chopped

2 tablespoons chili powder

2 teaspoons ground cumin

1 teaspoon dried oregano

1 teaspoon ground ancho chile pepper

1 (15-ounce) can organic no-salt-added red kidney beans, drained and rinsed

1 (15-ounce) can organic no-salt-added black beans, drained and rinsed

1 (14.5-ounce) can organic diced fire-roasted tomatoes

½ cup water

1 scoop chocolate vegan protein powder, dissolved in ⅓ cup water

½ teaspoon sea salt

¼ teaspoon freshly ground black pepper

Heat the oil in a Dutch oven over medium-high heat. Add the onion, garlic, and bell peppers, and cook, stirring occasionally, until slightly softened, 6 to 7 minutes. Add the chili powder, cumin, oregano, and ground ancho chile, and cook, stirring, for 30 seconds. Add the beans, tomatoes, and water; bring to a boil and reduce the heat to medium-low.

Simmer, covered, stirring occasionally, until slightly thickened, 22 to 24 minutes. Remove from the heat and stir in the dissolved protein powder, salt, and pepper.

## Nutrient Content per Serving

| | | | | | |
|---|---|---|---|---|---|
| Calories: | 267 | Fat: | 6 grams | Protein: | 16 grams |
| Fiber: | 16 grams | Saturated Fat: | 4 grams | Carbs: | 40 grams |
| Sodium: | 555 mg | | | | |

## QUINOA AND CHICKPEA TABBOULEH WITH MINT, PARSLEY, AND LEMON DRESSING

Quinoa and beans turn this variation on the classic Middle Eastern salad into a protein-packed meal. This can be made up to 4 hours ahead. Cover and refrigerate.

*Makes 4 servings*

1 cup quinoa
½ teaspoon sea salt
1 medium cucumber, peeled, seeded, and cut into ½-inch dice
2 medium plum tomatoes, seeded and chopped
1 (15-ounce) can organic no-salt-added chickpeas (garbanzo beans), drained and rinsed
2 green onions, chopped
¼ cup chopped fresh parsley
3 tablespoons chopped fresh mint
3 tablespoons lemon juice
2 tablespoons extra-virgin olive oil
¼ teaspoon freshly ground black pepper

Cook the quinoa with ¼ teaspoon of the salt according to the package directions. Transfer to a bowl and let cool for 10 minutes.

Add the cucumber, tomatoes, chickpeas, green onions, parsley, mint, lemon juice, oil, remaining ¼ teaspoon salt, and the pepper to the quinoa and mix well. Serve at room temperature or chilled.

## Nutrient Content per Serving

| | | | | | |
|---|---|---|---|---|---|
| **Calories:** | 348 | **Fat:** | 11 grams | **Protein:** | 12 grams |
| **Fiber:** | 9 grams | **Saturated Fat:** | 1 gram | **Carbs:** | 51 grams |
| **Sodium:** | 184 mg | | | | |

# SOUPS AND STEWS | 8

Yes, soup for you! Soup always sounds good, doesn't it? Proof: When's the last time you ate out and *didn't* ask about the soup of the day? If it's cold out, it's a must (hearty stew!), but even if it's not, sometimes that cool, light soup is irresistible. That's because there are no other meals that can bring together the delicate flavor combinations of soups. And we know that when they're prepared well, soups are not only delicious, they're healthy meals that can stand on their own.

Soups and stews are primarily water (yay, they hydrate!), with a healthy dose of vegetables and other nutrient-packed ingredients that fuel your body's fat-burning and disease-fighting machinery. The high vegetable content in many is a great source of fiber, too. You'll notice that most of mine are also beefed up with protein (pun intended) and flavored with herbs rather than added salt. That's because, as much as we love them, restaurant and store-bought varieties can be high in sodium, so if you're not sure about their ingredients, skip them and make these outstanding, flavorful, satisfying alternatives.

Don't dismiss soups and stews assuming they're time-consuming and complicated; that's simply not true, and these recipes prove it!

## HEARTY CHICKEN SOUP

Nothing heals colds and broken hearts like a bowl of homemade chicken soup! Choose free-range chicken to get the biggest nutrient boost out of this comforting dish.

*Makes 6 servings*

6 cups organic low-sodium chicken broth
1 large organic free-range bone-in, skinless chicken breast half (about 12 ounces)

2 organic free-range bone-in, skinless chicken thighs (about 10 ounces), trimmed

1 tablespoon olive oil

2 leeks (about 8 ounces), white and light green parts cut into ½-inch pieces

1 medium onion, chopped

8 ounces white mushrooms, sliced

2 celery stalks, sliced

1 carrot, sliced

1 parsnip, sliced

2 ounces quinoa linguine pasta, broken into 2-inch-long pieces

¾ teaspoon sea salt

¼ teaspoon freshly ground black pepper

Combine the broth, chicken breast, and chicken thighs in a Dutch oven. Bring to a boil over medium-high heat and immediately reduce the heat to medium-low. Cover, and simmer until the chicken is cooked through, 20 minutes. Transfer the chicken to a cutting board and let it cool for 10 minutes. Remove the meat from the bones and cut it into bite-sized pieces.

Heat the oil in a large nonstick skillet over medium-high heat. Add the leeks and onion; cook, stirring occasionally, until starting to soften, 2 to 3 minutes. Add the mushrooms and cook for 3 to 4 minutes. Add to the broth in the Dutch oven and stir in the celery, carrot, parsnip, and pasta. Bring to a simmer over medium heat and cook until the vegetables and pasta are tender, about 10 minutes. Stir in the chicken and cook until hot, about 2 minutes. Season with the salt and pepper.

## Nutrient Content per Serving

| | | | | | |
|---|---|---|---|---|---|
| Calories: | 221 | Fat: | 6 grams | Protein: | 20 grams |
| Fiber: | 3 grams | Saturated Fat: | 1 gram | Carbs: | 21 grams |
| Sodium: | 434 mg | | | | |

## MEXICAN CHICKEN TORTILLA SOUP

The crisp rice tortilla chips add a lovely crunch to this soup, and ground chipotle weighs in with a little kick.

*Makes 4 servings*

4 teaspoons olive oil or coconut oil

1 brown rice tortilla, cut in half, then into thin strips

1 medium onion, chopped

2 garlic cloves, minced

2 celery stalks, chopped

1 teaspoon ground cumin

1 teaspoon dried basil

¼ to ½ teaspoon ground chipotle pepper

1 (14.5-ounce) can organic diced fire-roasted tomatoes and their juice

4 cups organic low-sodium chicken broth

12 ounces cooked organic free-range boneless, skinless chicken breast, cut into cubes (2 cups)

2 tablespoons chopped fresh cilantro

1 tablespoon lime juice

½ teaspoon sea salt

1 avocado, cut into ½-inch dice

Heat 3 teaspoons of the oil in a Dutch oven over medium-high heat. Add the tortilla strips and cook, stirring, until crisp, 5 to 6 minutes. Transfer to a plate lined with a paper towel to drain.

Return the Dutch oven to the stove and heat the remaining 1 teaspoon oil over medium-high heat. Add the onion, garlic, celery, cumin, basil, and ground chipotle; cook, stirring occasionally, until the vegetables begin to soften, 2 to 3 minutes. Stir in the tomatoes and cook for 2 minutes. Pour in the broth, bring to a boil, and immediately reduce the heat to medium-low; cover and simmer for 25 minutes.

Stir in the chicken and cook until heated through, about 3 minutes. Remove from the heat and stir in the cilantro, lime juice, and salt.

Divide the soup among four bowls and top with the tortilla strips and avocado.

### Nutrient Content per Serving

| | | | | | |
|---|---|---|---|---|---|
| Calories: | 355 | Fat: | 16 grams | Protein: | 31 grams |
| Fiber: | 7 grams | Saturated Fat: | 3 grams | Carbs: | 20 grams |
| Sodium: | 711 mg | | | | |

## BLACK BEAN SOUP

For a completely vegetarian version, omit the bacon, use 1 tablespoon olive oil to cook the vegetables, and replace the chicken broth with vegetable broth. The beans may take anywhere from 1 to 2 hours, depending on their age.

*Makes 4 servings*

1 cup dried organic black beans, picked over and rinsed

4 slices nitrate-free bacon, chopped

1 medium onion, chopped

4 garlic cloves, minced

2 celery stalks, chopped

1 large jalapeño pepper, finely chopped

1 teaspoon dried oregano

1 bay leaf

6 cups organic low-sodium chicken broth

2 tablespoons chopped fresh cilantro

¼ teaspoon freshly ground black pepper

Place the beans in a large bowl and add enough cold water to cover by 3 inches; soak overnight. (Alternatively, place the beans in a large saucepan with enough water to cover by 4 inches, bring to a boil over high heat, and cook for 2 minutes. Remove from the heat and let stand, covered, for 1 hour.) Drain the beans.

Heat a Dutch oven over medium heat and add the bacon; cook, stirring occasionally, until crisp, 7 to 8 minutes. Transfer the bacon to a plate lined with a paper towel. Pour off all but 1 tablespoon bacon fat from the pan and return it to medium heat. Stir in the bacon, onion, garlic, celery, jalapeño, oregano, and bay leaf; cook, stirring occasionally, until the vegetables have softened, 6 to 7 minutes. Add the drained beans and the broth and bring to a boil; immediately reduce the heat to a gentle simmer and cook, partially covered, until the beans are very tender, 1 to 2 hours. Remove from the heat and let cool for 20 minutes.

Remove the bay leaf. Transfer the soup to a blender in batches, and puree. Return it to the Dutch oven and cook over medium heat until warmed through. Remove from the heat, and stir in the cilantro and black pepper.

## Nutrient Content per Serving

| | | | | | |
|---|---|---|---|---|---|
| Calories: | 217 | Fat: | 2 grams | Protein: | 15 grams |
| Fiber: | 11 grams | Saturated Fat: | 1 gram | Carbs: | 33 grams |
| Sodium: | 280 mg | | | | |

## MINESTRONE SOUP

This ancient Italian soup has many variations, but all, like this one, deliver the extensive rewards of the polyphenol-rich assortment of vegetables. Freeze it in portion-sized containers for a nearly instant "frozen dinner."

*Makes 4 servings*

4 teaspoons Malaysian red palm fruit oil

1 medium onion, chopped

4 garlic cloves, minced

2 celery stalks, chopped

1 carrot, chopped

1 teaspoon dried basil

½ medium fennel bulb, chopped (about ¾ cup)

1 medium zucchini (8 ounces), cut into ½-inch dice

4 cups organic low-sodium vegetable broth

1 (14.5-ounce) can organic diced tomatoes and their juice

3 ounces quinoa pasta shells (about ¾ cup)

4 cups baby spinach

1 (15-ounce) can organic no-salt-added cannellini beans, drained and rinsed

¾ teaspoon sea salt

¼ teaspoon freshly ground black pepper

Heat the oil in a Dutch oven over medium-high heat. Add the onion, garlic, celery, carrot, and basil; cook, stirring occasionally, until starting to soften, 2 to 3 minutes. Add the fennel and zucchini and cook for 3 minutes. Add the broth and tomatoes, bring to a boil, and immediately reduce the heat to medium. Simmer, uncovered, until the vegetables are crisp-tender, about 20 minutes.

Stir in the pasta, return to a simmer, and cook until the pasta is almost tender, about 8 minutes. Add the spinach and beans, return to a simmer, and cook until heated through, about 3 minutes. Season with the salt and pepper.

## Nutrient Content per Serving

| | | | | | |
|---|---|---|---|---|---|
| Calories: | 286 | Fat: | 6 grams | Protein: | 9 grams |
| Fiber: | 9 grams | Saturated Fat: | 2 grams | Carbs: | 49 grams |
| Sodium: | 703 mg | | | | |

## CREAMY SWEET POTATO SOUP

This soothing soup might be just the thing if you're feeling stressed. Sweet potatoes are a good source of magnesium, the relaxation mineral. Plus, it's extra soothing because it's as rich and creamy as if you had used dairy. *Mmmm.* Let the soup cool before pureeing it in the blender or food processor, in case it spills out the top. To make this a vegan-friendly soup, substitute vegetable broth for the chicken broth.

### Makes 4 servings

2 tablespoons coconut oil or Malaysian red palm fruit oil

1 medium onion, chopped

2 garlic cloves, minced

1 celery stalk, chopped

3 medium sweet potatoes (1½ pounds), peeled and cut into 1-inch pieces

3 cups organic low-sodium chicken broth

¼ teaspoon ground cinnamon

¾ cup unsweetened coconut milk (such as So Delicious)

½ teaspoon sea salt

¼ teaspoon freshly ground black pepper

Heat the oil in a Dutch oven over medium heat. Add the onion, garlic, and celery; cook, stirring occasionally, until tender, 7 to 8 minutes. Increase the heat to medium-high, add the sweet potatoes, broth, and cinnamon, and bring to a boil. Immediately reduce the heat to medium and simmer, uncovered, until the potatoes are tender, 18 to 20 minutes. Remove from the heat and let cool for 20 minutes.

Transfer the soup to a blender in batches, and puree. Return it to the Dutch oven, stir in the coconut milk, and cook over medium heat until warmed through, 4 to 5 minutes. Remove from the heat and stir in the salt and pepper.

## Nutrient Content per Serving

| | | | | | |
|---|---|---|---|---|---|
| Calories: | 179 | Fat: | 8 grams | Protein: | 4 grams |
| Fiber: | 4 grams | Saturated Fat: | 7 grams | Carbs: | 24 grams |
| Sodium: | 408 mg | | | | |

## KALE AND BEAN SOUP

By now you no doubt know that kale is considered a superfood, and for good reason. It's an off-the-charts source of vitamins A and C, and it's loaded with cancer-fighting phytonutrients. This soup freezes well, so double or triple the recipe to be sure more is just a thaw away.

*Serves 2 as a main course, 4 as a side*

1½ tablespoons olive oil

1 large shallot, chopped

1 medium onion, chopped

4 celery stalks, chopped

3 garlic cloves, minced

2 tablespoons chopped fresh sage

1 pound kale, woody stems removed, leaves chopped

3 cups organic low-sodium chicken broth

1 (14.5-ounce) can organic diced tomatoes and their juice

1 (15-ounce) can organic no-salt-added cannellini beans, rinsed and drained

½ teaspoon sea salt

¼ teaspoon freshly ground black pepper

Heat the oil in a Dutch oven over medium heat. Add the shallot, onion, celery, garlic, and sage; cook, stirring occasionally, until softened, 6 to 7 minutes. Increase the heat to medium-high and stir in the kale. Cook, stirring often, until the kale has wilted, about 3 minutes. Pour in the broth and tomatoes and bring to a boil. Immediately reduce the heat to medium-low, cover the pan, and simmer for 20 minutes.

Stir in the beans and cook until heated through, 2 to 3 minutes. Remove from the heat and season with the salt and pepper.

## Nutrient Content per Serving

| | | | | | |
|---|---|---|---|---|---|
| Calories: | 226 | Fat: | 7 grams | Protein: | 11 grams |
| Fiber: | 7 grams | Saturated Fat: | 1 gram | Carbs: | 32 grams |
| Sodium: | 544 mg | | | | |

## THAI COCONUT SHRIMP SOUP

There are different takes on coconut soups, but trust me, this one is just right. Not too sweet and not too spicy, and plenty of nutritious treats—from shrimp to mushrooms—in every spoonful. So warm and yummy!

Thai green curry paste is found in the Asian foods section of most supermarkets.

*Makes 4 servings*

3 (8-ounce) bottles clam juice
4 ounces white mushrooms, quartered
8 quarter-size slices fresh ginger
1 tablespoon fish sauce
1 stalk lemongrass, cut into 1-inch pieces
¾ teaspoon green curry paste
¾ teaspoon monk fruit extract
½ cup unsweetened coconut milk (such as So Delicious)
½ cup unsweetened full-fat canned organic, non-GMO coconut milk
1 pound wild shrimp, peeled and deveined
2 green onions, chopped
16 fresh basil leaves
1 tablespoon lime juice

Combine the clam juice, mushrooms, ginger, fish sauce, lemongrass, curry paste, and monk fruit extract in a large saucepan, and bring the mixture to a boil over medium-high heat. Reduce the heat to medium-low, cover the pan, and simmer for 15 minutes.

Stir in the coconut milks and cook until hot, about 5 minutes. Increase the heat to medium, stir in the shrimp, and cook until opaque, about 3 minutes. Remove from the heat and stir in the green onions, basil, and lime juice. Serve immediately.

## Nutrient Content per Serving

| | | | | | |
|---|---|---|---|---|---|
| Calories: | 144 | Fat: | 6 grams | Protein: | 19 grams |
| Fiber: | 0 grams | Saturated Fat: | 5 grams | Carbs: | 5 grams |
| Sodium: | 591 mg | | | | |

## LENTIL BACON SOUP

I love lentils for their high protein content and cholesterol-lowering fiber. And also, of course, for their earthy taste, which gets a smoky finish in this soup, thanks to the bacon.

*Makes 4 servings*

6 slices nitrate-free bacon, chopped
1 medium onion, finely chopped
3 garlic cloves, minced
3 celery stalks, finely chopped
1 carrot, finely chopped
1 teaspoon dried oregano
1 bay leaf
1 cup organic brown lentils, picked over and rinsed
4 cups organic low-sodium chicken broth
3 tablespoons tomato paste
½ teaspoon sea salt
¼ teaspoon freshly ground black pepper

Heat a Dutch oven over medium heat and add the bacon; cook, stirring occasionally, until crisp, 7 to 8 minutes. Use a slotted spoon or tongs to transfer the bacon to a plate lined with a paper towel to drain.

Pour off all but 2 tablespoons bacon fat from the pan and return it to medium heat. Stir in the onion, garlic, celery, carrot, oregano, and bay leaf; cook, stirring occasionally, until the vegetables are very tender, 14 to 15 minutes. Add the lentils, broth, and tomato paste, and bring to a boil. Immediately reduce the heat to medium-low, cover the pan, and simmer until the lentils are tender, 28 to 30 minutes. Remove the bay leaf, then stir in the bacon, salt, and pepper.

Nutrient Content per Serving

| | | | | | |
|---|---|---|---|---|---|
| Calories: | 264 | Fat: | 4 grams | Protein: | 19 grams |
| Fiber: | 13 grams | Saturated Fat: | 1 gram | Carbs: | 37 grams |
| Sodium: | 645 mg | | | | |

## GAZPACHO WITH LUMP CRAB

A classic, enhanced with the flavor and texture of vitamin $B_{12}$-rich lump crabmeat. This simple and elegant dish is served cold, which is especially nice in the warm summer months. If you prefer a thinner consistency, just add more water. You can also make this vegetarian by skipping the crabmeat.

*Makes 4 servings*

1½ pounds ripe plum tomatoes, seeded and chopped
1 seedless cucumber, peeled and finely chopped
1 medium red bell pepper, finely chopped
1 garlic clove, minced
1 small red onion, finely chopped
1 jalapeño pepper, finely chopped
1½ cups low-sodium vegetable juice, or 1½ cups water mixed with ¼ cup tomato paste
1½ tablespoons lime juice
½ cup ice water
1 tablespoon extra-virgin olive oil
3 tablespoons chopped fresh basil
1 tablespoon chopped fresh cilantro
2 teaspoons balsamic vinegar
½ teaspoon sea salt
¼ teaspoon freshly ground black pepper
½ avocado, cut into ¼-inch dice
1 pound lump crabmeat, picked over for shell fragments

Combine the tomatoes, cucumber, bell pepper, garlic, onion, jalapeño, vegetable juice, lime juice, and ice water in a bowl. Transfer 3 cups of the mixture to a blender, and puree. Pour the pureed soup back into the bowl and stir in the olive oil, basil, cilantro, vinegar, salt, and pepper. Cover with plastic wrap and chill for at least 2 hours.

Remove the soup from the refrigerator and stir in the avocado. Place some of the crabmeat in the bottom of each of four large soup bowls. Ladle in the soup, then top with the remaining crabmeat. Serve immediately.

## Nutrient Content per Serving

| | | | | | |
|---|---|---|---|---|---|
| Calories: | 325 | Fat: | 13 grams | Protein: | 30 grams |
| Fiber: | 8 grams | Saturated Fat: | 2 grams | Carbs: | 24 grams |
| Sodium: | 748 mg | | | | |

## MUSHROOM BISQUE

The variety of mushrooms in this bisque creates layers and depth of flavor. They also provide a spectrum of health benefits that range from improved immune function and resistance to free radicals to revved metabolism and weight loss. This soup can be frozen in individual portions.

*Makes 4 servings*

½ ounce dried porcini mushrooms
2 tablespoons coconut oil
1 pound white mushrooms, chopped
8 ounces assorted wild mushrooms, chopped
1 medium onion, chopped
2 celery stalks, chopped
1 carrot, chopped
1 shallot, chopped
2 garlic cloves, chopped
4 cups organic low-sodium vegetable broth
2 teaspoons coconut aminos
¼ teaspoon sea salt
¼ teaspoon freshly ground black pepper

Bring a small saucepan of water to a boil over high heat. Add the porcini mushrooms and boil for 5 minutes. Drain the mushrooms and chop.

Heat the oil in a Dutch oven over medium-high heat. Add the white, wild, and porcini mushrooms and cook, stirring occasionally, until softened, about 5 minutes. Stir in the onion, celery, carrot, shallot, and garlic; cook, stirring occasionally, until softened, 8 to 9 minutes. Pour in the broth and coconut aminos and bring to a boil. Immediately reduce the heat to medium-low, cover, and simmer for 20 minutes.

Remove from the heat and let cool for 10 minutes. Then transfer the mixture to a blender in batches, and puree. Return the soup to the Dutch oven and heat it over medium heat until hot, 2 to 3 minutes. Season with the salt and pepper.

## Nutrient Content per Serving

| | | |
|---|---|---|
| Calories: 162 | Fat: 8 grams | Protein: 5 grams |
| Fiber: 5 grams | Saturated Fat: 6 grams | Carbs: 19 grams |
| Sodium: 383 mg | | |

## MUSHROOM BEEF STEW

Stew always sounds comforting, with or without a warm blanket and a fire. This stew is rich, hearty, and flavorful—and it will make you wonder more than once how you could possibly be on a diet. Make the stew without wine until Cycle 3; just use an additional ½ cup beef broth in its place.

### Makes 4 servings

1 pound grass-fed beef round roast, cut into 1-inch cubes
¾ teaspoon sea salt
½ teaspoon freshly ground black pepper
2 tablespoons arrowroot
2 tablespoons macadamia nut oil
1 large onion, coarsely chopped (about 1½ cups)
8 ounces white mushrooms, sliced
4 ounces shiitake mushrooms, stemmed and sliced
1 tablespoon fresh thyme leaves
4 garlic cloves, minced
3 celery stalks, cut into 1-inch pieces
⅔ cup dry red wine
3 tablespoons tomato paste
2 cups organic low-sodium beef broth
1 small sweet potato (6 ounces), peeled and cut into ¾-inch cubes

Season the beef with ¼ teaspoon of the salt and ¼ teaspoon of the pepper in a medium bowl. Add the arrowroot and toss well to coat.

Heat 1 tablespoon of the oil in a Dutch oven over medium-high heat. Add the beef and cook, turning occasionally, until browned, 4 to 5 minutes. Transfer to a plate.

Return the Dutch oven to the stove and heat the remaining 1 tablespoon oil over medium heat. Add the onion, mushrooms, and thyme and cook, stirring occasionally, until slightly browned, 8 to 9 minutes. Stir in the garlic and celery and cook for 2 minutes. Stir in the wine and tomato paste and bring to a boil; cook for

1 minute. Add the broth and the reserved beef, and return to a boil. Immediately reduce the heat to medium-low, cover the pan, and simmer gently until the beef is nearly tender, about 40 minutes.

Stir in the sweet potato and the remaining ½ teaspoon salt and ¼ teaspoon pepper, and return to a gentle simmer. Cook until the beef and potato are tender, about 20 minutes.

### Nutrient Content per Serving

| | | | | | |
|---|---|---|---|---|---|
| Calories: | 373 | Fat: | 13 grams | Protein: | 30 grams |
| Fiber: | 4 grams | Saturated Fat: | 3 grams | Carbs: | 26 grams |
| Sodium: | 514 mg | | | | |

## SLOW COOKER COQ AU VIN

If you're like me, this dish always makes you think of Julia Child, even though it's been around for centuries. While the bacon adds a lovely smoky flavor, it can be completely omitted and oil used in place of the bacon fat. Also, when you're in Cycle 1, eliminate the wine and go with broth only.

*Makes 6 servings*

4 slices nitrate-free bacon, cut into 1-inch pieces
6 organic free-range bone-in, skinless chicken thighs (5 to 6 ounces each), trimmed
8 ounces white mushrooms, halved
2 cups frozen white pearl onions, thawed
3 celery stalks, cut into 1-inch pieces
2 carrots, cut into 1-inch pieces
3 garlic cloves, minced
¾ cup dry red wine
2 tablespoons tomato paste
½ cup organic low-sodium chicken broth
4 teaspoons arrowroot
2 sprigs thyme
1 bay leaf
¼ teaspoon sea salt
⅛ teaspoon freshly ground black pepper

Lightly oil a 6-quart slow cooker.
Cook the bacon in a large nonstick skillet over medium heat until crisp, 6 to 7 minutes. Drain on a plate lined with a paper towel.

Pour off all but 1 tablespoon bacon fat from the skillet and return it to the stove over medium-high heat. Add the chicken, in two batches if necessary, and cook until browned, turning once, about 4 minutes per side. Transfer to a plate.

Return the skillet to the heat, add the mushrooms, and cook until lightly browned, 3 to 4 minutes. Transfer the mushrooms to the slow cooker.

Return the skillet to medium-high heat. Add the onions, celery, carrots, and garlic and cook, stirring occasionally, until just starting to soften, about 3 minutes. Transfer the vegetables to the slow cooker and return the skillet to the heat. Pour in the wine, bring to a boil, and cook for 1 minute. Remove from the heat and whisk in the tomato paste, broth, and arrowroot; pour into the slow cooker and add the thyme sprigs and bay leaf. Place the chicken thighs on top of the vegetables and top with the reserved bacon. Cover and cook on low for 7 to 8 hours, until the chicken and vegetables are tender. Remove the sprigs and bay leaf and season with the salt and pepper just before serving.

## Nutrient Content per Serving

| | | | | | |
|---|---|---|---|---|---|
| Calories: | 214 | Fat: | 6 grams | Protein: | 19 grams |
| Fiber: | 2 grams | Saturated Fat: | 2 grams | Carbs: | 11 grams |
| Sodium: | 308 mg | | | | |

## WEEKNIGHT CIOPPINO

This is a fast, easy version of the beloved San Francisco seafood stew, and the health benefits abound—from the fatty acids in the seafood that help protect against heart disease and lower blood sugar to the antioxidants in the tomatoes. Discard any clams that don't open when cooked.

*Makes 4 servings*

1 tablespoon olive oil

1 medium onion, sliced

6 garlic cloves, minced

1 small fennel bulb, sliced (about 1 cup)

1 medium red bell pepper, cut into thin strips

1/8 teaspoon saffron threads

1/8 teaspoon crushed red pepper flakes

1 (14.5-ounce) can organic diced tomatoes and their juice

1 (8-ounce) bottle clam juice

2 tablespoons tomato paste

18 littleneck clams, scrubbed

12 ounces wild prawns, peeled and deveined

1 (6-ounce) wild halibut fillet, cut into 8 pieces

12 fresh basil leaves

Heat the oil in a large pot over medium-high heat. Add the onion, garlic, fennel, and bell pepper and cook, stirring occasionally, until starting to soften, 3 to 4 minutes. Crush the saffron threads lightly with your fingertips; add them and the red pepper flakes, and cook for 1 minute. Add the diced tomatoes, clam juice, and tomato paste; bring to a boil, and immediately reduce the heat to medium-low. Cover the pot and simmer for 20 minutes.

Add the clams and increase the heat to medium. Cover and cook until the clams open, 12 to 14 minutes. Use a slotted spoon to transfer the clams to four large bowls.

Add the prawns and halibut to the pot, and cook until the prawns are opaque and the halibut flakes easily, 3 to 4 minutes. Remove the pot from the heat and stir in the basil leaves. Ladle the mixture over the clams and serve immediately.

## Nutrient Content per Serving

| | | | | | |
|---|---|---|---|---|---|
| Calories: | 272 | Fat: | 5 grams | Protein: | 36 grams |
| Fiber: | 3 grams | Saturated Fat: | 1 gram | Carbs: | 19 grams |
| Sodium: | 924 mg | | | | |

## TURKEY CHILI

I extol the virtues of free-range turkey as a nearly perfect, inexpensive source of lean protein, and it's harder still to beat in this sassy chili. If you like it spicier, replace 1 teaspoon of the chili powder with 1 teaspoon hot Mexican chili powder.

*Makes 4 servings*

1 tablespoon Malaysian red palm fruit oil

1 medium onion, chopped

4 garlic cloves, minced

1 large green bell pepper, chopped

1 pound natural lean ground turkey

5 teaspoons chili powder

1 teaspoon smoked paprika

½ teaspoon dried oregano

2 (14.5-ounce) cans organic diced fire-roasted tomatoes and their juice

2 tablespoons tomato paste

1 (15-ounce) can organic no-salt-added red kidney beans, drained and rinsed

½ teaspoon sea salt

¼ teaspoon freshly ground black pepper

Heat the oil in a Dutch oven over medium-high heat. Add the onion, garlic, and bell pepper and cook, stirring occasionally, until the vegetables begin to soften, 2 to 3 minutes. Add the turkey and cook, breaking it into smaller pieces with a wooden spoon, until no longer pink, 5 to 6 minutes. Stir in the chili powder, paprika, and oregano and cook for 1 minute. Add the tomatoes and tomato paste, bring to a boil, and immediately reduce the heat to medium-low; cover and simmer, stirring occasionally, for 30 minutes or until slightly thickened.

Stir in the beans and cook for 5 minutes longer. Remove from the heat and stir in the salt and pepper.

## Nutrient Content per Serving

| | | | | | |
|---|---|---|---|---|---|
| Calories: | 309 | Fat: | 6 grams | Protein: | 35 grams |
| Fiber: | 12 grams | Saturated Fat: | 2 grams | Carbs: | 30 grams |
| Sodium: | 759 mg | | | | |

## LENTIL, KALE, AND SAUSAGE STEW

The protein-packed combination of sweet Italian sausage and lentils will warm your bones on wicked winter days. This rustic, savory soup keeps well in the refrigerator for up to 5 days and freezes beautifully.

*Serves 2 as a main course, or 4 as a starter*

1 tablespoon olive oil

1 medium onion, chopped

3 garlic cloves, minced

3 celery stalks, chopped

1 carrot, chopped

2 links fully cooked organic, nitrate-free sweet Italian sausage, halved lengthwise and sliced

8 ounces red or green kale, woody stems removed, leaves coarsely chopped

1 cup organic dry-sprouted green lentils (such as TruRoots)

4 cups organic low-sodium chicken broth

3 sprigs thyme

½ teaspoon sea salt

¼ teaspoon freshly ground black pepper

Heat the oil in a large saucepan over medium-high heat. Add the onion, garlic, celery, and carrot; cook, stirring occasionally, until somewhat softened, 5 to 6 minutes. Stir in the sausage and cook until the vegetables start to brown, about 3 minutes. Add the kale and cook, stirring, until wilted, 1½ to 2 minutes.

Add the lentils, broth, and thyme, and bring to a boil. Immediately reduce the heat to medium-low, cover the pan, and simmer until the lentils are tender, 22 to 25 minutes. Remove from the heat, remove thyme sprigs, and season with the salt and pepper.

## Nutrient Content per Serving

| | | | | | |
|---|---|---|---|---|---|
| Calories: | 345 | Fat: | 14 grams | Protein: | 21 grams |
| Fiber: | 9 grams | Saturated Fat: | 4 grams | Carbs: | 36 grams |
| Sodium: | 679 mg | | | | |

Even if a side dish by its very definition isn't the centerpiece of your plate, it does more than provide balance and color, or help you check off a box. Sides can be a way to bring a meal to life by introducing complementary flavors and nutrients that offset the main thing. I mean, clean, lean proteins are essential, but they don't deliver all the disease-fighting micronutrients that Orange-Scented Mashed Sweet Potatoes with Coconut (page 188) does. So try to suffer through the sides, will you? You're welcome!

## BUTTERNUT SQUASH "FRIES"

Giving up fries can be a final frontier for some of my clients. So don't! Pair these with one of my Lentil Nut (page 163) or Tex-Mex (page 134) burgers and collapse in bliss. Butternut squash is an off-the-charts source of vitamin A, and rich in fiber and phytonutrients that protect against heart disease. The key to getting a crisp exterior on the fries is to make sure there is plenty of room between the sticks in the roasting pan. If the pan is crowded, the squash will steam, which means squishy squash fries . . . not good!

*Makes 4 servings*

2 pounds butternut squash, peeled, seeded, and cut into 2 x ¼-inch sticks
4 teaspoons olive oil
¼ teaspoon sea salt

Preheat the oven to 450°F. Lightly oil a large baking sheet.

Combine the squash, oil, and salt in a large bowl and mix well. Arrange the squash sticks in a single layer, without touching, on the prepared baking sheet.

Roast the squash, turning occasionally, until browned, 23 to 25 minutes.

## Nutrient Content per Serving

| | | | | | |
|---|---|---|---|---|---|
| Calories: | 144 | Fat: | 5 grams | Protein: | 2 grams |
| Fiber: | 5 grams | Saturated Fat: | 1 gram | Carbs: | 27 grams |
| Sodium: | 154 mg | | | | |

## CONFETTI QUINOA

All quinoa has the same nutrient profile, so you can make a sacrifice-free swap of red quinoa for white if the former is your preference. This dish is equally good served hot or at room temperature.

*Makes 4 servings*

1 cup quinoa
¾ teaspoon sea salt
4 teaspoons coconut oil
1 large shallot, finely chopped
3 garlic cloves, minced
2 teaspoons chopped fresh thyme
1 medium red bell pepper, finely chopped
1 medium orange bell pepper, finely chopped
1 medium yellow bell pepper, finely chopped
1 teaspoon ground coriander
¼ cup unsalted sunflower seeds
1 tablespoon sherry vinegar
¼ teaspoon freshly ground black pepper

Cook the quinoa with ¼ teaspoon of the salt according to the package directions.

Heat the oil in a large nonstick skillet over medium-high heat. Add the shallot, garlic, and thyme and cook for 1 minute. Stir in the bell peppers and coriander and cook until crisp-tender, 3 to 4 minutes. Add the sunflower seeds and cook for 1 minute. Stir in the quinoa and cook, stirring, until well mixed and heated through, about 1 minute. Remove from the heat and stir in the vinegar, remaining ½ teaspoon salt, and pepper.

## Nutrient Content per Serving

| | | | | | |
|---|---|---|---|---|---|
| Calories: | 296 | Fat: | 11 grams | Protein: | 9 grams |
| Fiber: | 7 grams | Saturated Fat: | 5 grams | Carbs: | 41 grams |
| Sodium: | 452 mg | | | | |

## VEGETABLE FRIED RICE

If you have a (I hope not late-night!) craving for Chinese food, make this vegetable fried rice and avoid the sugar-spiking, nearly nutrition-less white rice fried in unhealthy oils. Believe it or not, day-old rice works best here; it's drier and stir-fries better.

*Makes 4 servings*

1½ tablespoons Malaysian red palm fruit oil or coconut oil
1 small onion, chopped (about ½ cup)
1 tablespoon grated fresh ginger
2 garlic cloves, minced
4 ounces snow peas, cut in half crosswise
1 medium plum tomato, seeded and chopped
3 cups cold cooked brown rice
2½ tablespoons coconut aminos
3 green onions, chopped

Heat the oil in a large nonstick skillet over medium-high heat. Add the onion, ginger, and garlic; cook, stirring, for 1 minute. Add the snow peas and cook until they are bright green, about 1 minute. Add the tomato and cook for 1 minute. Stir in the rice and cook, stirring, until it is heated through, about 2 minutes. Add the coconut aminos and green onions, and cook for 30 seconds.

### Nutrient Content per Serving

| | | | | | |
|---|---|---|---|---|---|
| Calories: | 250 | Fat: | 6 grams | Protein: | 5 grams |
| Fiber: | 4 grams | Saturated Fat: | 3 grams | Carbs: | 43 grams |
| Sodium: | 218 mg | | | | |

## SPICE ROASTED SWEET POTATOES

This fiber-rich dish is a healthier, more flavorful alternative to the popular potato side. And for a change-up, it can also be made with butternut squash.

*Makes 4 servings*

2 medium sweet potatoes (about 1 pound), peeled
4 teaspoons olive oil or Malaysian red palm fruit oil
½ teaspoon chili powder

½ teaspoon ground coriander

¼ teaspoon paprika

¼ teaspoon sea salt

¼ teaspoon freshly ground black pepper

Preheat the oven to 425°F. Lightly oil a large baking sheet.

Cut the potatoes in half lengthwise, then across into ½-inch-thick slices. Combine with the oil in a bowl and toss to coat.

Combine the chili powder, coriander, paprika, salt, and pepper in a small bowl; toss with the potatoes. Arrange the potatoes in a single layer on the prepared baking sheet.

Roast, turning occasionally, until browned and tender, 22 to 24 minutes.

### Nutrient Content per Serving

| | | | | | |
|---|---|---|---|---|---|
| Calories: | 114 | Fat: | 5 grams | Protein: | 1 gram |
| Fiber: | 3 grams | Saturated Fat: | 1 gram | Carbs: | 17 grams |
| Sodium: | 190 mg | | | | |

## ORANGE-SCENTED MASHED SWEET POTATOES WITH COCONUT

Tropical island flavors abound in this naturally sweet treat. How could you want plain old mashed ever again? And in addition to the amazing taste, there's genius in the chemistry: Healthy fat (coconut milk) increases the uptake of beta-carotene (sweet potatoes), which your body transforms into vitamin A.

*Makes 4 servings*

2 medium sweet potatoes (about 1 pound), peeled and cut into 1-inch pieces

2 tablespoons coconut butter

2 teaspoons grated orange zest

½ teaspoon sea salt

¼ teaspoon freshly ground black pepper

1 tablespoon unsweetened shredded coconut

Place the potatoes in a medium saucepan, add enough cold water to cover by 2 inches, and bring to a boil. Cook until the potatoes are fork-tender, 8 to 9 minutes; drain.

Return the potatoes to the saucepan and mash until smooth. Stir in the coconut butter, orange zest, salt, and pepper. Transfer to a serving bowl and sprinkle with the shredded coconut.

## Nutrient Content per Serving

| Calories: | 168 | Fat: | 7 grams | Protein: | 2 grams |
|---|---|---|---|---|---|
| Fiber: | 4 grams | Saturated Fat: | 7 grams | Carbs: | 23 grams |
| Sodium: | 353 mg | | | | |

## CUBAN-STYLE BLACK BEANS

Black beans are a staple in cuisines around the world, often as the main dish, though I prefer to use them as a side. Their high protein and fiber content supports digestive tract health, which in turn helps regulate blood sugar.

*Makes 4 servings*

1 tablespoon olive oil
1 medium onion, chopped
3 garlic cloves, minced
1 teaspoon ground cumin
½ teaspoon dried oregano
1 medium green bell pepper, chopped
2 medium plum tomatoes, seeded and chopped
2 teaspoons red wine vinegar
1 (15-ounce) can organic no-salt-added black beans and their juice
¼ teaspoon sea salt
¼ teaspoon freshly ground black pepper

Heat the oil in a medium saucepan over medium heat; add the onion, garlic, cumin, and oregano. Cook, stirring occasionally, until the vegetables begin to soften, 2 to 3 minutes. Add the bell pepper and cook for 2 minutes. Add the tomatoes and vinegar and cook until slightly wilted, about 2 minutes. Add the beans and their liquid, reduce the heat to medium-low, cover the pan, and simmer, stirring occasionally, until the vegetables are very tender, 10 to 12 minutes. Remove from the heat and season with the salt and pepper.

## Nutrient Content per Serving

| Calories: | 135 | Fat: | 4 grams | Protein: | 6 grams |
|---|---|---|---|---|---|
| Fiber: | 6 grams | Saturated Fat: | 1 gram | Carbs: | 20 grams |
| Sodium: | 161 mg | | | | |

## RED QUINOA WITH KALE, ONIONS, AND PINE NUTS

Quinoa is a health food rock star: It's a complete protein and high in fiber. Some brands of quinoa are prerinsed—which the package will tell you—but others are not. If it isn't, the quinoa must be rinsed to get rid of its bitter flavor.

*Makes 4 servings*

1 cup red quinoa
½ teaspoon sea salt
1 tablespoon Malaysian red palm fruit oil
1 extra-large onion, chopped (about 2 cups)
1 tablespoon chopped fresh rosemary
4 garlic cloves, minced
8 ounces kale, woody stems removed, leaves coarsely chopped
¼ cup pine nuts, toasted
¼ teaspoon freshly ground black pepper

Cook the quinoa with ¼ teaspoon of the salt according to the package directions.

Meanwhile, heat the oil in a large nonstick skillet over medium-high heat. Add the onion and rosemary and cook, stirring occasionally, until the onion begins to brown, 8 to 9 minutes. Add the garlic; cook for 2 minutes. Add the kale and cook until wilted and tender, about 3 minutes. Add the pine nuts and remaining ¼ teaspoon salt; cook for 1 minute.

Add the quinoa and cook until warmed through, about 1 minute. Remove from the heat and stir in the pepper.

### Nutrient Content per Serving

| | | | | | |
|---|---|---|---|---|---|
| Calories: | 302 | Fat: | 12 grams | Protein: | 10 grams |
| Fiber: | 6 grams | Saturated Fat: | 3 grams | Carbs: | 40 grams |
| Sodium: | 320 mg | | | | |

## CURRIED LENTILS

Don't you just love the rich flavor of Indian food? And here it is, right in your kitchen. This meal is high in protein (good news for vegans and vegetarians), and sprouting the lentils boosts their nutrient content and digestibility. Prepare this dish as a stand-alone meal or as a perfect fiber-rich side.

*Makes 4 servings*

¾ cup organic dry-sprouted green lentils (such as TruRoots)

4 teaspoons coconut oil or Malaysian red palm fruit oil

1 small onion, chopped

1 celery stalk, chopped

½ medium red bell pepper, chopped

2 garlic cloves, minced

½ teaspoon curry powder

2 tablespoons chopped fresh cilantro

¼ teaspoon sea salt

⅛ teaspoon cayenne pepper

Cook the sprouted lentils according to the package directions.

Heat the oil in a large nonstick skillet over medium-high heat. Add the onion, celery, and bell pepper; cook, stirring occasionally, until starting to soften, 2 to 3 minutes. Add the garlic and cook for 1 minute. Stir in the curry powder and cook until fragrant, about 30 seconds. Add the lentils and cook, stirring, until heated through, 1 to 2 minutes. Remove from the heat and stir in the cilantro, salt, and cayenne pepper.

## Nutrient Content per Serving

| | | | | | |
|---|---|---|---|---|---|
| Calories: | 166 | Fat: | 6 grams | Protein: | 8 grams |
| Fiber: | 6 grams | Saturated Fat: | 4 grams | Carbs: | 23 grams |
| Sodium: | 163 mg | | | | |

## CHICKPEAS WITH SPINACH, LEMON, AND TOMATOES

This dish has a Moroccan flair with all the flavors and heft to satisfy you, whether you're a vegetarian or an omnivore. Chickpeas, high in fiber and protein, balance the vitamin- and mineral-rich veggies with a pleasant light, nutty flavor.

*Makes 4 servings*

4 teaspoons coconut oil or Malaysian red palm fruit oil

10 cups (5 ounces) baby spinach

1 small onion, chopped

2 garlic cloves, minced

1 pint grape tomatoes, halved

¼ teaspoon curry powder

⅛ teaspoon monk fruit extract

1 (15-ounce) can organic no-salt-added chickpeas (garbanzo beans), drained and rinsed

2 teaspoons lemon juice

¼ teaspoon sea salt

¼ teaspoon freshly ground black pepper

Heat 1 teaspoon of the oil in a large nonstick skillet over medium-high heat. Add the spinach and cook, turning with kitchen tongs, until wilted, 1 to 1½ minutes. Transfer to a strainer to drain.

Return the skillet to the stove (after pouring out any residual liquid) and heat the remaining 3 teaspoons oil over medium-high heat. Add the onion and garlic and cook for 1 minute. Reduce the heat to medium and add the tomatoes, curry powder, and monk fruit extract; cook, stirring occasionally, until the tomatoes have softened, about 4 minutes. Add the chickpeas and cook for 1 minute. Add the spinach and cook until heated through, about 1 minute. Remove from the heat and stir in the lemon juice, salt, and pepper.

## Nutrient Content per Serving

| | | | | | |
|---|---|---|---|---|---|
| Calories: | 180 | Fat: | 6 grams | Protein: | 7 grams |
| Fiber: | 7 grams | Saturated Fat: | 4 grams | Carbs: | 27 grams |
| Sodium: | 229 mg | | | | |

## ROASTED ACORN SQUASH PUREE

Acorn squash (so called because it looks like a large acorn) is a good source of vitamin C, potassium, and fiber, but other squash, including butternut and kabocha, may be substituted in this puree.

*Makes 4 servings*

1 acorn squash (about 2¼ pounds), cut in half and seeds removed

1 tablespoon macadamia nut oil

Pinch of ground nutmeg

½ teaspoon sea salt

⅛ teaspoon freshly ground black pepper

Preheat the oven to 400°F. Lightly oil an 11 x 7-inch baking dish.

Place the squash, cut side down, in the prepared baking dish. Cover with aluminum foil and roast until very tender, 55 to 60 minutes. Remove from the oven and let cool for 10 minutes.

When the squash is cool enough to handle, use a spoon to scoop out the flesh and transfer it to a food processor. Puree the squash. Transfer the puree to a medium nonstick skillet over medium-high heat and cook, stirring, until it is somewhat drier, about 4 minutes. Remove from the heat and stir in the oil, nutmeg, salt, and pepper.

Nutrient Content per Serving

| | | | | | |
|---|---|---|---|---|---|
| Calories: | 129 | Fat: | 4 grams | Protein: | 2 grams |
| Fiber: | 8 grams | Saturated Fat: | 0 grams | Carbs: | 25 grams |
| Sodium: | 297 mg | | | | |

## TUSCAN WHITE BEANS WITH SAGE

The soft, sweet flavor of sage creates a delicious balance between the earthy beans and the garlic. And white beans are an awesome source of vegetarian protein. They're also low on the glycemic index, which means they won't spike your blood sugar—which in turn means you're not storing excess sugar as fat. For a vegan option, sub vegetable broth for the chicken broth.

*Makes 4 servings*

4 teaspoons olive oil

3 garlic cloves, minced

2 tablespoons chopped fresh sage

1 (15-ounce) can organic no-salt-added cannellini beans, drained and rinsed

⅔ cup organic low-sodium chicken broth

2 teaspoons grated lemon zest

¼ teaspoon sea salt

⅛ teaspoon freshly ground black pepper

Heat the oil in a large nonstick skillet over medium heat. Add the garlic and sage; cook, stirring occasionally, until slightly softened, 1½ to 2 minutes. Add the beans and cook for 1 minute. Pour in the broth, bring to a simmer, and cook until slightly thickened, 2 to 3 minutes. Remove from the heat and season with the lemon zest, salt, and pepper.

Nutrient Content per Serving

| | | | | | |
|---|---|---|---|---|---|
| Calories: | 125 | Fat: | 5 grams | Protein: | 5 grams |
| Fiber: | 4 grams | Saturated Fat: | 1 gram | Carbs: | 14 grams |
| Sodium: | 115 mg | | | | |

## ROASTED ROOT VEGETABLES WITH THYME

Root vegetables are rich in carotenoids, which are full of phytonutrients and antioxidants. And that's the good news—before you even think about how succulent "butternut" sounds. The vegetables are also delicious cold the next day or perfect as a salad with a little eggless mayo (see page 214).

*Makes 4 servings*

8 ounces butternut squash, peeled and cut into 1-inch chunks (about 2 cups)

1 large white turnip (8 ounces), peeled and cut into ¾-inch chunks

1 medium red onion, peeled and cut through the root into 8 wedges

1 small sweet potato (6 ounces), peeled and cut into ¾-inch chunks

4 teaspoons fresh thyme leaves

1 tablespoon Malaysian red palm fruit oil

⅛ teaspoon ground nutmeg

½ teaspoon sea salt

¼ teaspoon freshly ground black pepper

Preheat the oven to 425°F. Lightly oil a large baking sheet.

Combine the squash, turnip, onion, sweet potato, thyme, oil, nutmeg, salt, and pepper in a large bowl; toss well. Spread the vegetables out in a single layer on the prepared baking sheet.

Roast, stirring occasionally, until the vegetables are fork-tender and lightly browned, 33 to 35 minutes.

## Nutrient Content per Serving

| | | | | | |
|---|---|---|---|---|---|
| Calories: | 107 | Fat: | 4 grams | Protein: | 2 grams |
| Fiber: | 4 grams | Saturated Fat: | 2 grams | Carbs: | 19 grams |
| Sodium: | 341 mg | | | | |

## ROASTED BRUSSELS SPROUTS WITH HAZELNUTS

Brussels sprouts have made a comeback! And that's good news for your taste buds and your health, because these cruciferous vegetables pack a serious nutritional punch, fighting everything from cholesterol to inflammation. This dish can be made in advance and slightly undercooked, then popped into the oven just before serving to finish cooking and heat through.

*Makes 4 servings*

¼ cup raw hazelnuts

1¼ pounds Brussels sprouts, trimmed and halved

2 tablespoons macadamia nut oil or olive oil

½ teaspoon sea salt

⅛ teaspoon freshly ground black pepper

Preheat the oven to 350°F.

Spread the hazelnuts on a large baking sheet and place it in the oven. Bake until the nuts are lightly toasted, 10 to 12 minutes. Remove from the oven and let cool for 10 minutes; then coarsely chop.

Increase the oven temperature to 425°F.

Combine the Brussels sprouts, oil, salt, and pepper in a bowl. Transfer them to a large baking sheet and roast, stirring occasionally, until the Brussels sprouts are browned and crisp-tender, 20 to 22 minutes. Transfer to a bowl and toss with the chopped nuts.

### Nutrient Content per Serving

| | | | | | |
|---|---|---|---|---|---|
| Calories: | 185 | Fat: | 13 grams | Protein: | 6 grams |
| Fiber: | 6 grams | Saturated Fat: | 1 gram | Carbs: | 14 grams |
| Sodium: | 325 mg | | | | |

## EASY SPINACH-AND-GARLIC SAUTÉ

There's a reason "easy" is part of this recipe title. And if that encourages you to make it the first time, great; you'll make it again and again once you taste how the heart-healthy olive oil and garlic bring the taste of the spinach to life. Popeye was onto something here!

Substitute other greens if you'd like, although most will take a little longer than delicate spinach; kale, chard, and dandelion greens all make great sautés.

*Makes 4 servings*

2 tablespoons olive oil
6 garlic cloves, thinly sliced
⅛ teaspoon crushed red pepper flakes
1½ pounds fresh spinach
½ teaspoon sea salt
⅛ teaspoon freshly ground black pepper

Heat the oil in a large skillet over medium heat. Add the garlic and red pepper flakes and cook, stirring occasionally, until the garlic just starts to brown, 2 to 3 minutes. Add the spinach and cook, tossing with kitchen tongs, until it has wilted, 2 to 3 minutes. Remove from the heat and season with the salt and pepper.

### Nutrient Content per Serving

| | | | | | |
|---|---|---|---|---|---|
| Calories: | 109 | Fat: | 8 grams | Protein: | 5 grams |
| Fiber: | 4 grams | Saturated Fat: | 1 gram | Carbs: | 8 grams |
| Sodium: | 329 mg | | | | |

## CAULIFLOWER PUREE

Cauliflower's detoxification properties make this puree a satisfying, healthy alternative to mashed potatoes. To make a pesto version of the puree, simply stir in ⅓ cup Pesto Sauce (page 211).

*Makes 4 servings*

1 head cauliflower (about 2 pounds), stemmed and roughly chopped

3 cups water

½ cup unsweetened coconut milk (such as So Delicious), warmed

2 tablespoons extra-virgin olive oil

¾ teaspoon sea salt

¼ teaspoon freshly ground black pepper

Place the cauliflower in a medium saucepan, add the water, and bring to a boil over medium-high heat. Immediately reduce the heat to medium, cover the pan, and simmer gently until very tender, 10 to 12 minutes. Drain, and transfer the cauliflower to the bowl of a food processor; add the coconut milk and puree. Stir in the oil, salt, and pepper.

### Nutrient Content per Serving

| | | | | | |
|---|---|---|---|---|---|
| Calories: | 106 | Fat: | 8 grams | Protein: | 3 grams |
| Fiber: | 3 grams | Saturated Fat: | 2 grams | Carbs: | 8 grams |
| Sodium: | 481 mg | | | | |

## SHREDDED BRUSSELS SPROUTS WITH BACON

Shredding Brussels sprouts gives them an entirely different texture. When you allow more of the surface area to come in contact with the hot skillet, they begin to caramelize, which gives them a nuttier flavor. And all of the health benefits of this cruciferous vegetable remain when it's shredded.

*Makes 4 servings*

4 slices nitrate-free bacon

2 teaspoons olive oil

1 medium onion, chopped

4 garlic cloves, minced

1 teaspoon chopped fresh thyme

1½ pounds Brussels sprouts, very thinly sliced

1 tablespoon cider vinegar

¼ teaspoon sea salt

⅛ teaspoon freshly ground black pepper

Cook the bacon in a large nonstick skillet over medium heat until crisp, 6 to 7 minutes. Transfer to a plate lined with a paper towel to drain. Then chop the bacon.

Pour off all but 1 tablespoon of the bacon fat and return the skillet to medium heat. Add the olive oil, onion, garlic, and thyme and cook, stirring occasionally, until the onion is slightly softened, 2 to 3 minutes. Add the Brussels sprouts and vinegar and cook, stirring occasionally, until the sprouts are crisp-tender and lightly browned, 7 to 8 minutes. Remove from the heat and stir in the reserved bacon, the salt, and the pepper.

## Nutrient Content per Serving

| | | | | | | | |
|---|---|---|---|---|---|---|---|
| **Calories:** | 138 | **Fat:** | 5 grams | **Protein:** | 8 grams |
| **Fiber:** | 6 grams | **Saturated Fat:** | 1 gram | **Carbs:** | 18 grams |
| **Sodium:** | 342 mg | | | | |

## WILD MUSHROOMS AND ONIONS

The beef broth enhances the meaty flavor of this side dish, but you don't need it—the oyster mushrooms more than deliver on that front. So, for a vegan option, use vegetable broth instead.

*Makes 4 servings*

2 tablespoons olive oil

1 large Vidalia onion (or other sweet onion), thinly sliced (about 1½ cups)

8 ounces shiitake mushrooms, stemmed and sliced

6 ounces oyster mushrooms, sliced

6 ounces cremini mushrooms, sliced

1 teaspoon fresh chopped thyme

¼ teaspoon plus ⅛ teaspoon sea salt

3 garlic cloves, minced

¼ cup organic low-sodium beef broth

1 tablespoon balsamic vinegar

⅛ teaspoon freshly ground black pepper

Heat the oil in a large nonstick skillet over medium-high heat. Add the onion and cook until slightly softened, 2 to 3 minutes. Add the mushrooms, thyme, and ¼ teaspoon of the salt; cook, stirring occasionally, until the mushrooms give off their liquid and begin to brown, 11 to 12 minutes. Stir in the garlic and cook until the mushrooms are browned, 5 to 6 minutes. Add the broth and vinegar and cook, stirring, until evaporated, 1 to 2 minutes. Remove from the heat and season with the remaining ⅛ teaspoon salt and the pepper.

Nutrient Content per Serving

| | | | | | |
|---|---|---|---|---|---|
| Calories: | 146 | Fat: | 8 grams | Protein: | 4 grams |
| Fiber: | 4 grams | Saturated Fat: | 1 gram | Carbs: | 17 grams |
| Sodium: | 266 mg | | | | |

## ROASTED ASPARAGUS WITH LEMON ZEST

Make this your go-to vegetable on a busy weeknight. It's fast and easy, and it elegantly does the good things many veggies do for you while also giving you a dose of the detoxifying compound glutathione. Leftovers are great to add to a salad or have on the side with your lunch.

*Makes 4 servings*

1½ pounds asparagus, trimmed

1 tablespoon Malaysian red palm fruit oil

¼ teaspoon sea salt

⅛ teaspoon freshly ground black pepper

2 teaspoons grated lemon zest

2 teaspoons chopped fresh parsley

Preheat the oven to 425°F. Lightly oil a large baking sheet.

Combine the asparagus, oil, salt, and pepper in a medium bowl. Arrange the asparagus in a single layer on the prepared baking sheet.

Roast the asparagus, shaking the baking sheet once or twice, until tender, 10 to 12 minutes. Remove from the oven and toss with the lemon zest and parsley. Serve warm, at room temperature, or chilled.

Nutrient Content per Serving

| | | | | | |
|---|---|---|---|---|---|
| Calories: | 65 | Fat: | 4 grams | Protein: | 4 grams |
| Fiber: | 4 grams | Saturated Fat: | 2 grams | Carbs: | 7 grams |
| Sodium: | 149 mg | | | | |

## STIR-FRIED KALE WITH GINGER

In addition to an anti-inflammatory boost, piquant ginger adds bright flavor to the kale in this dish. If you're not sensitive to soy and you are in Cycle 3, you can replace the coconut aminos with 2 tablespoons wheat-free tamari.

*Makes 4 servings*

4 teaspoons Malaysian red palm fruit oil

1½ tablespoons grated fresh ginger

2 garlic cloves, minced

1½ pounds kale, woody stems removed, leaves coarsely chopped

1½ tablespoons coconut aminos

1 tablespoon rice vinegar

Heat the oil in a large nonstick skillet over medium-high heat. Add the ginger and garlic and cook, stirring, until fragrant, about 30 seconds. Add the kale and cook, turning with kitchen tongs, until slightly wilted, about 2 minutes. Add the coconut aminos and vinegar, and cook until tender, another 2 to 3 minutes.

## Nutrient Content per Serving

| | | | | | |
|---|---|---|---|---|---|
| Calories: | 122 | Fat: | 6 grams | Protein: | 6 grams |
| Fiber: | 3 grams | Saturated Fat: | 2 grams | Carbs: | 15 grams |
| Sodium: | 182 mg | | | | |

## GREEN BEANS WITH SHIITAKES AND SHALLOTS

Smoky, meaty shiitake mushrooms have been used medicinally in Asia for thousands of years. Their support of the immune system is well known, but they're also chock-full of metabolism-revving B vitamins and—heads up, vegetarians!—they're a good source of bioavailable iron.

*Makes 4 servings*

12 ounces green beans, trimmed

2 tablespoons macadamia nut oil or Malaysian red palm fruit oil

2 large shallots, thinly sliced

8 ounces shiitake mushrooms, stemmed and sliced

½ medium red bell pepper, thinly sliced

2 teaspoons coconut aminos

⅛ teaspoon sea salt

⅛ teaspoon freshly ground black pepper

Bring a large saucepan of lightly salted water to a boil over high heat. Add the green beans, cover the pan, and return to a boil; cook for 2 minutes. Drain, and rinse under cold water to stop the cooking; drain again.

Heat the oil in a large nonstick skillet over medium-high heat. Add the shallots and cook, stirring occasionally, until they begin to soften, 2 to 3 minutes. Add the mushrooms and bell pepper and cook, stirring occasionally, until the mushrooms are slightly browned, 6 to 7 minutes. Add the green beans and cook for 1 minute. Add the coconut aminos, salt, and pepper; cook, stirring, until hot, about 1 minute.

### Nutrient Content per Serving

| | | | | | |
|---|---|---|---|---|---|
| Calories: | 142 | Fat: | 8 grams | Protein: | 4 grams |
| Fiber: | 5 grams | Saturated Fat: | 1 gram | Carbs: | 17 grams |
| Sodium: | 144 mg | | | | |

## SWISS CHARD WITH OLIVES

The headline ingredients in this side bring together two nutritional powerhouses in a heart-healthy, anti-inflammatory combination. For a truly beautiful dish, use ruby chard, which has red veins and stems.

*Makes 4 servings*

1½ tablespoons olive oil or macadamia nut oil
⅓ cup pitted Kalamata olives, sliced
3 garlic cloves, minced
2 (1-pound) bunches Swiss chard, stems removed, leaves cut into thin strips (ribbons)
1 teaspoon grated lemon zest
¼ teaspoon sea salt

Heat the oil in a large nonstick skillet over medium-high heat. Add the olives and garlic and cook, stirring often, until fragrant and the garlic is just beginning to brown slightly, 1 to 1½ minutes. Add the chard and cook, turning with kitchen tongs, until wilted and tender, 4 to 5 minutes. Remove from the heat and stir in the lemon zest and salt.

### Nutrient Content per Serving

| | | | | | |
|---|---|---|---|---|---|
| Calories: | 99 | Fat: | 7 grams | Protein: | 3 grams |
| Fiber: | 3 grams | Saturated Fat: | 1 gram | Carbs: | 8 grams |
| Sodium: | 454 mg | | | | |

## SESAME SPINACH WITH SCALLIONS

Spinach is jam-packed with vitamins and minerals and cancer-fighting antioxidants. You don't need to dry the spinach before cooking it—the moisture clinging to the leaves helps steam it!

*Makes 4 servings*

1½ pounds baby spinach, rinsed but not dried

2 teaspoons Asian sesame oil

1 teaspoon macadamia nut oil

1 tablespoon grated fresh ginger

1 garlic clove, minced

3 green onions, chopped

2 teaspoons coconut aminos

⅛ teaspoon sea salt

2 teaspoons sesame seeds

Heat a large nonstick skillet over medium heat. Add the spinach and cook, turning with kitchen tongs, until wilted, about 2 to 3 minutes. Transfer to a strainer and let cool for 5 minutes, then squeeze out the excess liquid.

Return the skillet to the stove and heat the sesame and macadamia oils over medium-high heat. Add the ginger and garlic and cook, stirring, until fragrant, about 15 seconds. Add the green onions and cook, stirring, for 1 minute. Add the spinach and cook 1 minute, or until heated through. Add the coconut aminos and salt, cook for 30 seconds, and remove from the heat. Top with the sesame seeds and serve hot or at room temperature.

## Nutrient Content per Serving

| | | | | | | |
|---|---|---|---|---|---|---|
| **Calories:** | 117 | **Fat:** | 4 grams | **Protein:** | 5 grams |
| **Fiber:** | 8 grams | **Saturated Fat:** | 1 gram | **Carbs:** | 20 grams |
| **Sodium:** | 402 mg | | | | |

## ROASTED FENNEL AND ONIONS

Fennel has a distinctive licorice flavor that people tend to either love or hate. If you're someone who loves it, I've got good news: Fennel is one of the most outstanding antioxidant, anti-inflammatory, and immune-supporting plants you can put on your plate.

*Makes 4 servings*

2 medium fennel bulbs, trimmed and cut into ½-inch-thick wedges

2 medium onions, halved through the root end and cut into ½-inch-thick slices

4 teaspoons olive oil

½ teaspoon sea salt

¼ teaspoon freshly ground black pepper

Preheat the oven to 450°F. Lightly oil a large baking sheet.

Brush the fennel and the onions with the oil, and then season with the salt and pepper. Arrange the fennel in a single layer on the prepared baking sheet. Spread the onions in a single layer over the fennel.

Roast, turning occasionally, until the vegetables are very tender and the fennel is lightly browned, 28 to 30 minutes. Serve warm or at room temperature.

### Nutrient Content per Serving

| | | | | | |
|---|---|---|---|---|---|
| Calories: | 101 | Fat: | 5 grams | Protein: | 2 grams |
| Fiber: | 5 grams | Saturated Fat: | 1 gram | Carbs: | 14 grams |
| Sodium: | 353 mg | | | | |

## ROASTED CAULIFLOWER AND BROCCOLI

This seemingly simple side dish does a lot of nutritional heavy lifting, from fighting cancer to detoxifying. Be sure to use a baking pan with very low sides so the vegetables roast and don't steam.

*Makes 4 servings*

1 head cauliflower (about 1¾ pounds), cut into bite-sized florets (about 4 cups)

1 medium head broccoli, cut into bite-sized florets (about 4 cups)

2 tablespoons macadamia nut oil

¼ teaspoon sea salt

¼ teaspoon freshly ground black pepper

2 teaspoons grated orange zest

Preheat the oven to 425°F. Lightly oil a large rimmed baking sheet.

Combine the cauliflower, broccoli, oil, salt, and pepper in a large bowl; mix well. Place in a single layer on the prepared baking sheet.

Roast, tossing occasionally, until the cauliflower and broccoli are crisp-tender and lightly browned, 28 to 30 minutes. Remove from the oven, transfer to a bowl, and toss with the orange zest.

### Nutrient Content per Serving

| | | | | | |
|---|---|---|---|---|---|
| Calories: | 132 | Fat: | 8 grams | Protein: | 5 grams |
| Fiber: | 5 grams | Saturated Fat: | 1 gram | Carbs: | 14 grams |
| Sodium: | 219 mg | | | | |

## FRENCH BEANS WITH MACADAMIA NUTS

Haricots verts, also known as French beans, are a thinner, more delicate variety of green beans than the ones most of us are accustomed to. You've probably had them as a side dish to complement lean white meats, and these will do those meats one better. But did you know green beans contain vitamins that are healing? Eat your vegetables!

*Makes 4 servings*

1 pound haricots verts, trimmed
4 teaspoons olive oil
¼ cup raw macadamia nuts, coarsely chopped
3 garlic cloves, minced
¼ teaspoon salt
⅛ teaspoon freshly ground black pepper

Bring a large saucepan of lightly salted water to a boil over high heat. Add the haricots verts, cover the pan, return to a boil, and cook for 1 minute. Drain into a colander and rinse under cold water to stop the cooking; drain again.

Heat the oil in a large nonstick skillet over medium heat. Add the nuts and garlic; cook, stirring often, until the garlic starts to brown, 1½ to 2 minutes. Add the haricots verts and cook, tossing, until hot, 2 to 3 minutes. Remove from the heat and season with the salt and pepper.

### Nutrient Content per Serving

| | | | | | | |
|---|---|---|---|---|---|---|
| Calories: | 152 | Fat: | 11 grams | Protein: | 2 grams |
| Fiber: | 3 grams | Saturated Fat: | 2 grams | Carbs: | 9 grams |
| Sodium: | 146 mg | | | | |

## SPAGHETTI SQUASH ARRABBIATA

Swap carb-packed pasta for spaghetti squash and all you'll be missing is the sugar spike. Oh, and the gluten. This is a spicy, hot, and healthful version of spaghetti with tomato sauce. It's a great side dish, but you can turn it into a main course by topping it off with some clean, lean protein.

*Makes 4 servings*

1 medium spaghetti squash (about 2½ pounds), cut in half lengthwise and seeded
¼ teaspoon sea salt
2 teaspoons olive oil

¼ teaspoon crushed red pepper flakes

1⅓ cups Go-To-Marinara Sauce (page 209)

Preheat the oven to 350°F. Lightly oil a large baking sheet.

Place the squash, cut sides down, on the prepared baking sheet. Prick all over with the tip of a knife. Bake until very tender, 28 to 30 minutes. Remove from the oven and let cool for 5 minutes. Turn the squash over, and use the tines of a fork to scrape out the flesh—it will come out in long, thin spaghetti-like strands. You should have about 3 cups. Transfer the strands to a bowl and toss with the salt.

Heat the oil in a medium nonstick skillet over medium heat. Add the red pepper flakes and cook for 30 seconds. Add the marinara sauce and cook, stirring, until hot, 1 to 2 minutes. Serve the sauce over the squash.

## Nutrient Content per Serving

| | | | | | |
|---|---|---|---|---|---|
| Calories: | 143 | Fat: | 6 grams | Protein: | 2 grams |
| Fiber: | 4 grams | Saturated Fat: | 1 gram | Carbs: | 21 grams |
| Sodium: | 434 mg | | | | |

## SLOW-ROASTED PLUM TOMATOES

Let these tomatoes do their work of cleaning up free radicals and fighting inflammation while you focus on their incredible flavor. And you'll have no shortage of ways to do so. Place one cut-side-down over a piece of cooked fish, add them to salads or rice, or serve them on their own as a side dish.

*Makes 4 servings*

8 plum tomatoes (about 2 pounds), halved lengthwise

1½ tablespoons olive oil

1 teaspoon dried basil

¼ teaspoon garlic powder

½ teaspoon sea salt

¼ teaspoon freshly ground black pepper.

Preheat the oven to 325°F. Lightly oil a large baking sheet.

Combine the tomatoes, oil, basil, garlic powder, salt, and pepper in a large bowl; toss well to coat. Arrange the tomatoes, cut side up, in a single layer on the prepared baking sheet.

Bake until the tomatoes are very tender but still just hold their shape, about 1½ hours. Serve warm, room temperature, or cold. Store in a covered container in the refrigerator for up to 1 week.

### Nutrient Content per Serving

| | | | | | |
|---|---|---|---|---|---|
| Calories: | 89 | Fat: | 6 grams | Protein: | 2 grams |
| Fiber: | 3 grams | Saturated Fat: | 1 gram | Carbs: | 9 grams |
| Sodium: | 302 mg | | | | |

## BRAISED KALE

I want everyone to have access to the nutrient super-power of kale, so to make this preparation vegetarian-friendly, just use vegetable broth in place of the chicken broth.

*Makes 4 servings*

2 tablespoons olive oil

1 medium onion, sliced

3 garlic cloves, minced

1½ pounds kale, woody stems removed, leaves coarsely chopped

1 cup organic low-sodium chicken broth

¼ teaspoon sea salt

⅛ teaspoon freshly ground black pepper

Heat the oil in a Dutch oven over medium-high heat. Add the onion and garlic and cook until they are starting to soften, 2 to 3 minutes. Add the kale and broth and cook, stirring occasionally, until the kale has wilted, about 3 minutes. Cover, reduce the heat to medium, and simmer until the kale is tender, 6 to 7 minutes.

Uncover the pot, increase the heat to medium-high, and cook until the liquid is nearly evaporated, 1 to 2 minutes. Remove from the heat and season with the salt and pepper.

### Nutrient Content per Serving

| | | | | | |
|---|---|---|---|---|---|
| Calories: | 151 | Fat: | 8 grams | Protein: | 7 grams |
| Fiber: | 3 grams | Saturated Fat: | 1 gram | Carbs: | 16 grams |
| Sodium: | 218 mg | | | | |

## BALSAMIC ROASTED VEGETABLES

Think of this colorful side dish as delicious medicine by the forkful. It ensures that you get a wide variety of nutrients, exploding flavors, and lively textures in every bite.

*Makes 4 servings*

2 tablespoons olive oil

2 tablespoons balsamic vinegar

½ teaspoon dried basil

½ teaspoon sea salt

¼ teaspoon freshly ground black pepper

2 medium zucchini (12 ounces), halved lengthwise and cut into 1-inch pieces

2 medium yellow squash (12 ounces), halved lengthwise and cut into 1-inch pieces

2 Japanese eggplants (10 ounces), halved lengthwise and cut into 1-inch pieces

1 medium red onion, cut through the root into 8 wedges

1 large red bell pepper, cut into 1-inch pieces

Preheat the oven to 450°F. Lightly oil a large baking sheet.

Combine the oil, vinegar, basil, salt, and pepper in a small bowl. Combine the zucchini, yellow squash, eggplant, onion, and bell pepper in a separate bowl. Add the vinegar mixture to the vegetables and toss well. Transfer to the prepared baking sheet.

Roast, stirring occasionally, until the vegetables are tender and lightly browned, 33 to 35 minutes. Serve warm or at room temperature.

## Nutrient Content per Serving

| | | | | | | |
|---|---|---|---|---|---|---|
| Calories: | 140 | Fat: | 8 grams | Protein: | 4 grams |
| Fiber: | 5 grams | Saturated Fat: | 1 gram | Carbs: | 16 grams |
| Sodium: | 305 mg | | | | |

## CAULIFLOWER AND NUT STIR-FRY

One of cauliflower's nutritional claims to fame is that it has cancer-fighting power in the form of the phytochemical sulforaphane. This stir-fry can be served hot or at room temperature. And it can be made ahead, but don't stir in the fresh basil until just before serving.

*Makes 4 servings*

2 tablespoons coconut oil

1 medium red onion, chopped

3 garlic cloves, minced

1 small head cauliflower (about 1½ pounds), cut into bite-sized florets (4 to 5 cups)

¼ cup pine nuts

¼ cup water

2 tablespoons chopped fresh basil

¼ teaspoon sea salt

⅛ teaspoon freshly ground black pepper

Heat the oil in a large nonstick skillet over medium-high heat. Add the onion and garlic and cook until the vegetables just begin to soften, 2 to 3 minutes. Add the cauliflower and pine nuts and cook, stirring often, for 2 minutes. Pour in the water and cook, stirring, until it evaporates and the cauliflower is crisp-tender, 4 to 5 minutes. Remove from the heat and stir in the basil, salt, and pepper.

## Nutrient Content per Serving

| | | | | | | |
|---|---|---|---|---|---|---|
| **Calories:** | 156 | **Fat:** | 13 grams | **Protein:** | 3 grams |
| **Fiber:** | 3 grams | **Saturated Fat:** | 7 grams | **Carbs:** | 8 grams |
| **Sodium:** | 171 mg | | | | |

## GRILLED MARINATED PORTOBELLO MUSHROOMS

These meaty and flavorful mushrooms are a hearty side dish on their own, or great sliced and served over rice or in a salad. And like many other mushrooms, they're high in antioxidants and polyphenols, and a good source of fiber.

*Makes 4 servings*

2 garlic cloves, minced

2 tablespoons balsamic vinegar

1 tablespoon red wine vinegar

2 teaspoons Dijon mustard

2 teaspoons fresh thyme

½ teaspoon dried basil

¼ teaspoon crushed red pepper flakes

4 large portobello mushroom caps (about 1¼ pounds)

¼ teaspoon sea salt

Combine the garlic, balsamic and red wine vinegars, mustard, thyme, basil, and red pepper flakes in a bowl. Wipe the mushroom caps to remove any soil. Brush the mushrooms with the garlic mixture and let stand for 30 minutes.

Preheat the grill for direct medium heat.

Season the mushrooms with the salt, and place on the grill directly over the heat. Grill until the mushrooms are well marked and tender, 5 to 6 minutes per side. Serve warm or at room temperature.

## Nutrient Content per Serving

| | | | | | |
|---|---|---|---|---|---|
| Calories: | 44 | Fat: | 1 gram | Protein: | 3 grams |
| Fiber: | 2 grams | Saturated Fat: | 0 grams | Carbs: | 8 grams |
| Sodium: | 221 mg | | | | |

## ITALIAN-STYLE ESCAROLE

Escarole is a type of endive that's rich in blood sugar–balancing fiber, folic acid, and vitamins A and C. Its slightly bitter flavor is mediated here by the rich smokiness of the bacon.

*Makes 4 servings*

3 slices nitrate-free bacon, chopped
1 tablespoon olive oil
1 medium onion, chopped
5 garlic cloves, sliced
1½ pounds escarole, woody stems removed, leaves cut into 2-inch pieces
¼ teaspoon sea salt

Cook the bacon in a large nonstick skillet until crisp, 6 to 7 minutes. Transfer it to a plate lined with a paper towel to drain.

Pour off the bacon fat in the skillet. Return the skillet to the stove, add the oil, and heat it over medium heat. Add the onion and garlic and cook, stirring occasionally, until lightly browned, 4 to 5 minutes. Stir in the escarole and cook, stirring occasionally, until wilted, 2 to 3 minutes. Add the bacon and cook until the escarole is tender, about 1 minute. Season with the salt.

## Nutrient Content per Serving

| | | | | | |
|---|---|---|---|---|---|
| Calories: | 102 | Fat: | 6 grams | Protein: | 4 grams |
| Fiber: | 6 grams | Saturated Fat: | 1 gram | Carbs: | 10 grams |
| Sodium: | 302 mg | | | | |

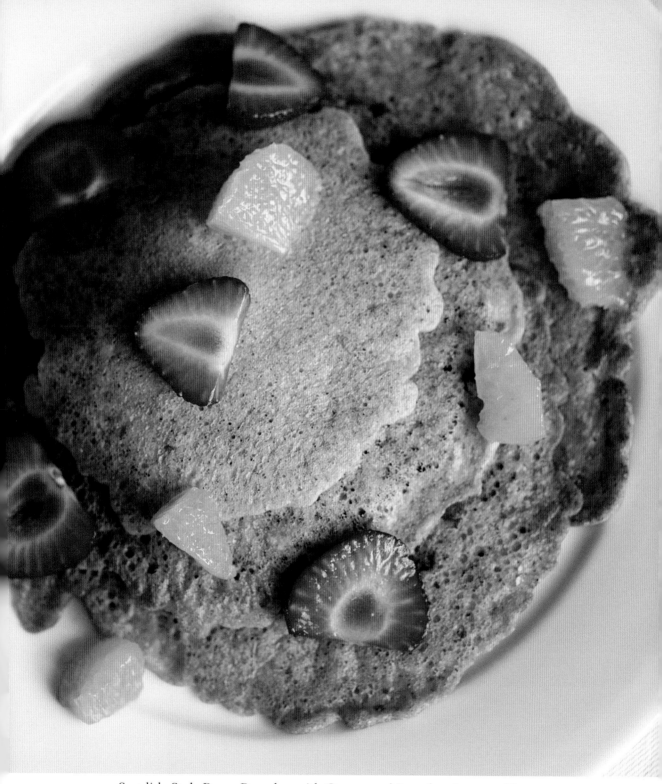

Swedish-Style Pecan Pancakes with Orange and Strawberries, page 89

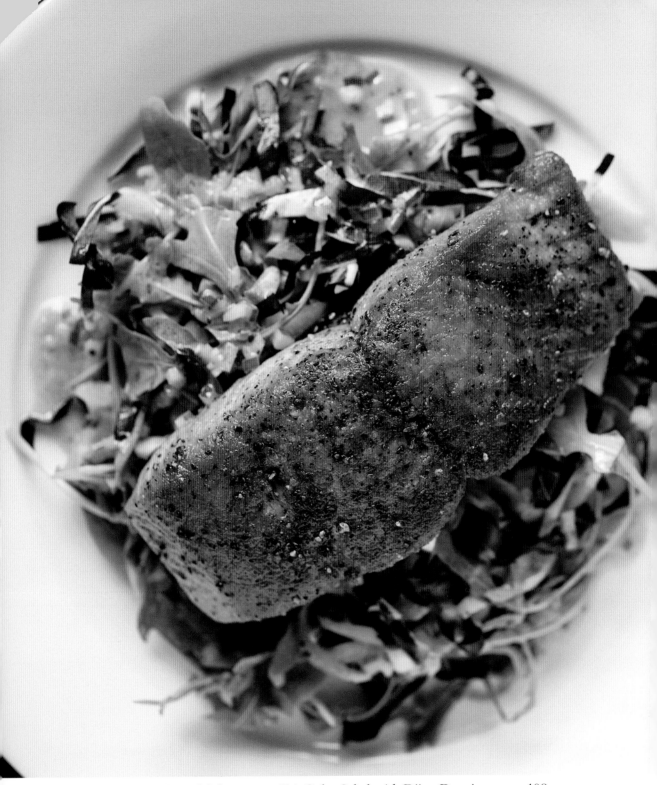

Pan-Seared Salmon over Tri-Color Salad with Dijon Dressing, page 108

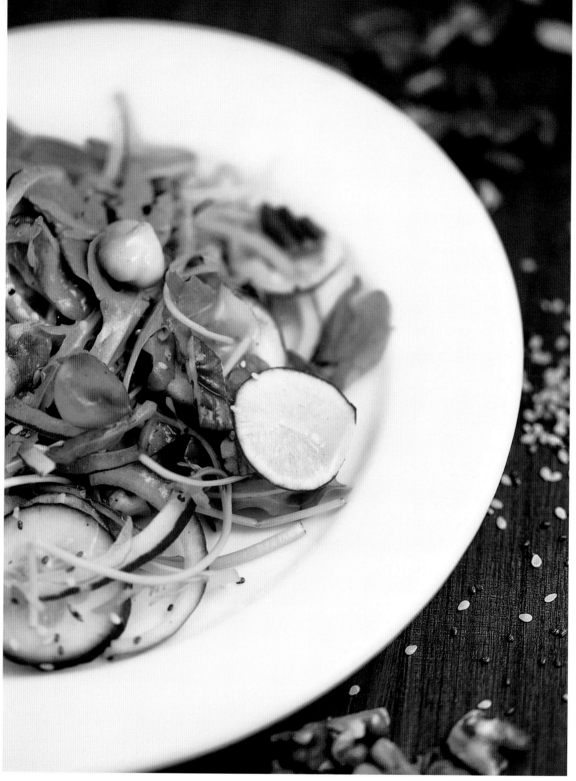

Cucumber and Radish Salad with Arugula, Nuts, and Seeds, page 113

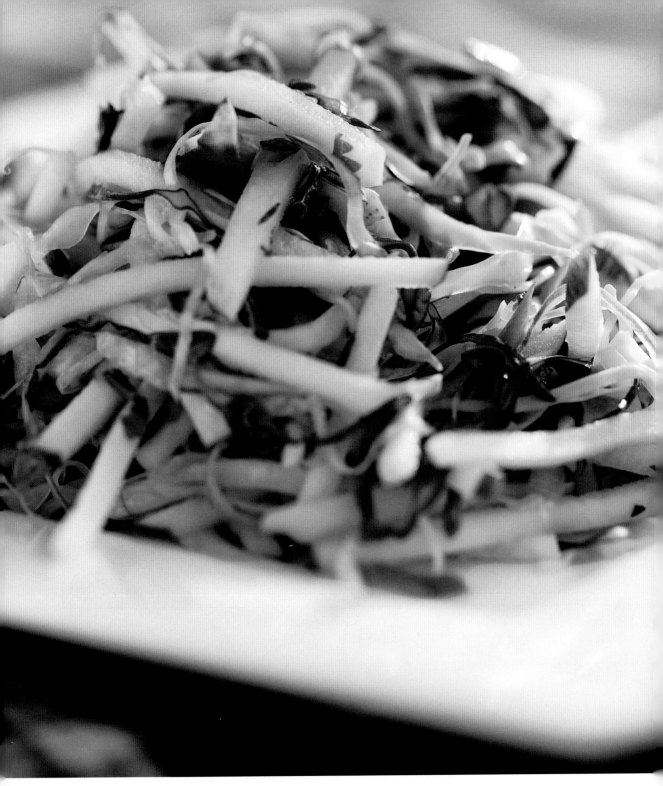

Jicama, Apple, and Pear Slaw, page 114

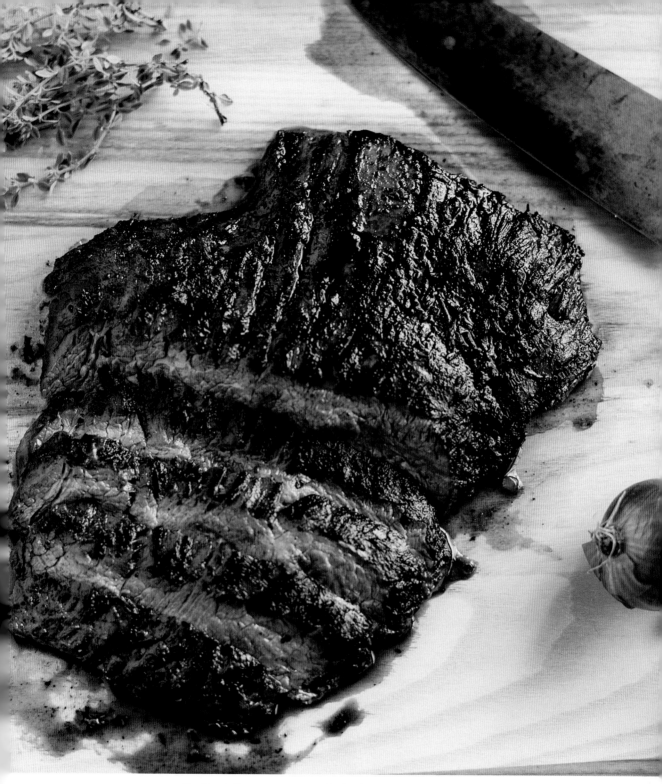

Shallot-Thyme Marinated Flank Steak, page 132

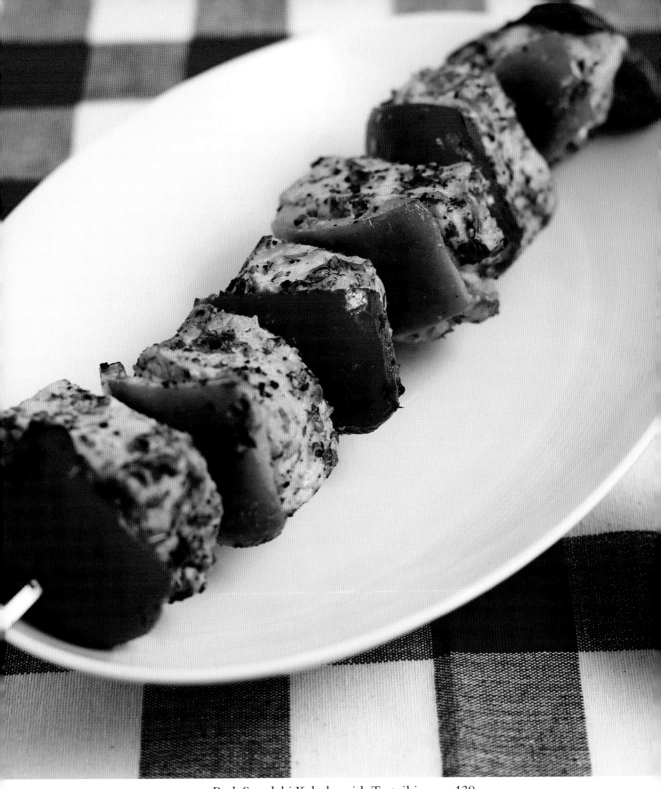

Pork Souvlaki Kabobs with Tzatziki, page 139

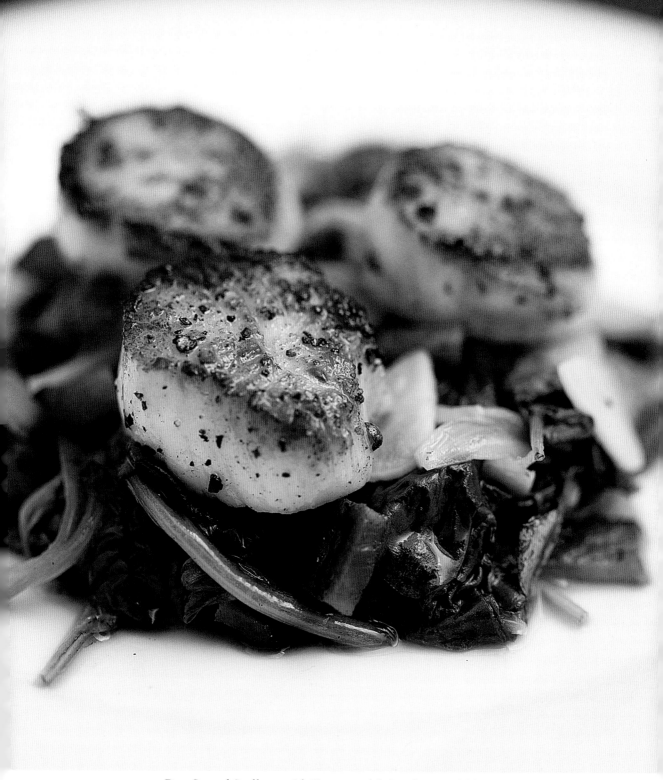

Pan-Seared Scallops with Bacon and Spinach, page 155

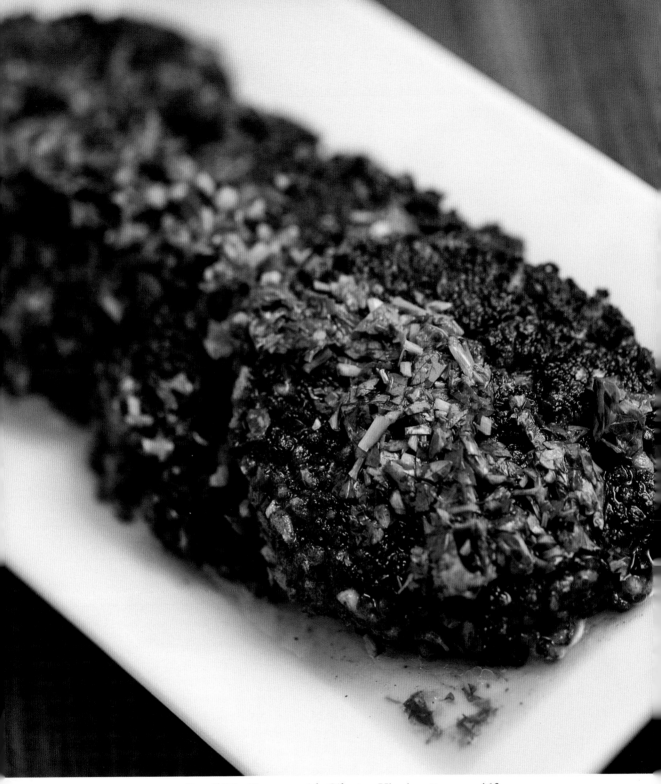

Lentil Nut Burgers with Cilantro Vinaigrette, page 163

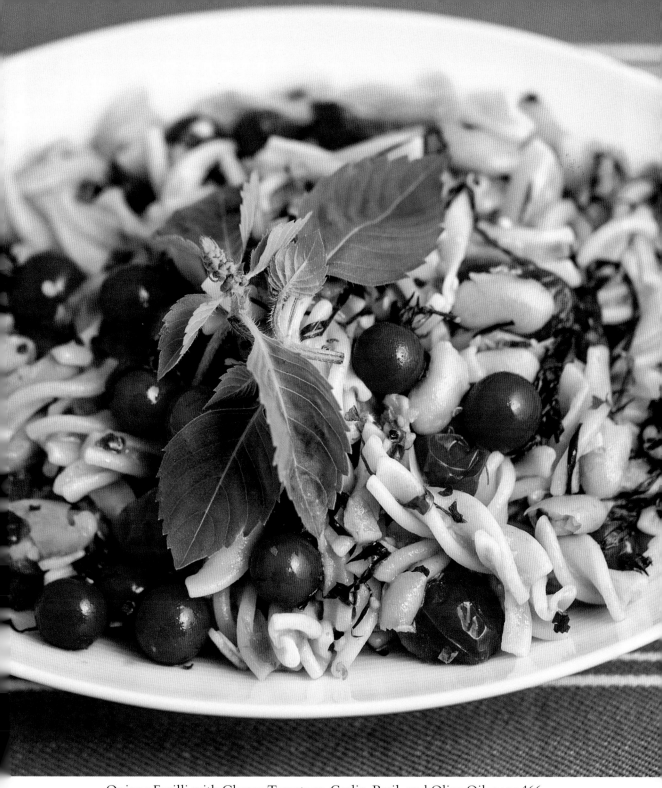

Quinoa Fusilli with Cherry Tomatoes, Garlic, Basil, and Olive Oil, page 166

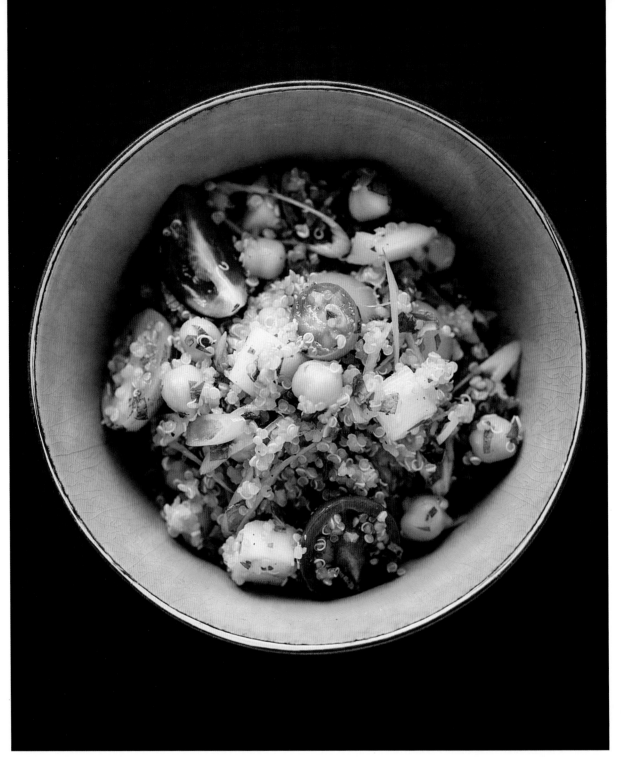

Quinoa and Chickpea Tabbouleh with Mint, Parsley, and Lemon Dressing, page 167

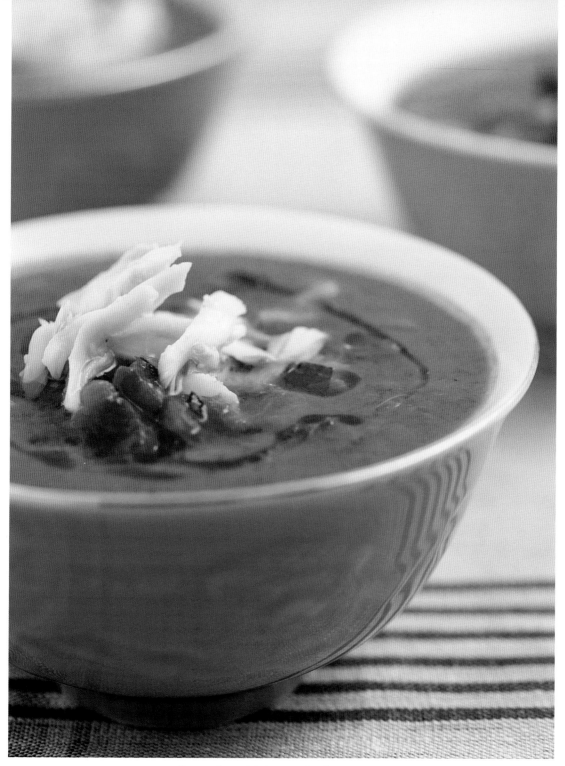

Gazpacho with Lump Crab, page 177

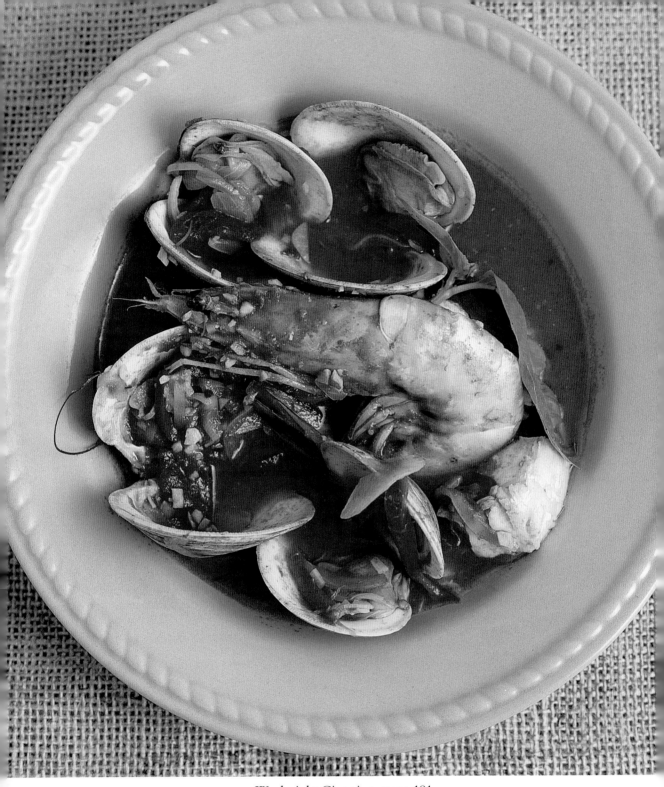

Weeknight Cioppino, page 181

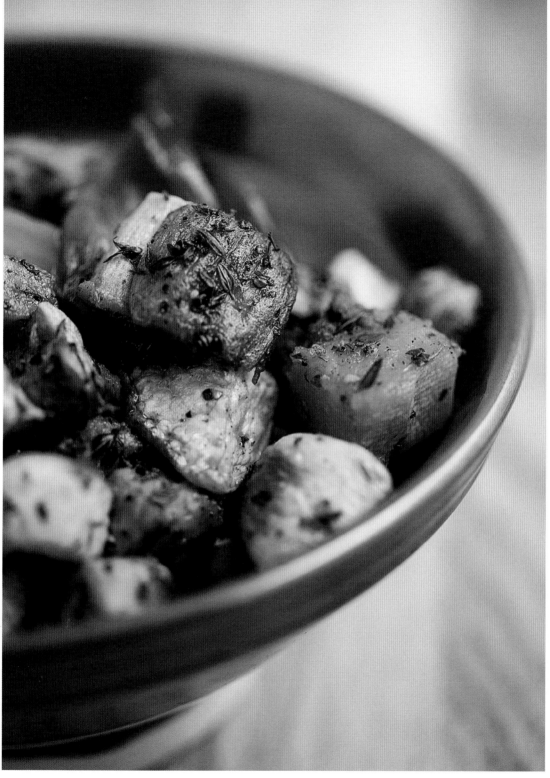

Roasted Root Vegetables with Thyme, page 193

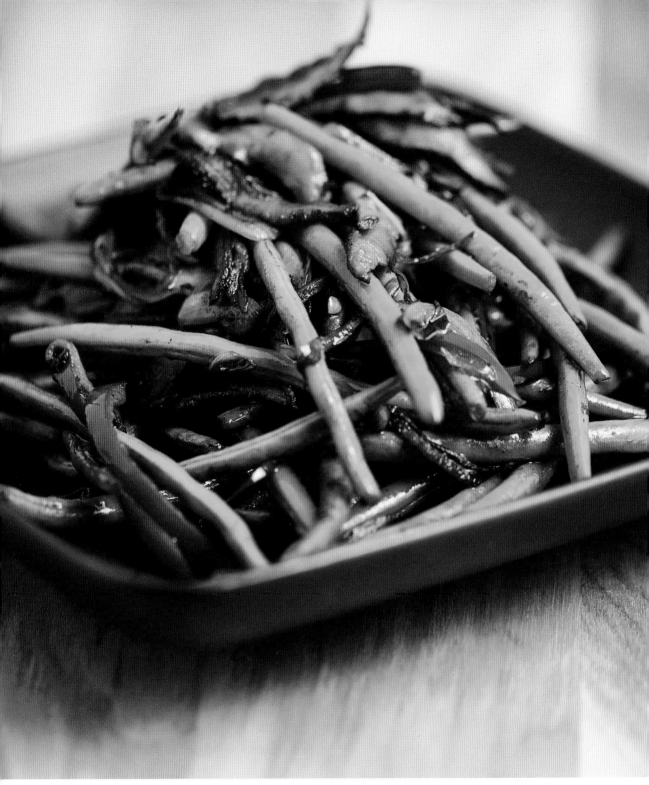

Green Beans with Shiitakes and Shallots, page 199

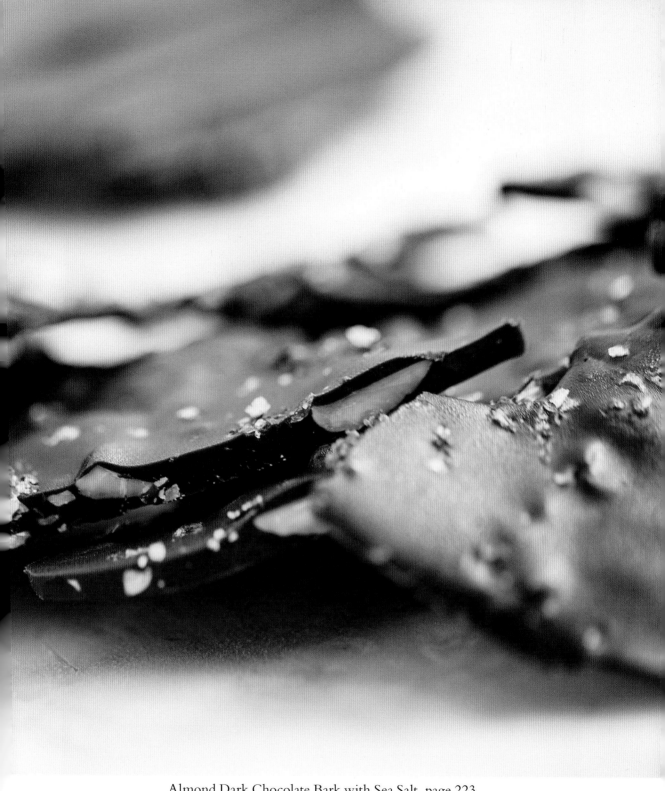

Almond Dark Chocolate Bark with Sea Salt, page 223

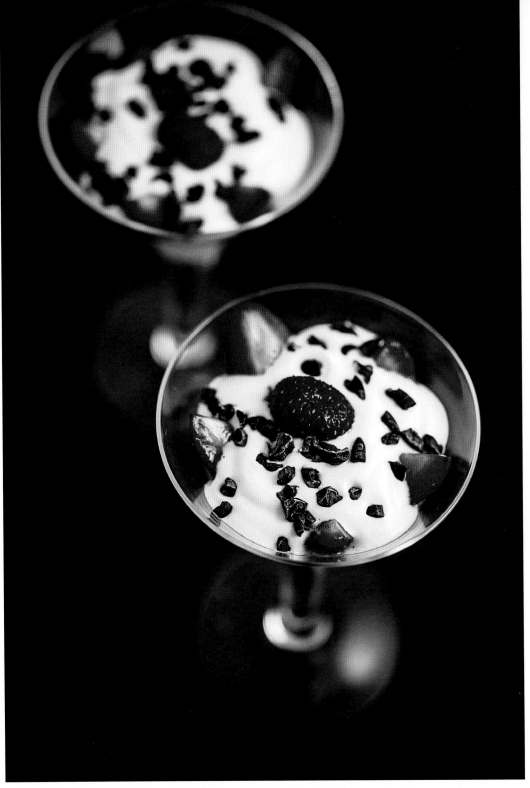

Strawberries and Cream, page 224

# SAUCES, RUBS, AND DRESSINGS 10

Sauces, rubs, and dressings usually drive healthy food straight into the intersection of Crash and Burn. They're often diet-sabotaging cocktails of high sugar and gluten, which add calories and bring a pro-inflammatory sledgehammer down on your meal. With these recipes, though, you can slather worry-free, knowing that in addition to enhancing the taste of your food, you're actually supporting your fast fat loss goals and health. Yay!

## GO-TO MARINARA SAUCE

There's something about homemade marinara that vaults pasta to the top of the comfort food pile. And this one is healthy to boot. To crush the fennel seeds, place them in a plastic bag and roll with a rolling pin or wine bottle. To store the sauce, cool it completely and refrigerate it, or spoon it into portion-sized serving containers and freeze until you're ready to use.

*Makes 3 cups*

2 tablespoons olive oil
1 medium onion, chopped
1 celery stalk, finely chopped
1 medium carrot, finely chopped
3 garlic cloves, minced
1 teaspoon dried basil
½ teaspoon dried oregano
½ teaspoon fennel seeds, crushed
1 (28-ounce) can organic diced tomatoes, with juice
¼ cup tomato paste
¼ cup fresh basil, chopped

½ teaspoon sea salt

¼ teaspoon freshly ground black pepper

Heat the oil in a medium saucepan over medium-high heat. Add the onion, celery, carrot, garlic, dried basil, oregano, and fennel seeds and cook, stirring occasionally, until the vegetables are slightly softened, 3 to 4 minutes. Stir in the diced tomatoes and tomato paste and bring to a boil. Immediately reduce the heat to medium-low, cover the pan, and simmer, stirring occasionally, until thickened, about 30 minutes. Remove from the heat and stir in the fresh basil, salt, and pepper.

## Nutrient Content per Serving (½ cup)

| | | | | | |
|---|---|---|---|---|---|
| Calories: | 101 | Fat: | 5 grams | Protein: | 2 grams |
| Fiber: | 2 grams | Saturated Fat: | 1 gram | Carbs: | 12 grams |
| Sodium: | 434 mg | | | | |

## ALL-PURPOSE FINGER-LICKIN'-GOOD BARBECUE SAUCE

I know, you can hardly believe your eyes—barbecue sauce! Smoked paprika, which is now in most grocery stores, lends a distinctive smoky flavor without resorting to unnatural substances like those found in liquid smoke. You can refrigerate this sauce for up to 3 weeks or freeze it.

*Makes 3 cups*

1 (28-ounce) can organic crushed tomatoes and their juice

½ cup cider vinegar

3 tablespoons chili powder

2 tablespoons smoked paprika

2 tablespoons monk fruit extract

2 teaspoons coconut aminos

1 teaspoon ground cumin

1 teaspoon garlic powder

½ teaspoon ground allspice

¾ teaspoon sea salt

¾ teaspoon ground black pepper

Combine the tomatoes, vinegar, chili powder, paprika, monk fruit extract, coconut aminos, cumin, garlic powder, and allspice in a medium saucepan and bring to a simmer over medium heat. Cook, stirring occasionally, until the sauce is very thick, 20 to 22 minutes. Remove from the heat and season with the salt and pepper.

Nutrient Content per Serving (3 Tablespoons)

| | | | | | |
|---|---|---|---|---|---|
| Calories: | 21 | Fat: | 0 grams | Protein: | 1 gram |
| Fiber: | 1 gram | Saturated Fat: | 0 grams | Carbs: | 6 grams |
| Sodium: | 273 mg | | | | |

## PESTO SAUCE

Pesto sauce originated in northern Italy, and I, for one, am grateful. The simplicity of this ingredients list belies the nutritious power of pesto—it's heart-healthy and can lower your risk of chronic disease. Because pesto is so flavorful, you often need less of it than you do of other sauces. Feel free to add another garlic clove or two and to increase the sea salt up to 1 teaspoon if you like a bit more of a punch! This sauce keeps well in the fridge for 1 week and in the freezer for 1 month.

*Makes ¾ cup*

3 cups loosely packed fresh basil
1 garlic clove
3 tablespoons pine nuts
1 tablespoon chia seeds
⅓ cup olive oil
¼ teaspoon sea salt

Combine the basil, garlic, pine nuts, and chia seeds in the bowl of a food processor, and process until finely chopped. With the machine running, add the oil in a steady stream. Turn off the machine and stir in the salt.

Nutrient Content per Serving (1 Tablespoon)

| | | | | | |
|---|---|---|---|---|---|
| Calories: | 154 | Fat: | 16 grams | Protein: | 1 gram |
| Fiber: | 1 gram | Saturated Fat: | 2 grams | Carbs: | 2 grams |
| Sodium: | 99 mg | | | | |

## HOMEMADE KETCHUP

We all know that ketchup is indispensable in our culinary arsenal. But store-bought brands are often drowning in sugar. This sweet and tangy alternative still delivers all the antioxidant benefit of the lycopene from the tomatoes, but with only natural sweetness. This condiment keeps well for about 3 weeks in the refrigerator.

*Makes about 2 cups*

2 (6-ounce) cans organic tomato paste

1 (8-ounce) can organic tomato sauce

⅓ cup cider vinegar

½ cup water

2 teaspoons monk fruit extract

1 teaspoon onion powder

½ teaspoon garlic powder

½ teaspoon ground allspice

⅛ teaspoon ground cinnamon

½ teaspoon sea salt

¼ teaspoon freshly ground black pepper

Combine the tomato paste, tomato sauce, vinegar, water, monk fruit extract, onion powder, garlic powder, allspice, cinnamon, salt, and pepper in a small saucepan over medium heat. Bring to a simmer and immediately reduce the heat to medium-low. Cover the pan and simmer gently, stirring occasionally, until thickened, about 15 minutes. Let the ketchup cool completely before refrigerating.

### Nutrient Content per Serving (1 Tablespoon)

| | | | | | |
|---|---|---|---|---|---|
| Calories: | 26 | Fat: | 0 grams | Protein: | 1 gram |
| Fiber: | 1 gram | Saturated Fat: | 0 grams | Carbs: | 6 grams |
| Sodium: | 186 mg | | | | |

## NUTTY CRANBERRY-ORANGE SAUCE

The natural sweetness of this sauce makes it mouthwatering, whether it's on poultry or in a sandwich as a spread. And you'll get to try both—you can refrigerate it for up to 1 week.

*Makes 1½ cups*

2 cups fresh or frozen cranberries

½ cup fresh or frozen raspberries

¾ cup water

3 tablespoons monk fruit extract

⅓ cup walnuts, coarsely chopped

1 tablespoon grated orange zest

Combine the cranberries, raspberries, water, and monk fruit extract in a medium saucepan over medium-high heat, and bring to a boil. Immediately reduce the heat to medium and cook, stirring occasionally, until all of the cranberries have popped and the mixture has thickened slightly, 6 to 8 minutes. Remove from the heat and stir in the walnuts and orange zest. Let cool completely and then chill for at least 3 hours before serving.

## Nutrient Content per Serving (1 Tablespoon)

| | | | | | |
|---|---|---|---|---|---|
| Calories: | 69 | Fat: | 4 grams | Protein: | 2 grams |
| Fiber: | 1 gram | Saturated Fat: | 0 grams | Carbs: | 12 grams |
| Sodium: | 10 mg | | | | |

## BARBECUE SPICE RUB

This smoky blend is perfect for grilled meat, poultry, or fish. Double or triple the recipe and keep the rub in a sealed jar in your spice cabinet.

*Makes about 6 tablespoons*

2 tablespoons smoked paprika

1 tablespoon chili powder

2 teaspoons ground cumin

1 teaspoon garlic powder

1 teaspoon sea salt

½ teaspoon freshly ground black pepper

Combine all the ingredients in a small bowl and mix well.

## Nutrient Content per Serving (1 Tablespoon)

| | | | | | |
|---|---|---|---|---|---|
| Calories: | 19 | Fat: | 0 grams | Protein: | 0 grams |
| Fiber: | 1 gram | Saturated Fat: | 0 grams | Carbs: | 4 grams |
| Sodium: | 390 mg | | | | |

## BLACKENING SPICE RUB

Use this fiery blend on meat, chicken, and robust fish like salmon and halibut. You can double or triple the recipe and keep the rub in a jar in your spice cabinet.

*Makes about 6 tablespoons*

2 tablespoons paprika
2 teaspoons ground cumin
1 teaspoon ground coriander
1 teaspoon ground thyme
1 teaspoon dried oregano
1 teaspoon sea salt
1 teaspoon cayenne pepper

Combine all the ingredients in a small bowl and mix well.

### Nutrient Content per Serving (1 Tablespoon)

| | | | | | |
|---|---|---|---|---|---|
| Calories: | 12 | Fat: | 0 grams | Protein: | 0 grams |
| Fiber: | 1 gram | Saturated Fat: | 0 grams | Carbs: | 2 grams |
| Sodium: | 390 mg | | | | |

## CREAMY EGGLESS MAYO

This eggless mayo is as rich and delicious as store-bought mayo, and can be used in all the same ways. But just look at the ingredients list! It's made with only healthy items. It keeps well in the refrigerator for up to 3 weeks.

*Makes ¾ cup*

¼ cup unsweetened coconut milk (such as So Delicious)
½ cup raw cashews
1 tablespoon lemon juice
1 tablespoon Dijon mustard
½ teaspoon sea salt
½ cup macadamia nut oil

Combine the coconut milk, cashews, lemon juice, mustard, and salt in a blender, and puree. With the blender running, add the oil in a slow, steady stream until the mixture is thick and creamy.

### Nutrient Content per Serving (1 Tablespoon)

| | | | | | |
|---|---|---|---|---|---|
| Calories: | 226 | Fat: | 23 grams | Protein: | 2 grams |
| Fiber: | 1 gram | Saturated Fat: | 3 grams | Carbs: | 4 grams |
| Sodium: | 255 mg | | | | |

## AVOCADO MAYO VARIATION

Great on burgers. This can be kept, refrigerated, for about 4 days.

*Makes about 1 cup*

Add ½ avocado to the blender with the Creamy Eggless Mayo ingredients.

### Nutrient Content per Serving (1 Tablespoon)

| | | | | | |
|---|---|---|---|---|---|
| Calories: | 189 | Fat: | 19 grams | Protein: | 2 grams |
| Fiber: | 1 gram | Saturated Fat: | 2 grams | Carbs: | 4 grams |
| Sodium: | 192 mg | | | | |

## SHALLOT-CHAMPAGNE VINAIGRETTE

This vinaigrette is so much more flavorful than your average vinegar-and-oil emulsion, but it's just as easy to make. Your palate deserves to experience this, so why not kick it up a notch? The recipe can be doubled or tripled and kept on hand in the refrigerator as your go-to salad dressing.

*Makes ¾ cup*

2 small shallots, finely chopped (about 3 tablespoons)
2 tablespoons champagne vinegar
2 teaspoons Dijon mustard
1 teaspoon capers, drained and chopped
½ teaspoon sea salt
¼ teaspoon freshly ground black pepper
½ cup extra-virgin olive oil

Combine the shallots, vinegar, mustard, capers, salt, and pepper in a small bowl. Whisk in the olive oil in a slow, steady stream until well combined.

### Nutrient Content per Serving (1 Tablespoon)

| | | | | | |
|---|---|---|---|---|---|
| Calories: | 175 | Fat: | 19 grams | Protein: | 0 grams |
| Fiber: | 0 grams | Saturated Fat: | 3 grams | Carbs: | 2 grams |
| Sodium: | 247 mg | | | | |

## SESAME-GINGER VINAIGRETTE

Make this your go-to Asian-flavored dressing for meat, chicken, fish, salads, marinades, and as a sauce over brown rice. The tamari is made from soybeans, but it has little or no wheat. For a Cycle 1 version, switch from 1 tablespoon tamari to 1 tablespoon coconut aminos. The dressing can be refrigerated for up to 1 week.

*Makes about ½ cup*

2 tablespoons rice vinegar

1½ teaspoons finely minced fresh ginger

1 tablespoon reduced-sodium wheat-free tamari

¼ teaspoon monk fruit extract

1 tablespoon Asian sesame oil

3 tablespoons Malaysian red palm fruit oil

3 tablespoons finely chopped green onions

1 tablespoon sesame seeds

⅛ teaspoon sea salt

Combine the vinegar, ginger, tamari, and monk fruit extract in a small bowl. Whisk in the oils until well combined. Stir in the green onions, sesame seeds, and salt.

### Nutrient Content per Serving (1 Tablespoon)

| | | | | | | |
|---|---|---|---|---|---|---|
| Calories: | 144 | Fat: | 15 grams | Protein: | 1 gram |
| Fiber: | 0 grams | Saturated Fat: | 6 grams | Carbs: | 2 grams |
| Sodium: | 249 mg | | | | |

## TOASTED MACADAMIA NUT DRESSING

Macadamia nuts have a buttery taste and are a rich source of heart-healthy energy. Keep this dressing in a tightly covered container in the refrigerator for up to 3 weeks.

*Makes ½ cup*

⅓ cup macadamia nut oil

¼ cup raw macadamia nuts

2 tablespoons white wine vinegar

1 teaspoon Dijon mustard

⅛ teaspoon monk fruit extract

½ teaspoon sea salt

⅛ teaspoon freshly ground black pepper

Heat 1 tablespoon of the oil in a small skillet over medium heat. Add the macadamia nuts and cook, stirring occasionally, until lightly toasted, 4 to 5 minutes. Transfer to a bowl and let cool. Coarsely chop the nuts.

Combine the remaining oil, the vinegar, mustard, monk fruit extract, salt, and pepper in another bowl. Stir in the cooled nuts and any oil that accumulated at the bottom of the bowl.

### Nutrient Content per Serving (1 Tablespoon)

| | | | | | |
|---|---|---|---|---|---|
| **Calories:** | 230 | **Fat:** | 25 grams | **Protein:** | 1 gram |
| **Fiber:** | 1 gram | **Saturated Fat:** | 3 grams | **Carbs:** | 2 grams |
| **Sodium:** | 320 mg | | | | |

I bet your experience is a lot like mine—most every diet you've ever tried starts with a focus on dessert, and promptly eliminates it. That only ensures that dessert is all you can think about, especially if you have a sweet tooth. And if you do, it turns out there could be a scientific reason you simply can't resist the siren call of those treats.

Researchers at Columbia University found that when obese people were shown pictures of high-calorie foods, it activated the areas of the brain associated with reward, memory, and emotion, making it harder for them to refuse sweet or salty treats. The reaction in non-obese people was much more subtle. So, if you have a Pavlovian response to fudge brownies, are you doomed to overindulge? No!

Here's the good news: Genetic factors certainly play a role in how you eat and how much you weigh, but your genes don't have to be your destiny. You can retrain your taste buds and rethink how you eat, and soon you'll be loving the natural sweetness of berries and other good-for-you sweets.

Remember, the Virgin Diet is a giver, not a taker, and it's certainly not about deprivation. You'll be blown away by these sensational desserts (I call them "Sweets with Benefits"). They'll satisfy your sweet tooth, and they won't spike your blood sugar or upend your weight loss goals. You'll notice that they even manage to slip in some nutrients, so indulge guilt-free. What's the point of having your cake if you can't eat it? Never understood that.

## COCONUT ICE CREAM

You don't need dairy in order to have creamy, rich ice cream! Enjoy this luscious dessert knowing coconut milk's healthy fats are supporting your fast fat loss, and that its lauric acid is good for your immune system health. Be sure to use full-fat, not light, coconut milk; I insist!

*Makes about 9 servings*

2 cups unsweetened full-fat canned organic, non-GMO coconut milk

¼ cup coconut butter

1½ tablespoons monk fruit extract

1 tablespoon lime juice

1 teaspoon coconut extract

Combine the coconut milk, coconut butter, monk fruit extract, lime juice, and coconut extract in a blender; puree. Transfer to a bowl and refrigerate until cold, about 1 hour.

Pour the coconut mixture into an ice cream maker and freeze according to the manufacturer's directions. Transfer to a covered container and allow to harden in your freezer. Let the ice cream stand at room temperature for 5 to 10 minutes to soften slightly before serving.

## Nutrient Content per Serving

| | | | | | |
|---|---|---|---|---|---|
| **Calories:** | 147 | **Fat:** | 15 grams | **Protein:** | 1 gram |
| **Fiber:** | 0 grams | **Saturated Fat:** | 14 grams | **Carbs:** | 4 grams |
| **Sodium:** | 13 mg | | | | |

## MOCHA PROTEIN POPSICLES

The perfect pick-me-up. Instant espresso (about 2 teaspoons dissolved in 3 ounces of water) works just as well as brewed coffee in these refreshing protein popsicles.

*Makes 6 servings*

2 scoops chocolate vegan protein powder

10 ounces unsweetened coconut milk (such as So Delicious)

3 ounces brewed espresso or strong coffee

1 teaspoon ground cinnamon

Whisk together the protein powder, coconut milk, espresso, and cinnamon in a bowl until well blended. Pour into 6 popsicle molds and freeze overnight.

Dip the molds into warm water to remove the popsicles. Store in a resealable plastic container in the freezer.

## Nutrient Content per Serving (1 Popsicle)

| | | | | | |
|---|---|---|---|---|---|
| **Calories:** | 39 | **Fat:** | 2 grams | **Protein:** | 4 grams |
| **Fiber:** | 1 gram | **Saturated Fat:** | 1 gram | **Carbs:** | 3 grams |
| **Sodium:** | 62 mg | | | | |

## CHOCOLATE AVOCADO MOUSSE WITH CACAO NIBS

While the idea of avocado in a dessert may surprise you, you'll be even more surprised at how incredibly addictive this rich, creamy mousse is. And this decadent treat won't spike your blood sugar, unlike its counterpart.

*Makes 4 servings*

2 ounces dark chocolate, 70 percent cacao or higher, chopped
1 avocado
¾ cup plain cultured coconut milk (such as So Delicious)
1½ teaspoons monk fruit extract
4 teaspoons cacao nibs

Place three-fourths of the chocolate in a microwave-safe bowl and microwave in 15-second intervals, stirring after each, until just melted. Stir in the remaining chocolate until melted and smooth; let cool for 3 minutes.

Combine the avocado, cultured coconut milk, and monk fruit extract in a medium bowl. Beat with an electric mixer on the highest setting until well combined. Add the melted chocolate and beat it in until the mixture is light and fluffy. Divide among four bowls and refrigerate for at least 20 minutes.

Just before serving, sprinkle with the cacao nibs.

### Nutrient Content per Serving

| | | | | | |
|---|---|---|---|---|---|
| Calories: | 215 | Fat: | 17 grams | Protein: | 2 grams |
| Fiber: | 7 grams | Saturated Fat: | 7 grams | Carbs: | 19 grams |
| Sodium: | 9 mg | | | | |

## BLUEBERRY SORBET

Blueberries are loaded with antioxidants that boost brain health by (among other things) improving memory and slowing cognitive decline. Still, doesn't it seem a little unfair to be getting the benefit of these brain berries in a dessert? No, I don't think so, either.

*Makes about 8 servings*

4 cups fresh or frozen blueberries, thawed if frozen
2 tablespoons lemon juice
2 tablespoons monk fruit extract
½ cup water

Combine the blueberries, lemon juice, monk fruit extract, and water in a blender, and puree.

Pour the blueberry puree into an ice cream maker and freeze according to the manufacturer's directions. Transfer it to a covered container and allow to harden in your freezer.

Let the sorbet stand at room temperature for 5 to 10 minutes to soften slightly before serving.

## Nutrient Content per Serving

| | | | | | |
|---|---|---|---|---|---|
| Calories: | 43 | Fat: | 0 grams | Protein: | 1 gram |
| Fiber: | 2 grams | Saturated Fat: | 0 grams | Carbs: | 14 grams |
| Sodium: | 2 mg | | | | |

## PEACH-AND-BERRY COCONUT CRISP

If you ever make the mistake of looking at the ingredients list for a crisp, you may never be able to enjoy it again. That's not a bad thing—it's usually loaded with sugar. Make this instead and you're back in business. This crisp can also be baked in individual ramekins.

*Makes 4 servings*

### Filling

2 cups sliced fresh or frozen peaches, thawed and drained if frozen
2 cups fresh or frozen mixed berries, thawed and drained if frozen
2 tablespoons granulated stevia extract
2 teaspoons arrowroot
¼ teaspoon almond extract
⅛ teaspoon ground nutmeg

### Topping

¾ cup gluten-free baking flour, such as Bob's Red Mill All-Purpose Baking Flour
¼ cup gluten-free oats
¼ cup unsweetened coconut flakes
4 teaspoons granulated stevia extract
3 tablespoons coconut butter

Preheat the oven to 350°F. Lightly brush a 4-cup baking dish with coconut oil.

Combine the peaches, berries, stevia extract, arrowroot, almond extract, and nutmeg in a medium bowl; mix well and transfer to the prepared baking dish.

Combine the flour, oats, coconut flakes, and stevia extract in a bowl. Add the coconut butter and work it into the mixture with your fingertips until you can form small clumps by pressing the mixture together. Sprinkle the topping (in small clumps) over the filling.

Bake until the filling is bubbly and thick, 33 to 35 minutes. Let cool for at least 10 minutes before serving.

## Nutrient Content per Serving

| | | | | | |
|---|---|---|---|---|---|
| Calories: | 326 | Fat: | 15 grams | Protein: | 5 grams |
| Fiber: | 6 grams | Saturated Fat: | 13 grams | Carbs: | 46 grams |
| Sodium: | 3 mg | | | | |

## ALMOND DARK CHOCOLATE BARK WITH SEA SALT

Dark chocolate has flavonoids that increase blood flow to your heart and lower blood pressure. It can also improve insulin sensitivity, and we know it improves mood!

*Makes 12 servings*

⅓ cup raw almonds
4 ounces dark chocolate, 70 percent or higher cacao, chopped
⅛ teaspoon coarse sea salt

Preheat the oven to 350°F. Line a baking sheet with parchment paper.

Place the nuts in a single layer on a second, large baking sheet. Bake until lightly toasted, 6 to 7 minutes. Remove from the oven and let cool for 10 minutes. Coarsely chop and reserve.

Place three-fourths of the chocolate in a microwave-safe bowl and microwave in 15-second intervals, stirring after each, until just melted. Stir in the remaining chocolate until melted. Add the chopped nuts. Pour the mixture onto the prepared baking sheet and spread into a thin 12-inch-diameter round. Sprinkle with the sea salt and refrigerate until the chocolate is set, 20 to 25 minutes. Break the chocolate bark into smaller pieces and store in a covered container in a cool place.

## Nutrient Content per Serving

| | | | | | |
|---|---|---|---|---|---|
| Calories: | 77 | Fat: | 6 grams | Protein: | 2 grams |
| Fiber: | 1 gram | Saturated Fat: | 2 grams | Carbs: | 5 grams |
| Sodium: | 22 mg | | | | |

## STRAWBERRIES AND CREAM

This dessert will make you feel like you're enjoying the festivities at Wimbledon. The parfaits can be made up to 2 hours in advance of serving, and you can use any berry without sacrificing even a little bit of the nutrition.

*Makes 4 servings*

1 cup plain cultured coconut milk (such as So Delicious)
¾ teaspoon monk fruit extract
¼ teaspoon almond extract
1 quart strawberries, hulled and quartered
2 teaspoons white balsamic vinegar
2 teaspoons cacao nibs

Combine the cultured coconut milk, ½ teaspoon of the monk fruit extract, and the almond extract in a bowl and beat well with a wire whisk.

Combine the strawberries, vinegar, and remaining ¼ teaspoon monk fruit extract in a separate bowl. Divide the strawberries among four parfait glasses, and then spoon the coconut milk mixture over the top. Sprinkle with the cacao nibs and serve.

### Nutrient Content per Serving

| | | | | | |
|---|---|---|---|---|---|
| Calories: | 119 | Fat: | 4 grams | Protein: | 1 gram |
| Fiber: | 5 grams | Saturated Fat: | 3 grams | Carbs: | 22 grams |
| Sodium: | 3 mg | | | | |

# THREE-WEEK VIRGIN DIET MEAL PLANS

If there's one thing I'm proudest to share, it's that I know the Virgin Diet can help you. How can I be so sure? Because I've designed the Virgin Diet to cast a wide net in its impact on your weight and health; it uses basic principles in targeting food intolerance to reverse the symptoms of a long list of common disorders. That means no matter what the source of your weight gain or inability to lose it, you're going to be thrilled to finally have discovered the one diet that liberates you from the long struggle and frustration you've endured. The beauty of the Virgin Diet's design is in its nuance; depending on the condition or issue you'd like to tackle, you can make slight adjustments specifically for your situation to amplify your results.

That's especially true if you have weight loss resistance, a condition other diets often ignore or can't address. Weight loss resistance can have its roots in anything from metabolic imbalance to caffeine overload, and can cause symptoms that range from gas and bloating to debilitating fatigue. And you can be pretty sure it's what's ailing you if you just can't lose fat, especially the obstinate paunch that clings to your middle, even when you're obsessively cutting calories, downing supplements, and working out like mad.

I've included the top 7 most requested meal plans in this book; they fine-tune the Virgin Diet specifically to help you home in on your target issue. But if you don't

see yourself in these meal plans, there are many more in the bonus material at www
.thevirgindietcookbook.com/bonus. They take aim at conditions like hypertension,
menopause, osteoporosis, sports performance, and even entertaining (yes, I consider
that a condition!). Seize on one or follow a few, because if you're a vegetarian in a
family on the go and on a budget, you have some options!

So take comfort in knowing the freedom that comes with weight loss and energizing health is on the way. And the sooner you get started, the sooner it'll be yours for
the rest of your life!

# THE BASICS | 12

Between picking your kids up from soccer practice, juggling a call from your boss, texting with your spouse about who's going to get the dry cleaning, and racing to find a party gift before the store closes, you don't always have the time to think about eating well until it's time to eat.

Sometimes you just need things to be easy. You do enough thinking and figuring and managing all day long, so it's not too much to ask that putting your meals together shouldn't require a postgraduate degree.

That's why I'm never surprised when my clients say that, yes, they're impressed by the science and the success stories, but they just want basics. They want everything laid out to take the guesswork out of the Virgin Diet.

If you're one of those people . . . well, you asked for it, you got it. That's exactly why I created this basic meal plan.

## HOW THE VIRGIN DIET CAN HELP

Consider this basic plan a guide. It's all about making it easy for you to follow the Virgin Diet, so flexibility is the key. Feel free to move things around. Maybe on super-hectic days you want to substitute a shake for two meals, or you want to do dinner for breakfast (who says wild salmon and shaved Brussels sprouts have to wait? It's 5 o'clock somewhere!). As long as you stay within the Virgin Diet rules, feel free to improvise.

And that means you can even have dessert (yes, you read that right!). But remember, desserts should count as part of your Virgin Diet Plate. Eat them accordingly; the dessert police are watching.

I've designed other meal plans in this book to address specific conditions, so please consult those protocols when you need something more tailored to a particular issue.

## STEP IT UP WITH THESE STRATEGIES

**1. Make a shake for breakfast.** I've had clients do nothing other than substitute a shake for breakfast and lose fat. Now, I'm not suggesting you can enjoy a shake for breakfast, then make your meals free-for-alls and expect to burn fat. But it does show how effective a protein shake can be for fast and lasting fat loss. Blend plant-based (but not soy) protein powder with berries, kale or other leafy greens, flaxseeds or chia seeds, and unsweetened coconut or almond milk for a satisfying, filling breakfast that takes minutes to make but keeps you full for hours.

**2. Eat by the Virgin Diet Plate.** My Plate formula takes the guesswork out of meals: You know exactly which satisfying, fat-burning foods to choose, and in which proportions. Load your plate with lean protein, leafy green and cruciferous veggies, slow-release high-fiber starches, and healthy fat. The varieties are endless, and once you get the hang of it, every meal becomes an opportunity to choose the healthiest, most nutrient-dense foods.

**3. Address food intolerances.** During Cycle 1 of the Virgin Diet, you will completely eliminate gluten, soy, dairy, eggs, peanuts, corn, and sugar and artificial sweeteners. Even a little of these foods during Cycle 1 can sabotage your success. In Cycle 2, you will challenge eggs, gluten, soy, and dairy (one a week) to see which you can handle and which you need to keep out of your diet forever.

**4. Get optimal nutrients.** On the Virgin Diet you eat only the healthiest, most nutrient-rich foods. But field-to-table transit times, mineral depletion in topsoil, and numerous other obstacles mean that even with these foods you might not be getting the vitamins, minerals, and antioxidants you need for lasting fat loss and optimal health. I recommend taking professional-quality multivitamin/mineral, antioxidant, and essential fatty acid supplements to meet your quota.

**5. Bump up your D.** Just about everyone tests low on vitamin D, a crucial nutrient (actually a hormone) that, among its many benefits, supports bone health and fat loss. Take a 25-hydroxy vitamin D test and work with a practitioner to get your range within 60 to 80 ng/ml. Once you're there, maintain optimal D levels by taking a 2,000 to 5,000 IU daily supplement, especially if you can't get a little sunscreen-free sun time every day.

**6. Consider a digestive enzyme.** Stress and age can deplete your body's ability to make digestive enzymes. That means you suffer with low nutrient absorption, incomplete food breakdown, and gut-health issues. If you're dealing with chronic stress (who isn't these days?) or you're over 30, I highly recommend taking digestive enzymes with your meals (see "Virgin Diet Supplements" in the Resources section).

**7. Get 7 to 9 hours of sleep every night.** When you don't get enough sleep, you crash your fat-burning hormones and set yourself up to be a caffeinated mess. Prepare for sleep: About an hour before bedtime turn off the electronics, take a hot bath, and enjoy a trashy novel with a cup of chamomile tea. Consider herbal sleep formulas if you need them.

**8. Control stress levels.** Ramped-up stress levels raise cortisol, a hormone that stores fat and breaks down muscle when it stays elevated. For fat loss and lasting health, stress management is essential, not a luxury. If a massage isn't in your budget, set a tea date with your bestie—she always cheers you up!—or take your dog for a long walk.

## WEEK 1 MEAL PLAN

**Day 1**
Breakfast: Mixed Berry and Avocado Protein Shake (page 93)
Lunch: Peach-Berry-Almond Protein Shake (page 95)
Optional Snack: Babaganoush (page 118) with rice chips or crudités
Dinner: Coconut Red Curry Chicken (page 144); Vegetable Fried Rice (page 187);
    mixed green salad with Toasted Macadamia Nut Dressing (page 216)

**Day 2**
Breakfast: Chocolate-Cherry-Chia Protein Shake (page 94)
Lunch: Grilled Pesto Chicken Wrap (page 100)
Optional Snack: Roasted Red Pepper Hummus (page 118) with crudités
Dinner: Green Coconut Protein Shake (page 94)

**Day 3**

Breakfast: Strawberry "Milkshake" Protein Shake (page 95)

Lunch: Seafood Salad with Italian Salsa Verde (page 110)

Optional Snack: Smoky Black Bean Hummus (page 119) with crudités

Dinner: Peach–Berry–Almond Protein Shake (page 95)

**Day 4**

Breakfast: Rise and Shine Mocha Espresso Protein Shake (page 96)

Lunch: Mixed Berry and Avocado Protein Shake (page 93)

Optional Snack: Kale Chips with Cumin and Sea Salt (page 120)

Dinner: Broiled Rosemary-and-Fennel Lamb Chops (page 140); Roasted
    Asparagus with Lemon Zest (page 198); Tuscan White Beans with Sage
    (page 193)

**Day 5**

Breakfast: Nutty Chai Breakfast Blast Shake (page 97)

Lunch: Chicken Tostadas (page 142)

Optional Snack: Avocado-Lime Black Bean Salsa (page 120) with crudités

Dinner: Chocolate-Cherry-Chia Protein Shake (page 94)

**Day 6**

Breakfast: Rise and Shine Mocha Espresso Protein Shake (page 96)

Lunch: Strawberry "Milkshake" Protein Shake (page 95)

Optional Snack: Roasted Jalapeño Guacamole with Toasted Pumpkin Seeds
    (page 121), with rice chips or crudités

Dinner: Kale and Bean Soup (page 174); Halibut en Papillote (page 158);
    Roasted Cauliflower and Broccoli (page 202)

**Day 7**

Breakfast: Nutty Chai Breakfast Blast Shake (page 97)

Lunch: Turkey Chili (page 182); mixed greens with your choice of vinaigrette

Optional Snack: Classic Tapenade on Endive (page 122)

Dinner: Peach-Berry-Almond Protein Shake (page 95)

# WEEK 1 SHOPPING LIST

### Proteins

Cooked chicken breast

Grass-fed lean bone-in loin lamb chops

Natural lean ground turkey

Organic free-range boneless, skinless chicken breast halves

Wild halibut fillets

Wild prawns or shrimp

Wild sea scallops

Wild squid

### Vegetables/Fruits/Herbs

| | | |
|---|---|---|
| Apples | Fresh rosemary | Medium red onions |
| Asparagus | Fresh sage | Mixed greens for salads |
| Avocados | Garlic cloves | Orange |
| Baby kale | Grape tomatoes | Plum tomatoes |
| Baby spinach | Green onions | Shallots |
| Belgian endive | Kale | Small fennel bulb |
| Carrots | Large green bell pepper | Small green pepper |
| Cauliflower | Lemons | Small jalapeño peppers |
| Celery | Limes | Small onion |
| Eggplants | Medium fennel bulbs | Small red bell pepper |
| Fresh basil | Medium head broccoli | Snow peas |
| Fresh cilantro | Medium jalapeño pepper | Vegetables for crudités |
| Fresh ginger | Medium onions | |
| Fresh parsley | Medium red bell pepper | |

### Grains/Nuts/Seeds

Brown rice tortillas

Macadamia nuts

Pine nuts

Raw pumpkin seeds

Milks

Plain cultured coconut milk
Unsweetened almond milk
Unsweetened coconut milk

# WEEK 2 MEAL PLAN

### Day 1

Breakfast: Blueberry Power Muffin (page 87) with a side of nitrate-free chicken breakfast sausage.

Lunch: Chocolate-Cherry-Chia Protein Shake (page 94)

Optional Snack: Classic Tapenade on Endive (page 122)

Dinner: Scallion Shrimp Stir-Fry with Snow Peas (page 154); Sesame Spinach with Scallions (page 200), over steamed quinoa or brown rice (optional)

### Day 2

Breakfast: Green Coconut Protein Shake (page 94)

Lunch: Lentil, Kale, and Sausage Stew (page 183; double portion)

Optional Snack: Roasted Artichoke Dip (page 123) with rice chips

Dinner: Chicken Sloppy Joes over Brown Rice (page 144); Swiss Chard with Olives (page 200)

### Day 3

Breakfast: Swedish-Style Pecan Pancakes with Orange and Strawberries (page 89), with a side of nitrate-free bacon

Lunch: Flank Steak Bistro Chopped Salad (page 105)

Optional Snack: Romesco Dip (page 126) with crudités or rice chips

Dinner: Mixed Berry and Avocado Protein Shake (page 93)

### Day 4

Breakfast: Rise and Shine Mocha Espresso Protein Shake (page 96)

Lunch: Mexican Chicken Tortilla Soup (page 170); mixed green salad with Toasted Macadamia Nut Dressing (page 216)

Optional Snack: Cinnamon Roasted Pecans (page 123)

Dinner: Dijon-and-Almond-Crusted Halibut with Lemon and Parsley (page 156); Roasted Acorn Squash Puree (page 192); Roasted Asparagus with Lemon Zest (page 198)

### Day 5

Breakfast: Bacon-and-Mushroom Sweet Potato Hash (page 91)

Lunch: Strawberry "Milkshake" Protein Shake (page 95)

Optional Snack: Smoked Paprika and Cayenne Roasted Almonds (page 124)

Dinner: Easy Pasta Bolognese (page 135); mixed green salad with Shallot-Champagne Vinaigrette (page 215)

### Day 6

Breakfast: Nutty Chai Breakfast Blast Shake (page 97)

Lunch: Vietnamese Chicken-and-Cabbage Salad (page 109)

Optional Snack: Babaganoush (page 118) with crudités or rice chips

Dinner: Lemon and Herb Broiled Sole (page 158); Chickpeas with Spinach, Lemon, and Tomatoes (page 191)

### Day 7

Breakfast: Hot Quinoa Flake Cereal with Warm Berry Compote (page 90)

Lunch: Chicken Salad Wrap (page 101) with crudités

Optional Snack: Sea Salt and Black Pepper Cashew Cheese (page 125) with rice chips

Dinner: Green Coconut Protein Shake (page 94)

## WEEK 2 SHOPPING LIST

### Proteins

Cooked organic free-range boneless, skinless chicken breast

Grass-fed flank steak

Grass-fed lean ground beef

Nitrate-free bacon

Nitrate-free chicken breakfast sausages

Nitrate-free fully cooked organic sweet Italian sausage

Organic free-range boneless, skinless chicken breast halves
Organic free-range lean ground chicken
Wild shrimp
Wild sole fillets
Wild halibut fillets

## Vegetables/Fruits/Herbs

Acorn squash
Apples
Asparagus
Avocados
Baby arugula
Baby kale
Baby spinach
Belgian endive
Carrots
Celery
Eggplants
Fresh basil
Fresh blueberries (or use frozen)
Fresh cilantro

Fresh ginger
Fresh parsley
Fresh rosemary
Fresh strawberries
Fresh thyme
Garlic cloves
Grape tomatoes
Green onions
Lemons
Limes
Medium cucumbers
Medium green bell pepper
Medium onions
Medium plum tomato
Medium red bell peppers

Medium red onion
Medium Vidalia or other sweet onion
Orange
Radishes
Red cabbage
Red or green kale
Romaine lettuce
Small onion
Small red onions
Small shallots
Small sweet potato
Snow peas
Swiss chard
White mushrooms

## Grains/Nuts/Seeds

Brown rice tortillas
Pecans
Raw almonds
Raw cashews
Sliced raw almonds

Slow-roasted almonds
Slow-roasted cashews
Slow-roasted pecans
Macadamia nuts
Walnuts

## Milks

Unsweetened almond milk
Unsweetened coconut milk

## WEEK 3 MEAL PLAN

**Day 1**

Breakfast: Rise and Shine Mocha Espresso Protein Shake (page 96)

Lunch: Hearty Chicken Soup (page 169); mixed green salad with Shallot-Champagne Vinaigrette (page 215)

Optional Snack: Freeze-Dried Fruit, Nut, and Seed Mix (page 127)

Dinner: Grass-Fed Beef Tenderloin Steaks with Sautéed Shiitakes (page 131); Butternut Squash "Fries" (page 185); Easy Spinach-and-Garlic Sauté (page 195)

**Day 2**

Breakfast: Mixed Berry and Avocado Protein Shake (page 93)

Lunch: Seared Ahi Tuna over Asian Slaw (page 107)

Optional Snack: Homemade Almond Butter (page 128) with apple slices

Dinner: Grilled Dijon-Lemon Lamb Kabobs (page 140); Spice Roasted Sweet Potatoes (page 187); Balsamic Roasted Vegetables (page 205)

**Day 3**

Breakfast: Hot Quinoa Flake Cereal with Warm Berry Compote (page 90)

Lunch: Peach-Berry-Almond Protein Shake (page 95)

Optional Snack: Babaganoush (page 118) with rice chips

Dinner: Salmon Puttanesca (page 161); Easy Spinach-and-Garlic Sauté (page 195)

**Day 4**

Breakfast: Strawberry "Milkshake" Protein Shake (page 95)

Lunch: Tex-Mex Turkey Wrap with Salsa, Avocado, and Arugula (page 104), with crudités

Optional Snack: Cinnamon Roasted Pecans (page 123)

Dinner: BBQ Glazed Chicken (page 143); Jicama, Apple, and Pear Slaw (page 114); Cauliflower Puree (page 196)

**Day 5**

Breakfast: Bacon-and-Mushroom Sweet Potato Hash (page 91)

Lunch: Chocolate-Cherry-Chia Protein Shake (page 94)

Optional Snack: Roasted Artichoke Dip (page 123) with crudités or rice chips

Dinner: Scallion Shrimp Stir-Fry with Snow Peas (page 154) and Vegetable Fried Rice (page 187)

### Day 6

Breakfast: Nutty Chai Breakfast Blast Shake (page 97)

Lunch: Pan-Seared Salmon over Tri-Color Salad with Dijon Dressing (page 108)

Optional Snack: Classic Tapenade on Endive (page 122)

Dinner: Shallot-Thyme Marinated Flank Steak (page 132); Wild Mushrooms and Onions (page 197); Roasted Root Vegetables with Thyme (page 193)

### Day 7

Breakfast: Blueberry Power Muffin (page 87) with a side of nitrate-free chicken breakfast sausage

Lunch: Asian Chicken in Lettuce Cups (page 146)

Optional Snack: Smoked Paprika and Cayenne Roasted Almonds (page 124)

Dinner: Green Coconut Protein Shake (page 94)

## WEEK 3 SHOPPING LIST

### Proteins

Ahi tuna steaks

Deli-sliced nitrate-free turkey breast

Grass-fed beef tenderloin steaks

Grass-fed flank steak

Grass-fed lean boneless leg of lamb

Nitrate-free bacon slices

Nitrate-free chicken breakfast sausage

Organic free-range bone-in, skinless chicken breast halves

Organic free-range bone-in, skinless chicken thighs

Organic free-range lean ground chicken

Shrimp

Wild salmon fillets, such as king or sockeye

### Vegetables/Fruits/Herbs

Apples

Avocado

Baby arugula

Baby kale

Baby spinach

Belgian endive

Boston lettuce

Butternut squash

Carrots

Cauliflower
Celery
Cremini mushrooms
Eggplants
Fresh basil
Fresh blueberries (or use frozen)
Fresh cilantro
Fresh ginger
Fresh marjoram
Fresh parsley
Fresh spinach
Fresh strawberries
Fresh tarragon
Fresh thyme
Garlic cloves
Grape tomatoes
Green cabbage

Green onions
Jalapeño pepper
Japanese eggplants
Jicama
Large red bell pepper
Large Vidalia or other sweet onion
Leeks
Lemons
Limes
Medium onion
Medium red bell pepper
Medium red onions
Medium sweet potatoes
Medium Vidalia or other sweet onion
Medium yellow squash
Medium zucchini

Napa cabbage
Oyster mushrooms
Parsnip
Pear
Plum tomatoes
Radicchio
Red cabbage
Shallots
Shiitake mushrooms
Small onions
Small red onion
Small shallots
Small sweet potatoes
Snow peas
White turnip
White mushrooms

### Grains/Nuts/Seeds

Brown rice tortillas
Raw almonds
Raw cashews
Raw pumpkin seeds

Raw sunflower seeds
Slow-roasted almonds
Slow-roasted cashews
Slow-roasted pecans

### Milks

Unsweetened almond milk
Unsweetened coconut milk

## STAPLES LIST

If you were painting a masterpiece (hint: it's you), you'd make certain every paint color and every brushstroke got the attention it deserved. Fill your fridge, freezer, and pantry with just as much care—what you put in them is going to contribute significantly to the way you look and feel on your journey. These staples, and the weekly shopping lists, are what you need to position yourself for a win on this diet, so keep the basics stocked.

### Protein Powders

Chai vegan protein powder

Chocolate vegan protein powder

Vanilla vegan protein powder

### Oils and Vinegars

Asian sesame oil

Coconut butter

Coconut oil

Extra-virgin olive oil

Macadamia nut oil

Malaysian red palm fruit oil

Olive oil

Balsamic vinegar

Champagne vinegar

Cider vinegar

Sherry vinegar

White balsamic vinegar

White wine vinegar

### Spices

Arrowroot

Cayenne pepper

Chili powder

Cinnamon

Coriander

Crushed red pepper flakes

Curry powder

Dried oregano

Freshly ground black pepper

Garlic powder

Ground allspice

Ground chipotle pepper

Ground dried cumin

Nutmeg

Onion powder

Sea salt

Smoked paprika

Sweet paprika

### Extracts

Almond extract

Coconut extract

Monk fruit extract

Stevia extract

Vanilla extract

## Grains/Seeds/Legumes

Brown rice

Bob's Red Mill Gluten-Free All-
Purpose Baking Flour

Chia seeds

Fennel seeds

Flaxseeds

Organic sprouted green lentils

Quinoa flakes cereal

Quinoa linguine pasta

Rice chips

Sesame seeds

## Jarred and Canned

Anchovies in oil

Capers

Cashew butter

Chili garlic sauce

Coconut aminos

Dijon mustard

Fish sauce

Kalamata olives

Organic low-sodium beef broth

Organic low-sodium chicken broth

Organic tahini paste

Picholine olives

Red curry paste (such as Thai Kitchen)

Roasted red peppers

Tabasco sauce

(6-oz) cans organic tomato paste

(8-oz) cans organic tomato sauce

(14.5-oz) cans fire-roasted diced
tomatoes

(14.5-oz) cans organic diced tomatoes

(15-oz) cans organic no-salt-added
black beans

(15-oz) cans organic no-salt-added
cannellini beans

(15-oz) cans organic no-salt-added
chickpeas (garbanzo beans)

(15-oz) cans organic no-salt-added red
kidney beans

(16-oz) cans organic low-fat refried
black beans

(28-oz) cans organic crushed tomatoes

(28-oz) cans organic diced tomatoes

## Frozen

Artichoke hearts

Organic blueberries

Organic dark cherries

Organic mixed berries

Organic peaches

Organic strawberries

## Miscellaneous

Aluminum-free baking powder
Baking soda
Instant espresso/coffee powder
Organic freeze-dried blueberries
Organic freeze-dried raspberries
Organic freeze-dried strawberries

# FAST WEIGHT LOSS 13

There are certain times in your life when you need to lose fat *fast*. Maybe you need to get into a bridal gown in 3 weeks, or you want to look fabulous for an upcoming high school reunion or beach vacation. Or you finally scored a hot date with the barista you've flirted with for ages, so you need to ditch those pesky pounds and fit into your new skinny jeans by Saturday night.

That probably means you think you have to resort to starving yourself and working out like a fiend. Worse, you're resigned to putting the weight right back on, because everybody's told you that to lose weight and keep it off, you have to be more of a tortoise than a hare.

For the longest time, nutrition and fitness experts believed that, too—that slow and steady wins the fat-loss race. Then a few studies knocked that myth on its head. One in the *International Journal of Behavioral Medicine*[1] found that fast fat burners lost more weight and kept it off better than slow fat burners. A more recent study in the *New England Journal of Medicine*[2] took it further and confirmed that fast fat loss can become safe, *permanent* fat loss. Great news!

## HOW THE VIRGIN DIET CAN HELP

Here's the secret for *healthy* fast fat loss: You need the right plan. Ultra-low-calorie diets, juice cleanses, and other fad diets can create more metabolic damage than long-term fat loss.

1. L. M. Nackers, K. M. Ross, and M. G. Perri, "The association between rate of initial weight loss and long-term success in obesity treatment: Does slow and steady win the race?" *International Journal of Behavioral Medicine* 17, no. 3 (2010): 161–67.

2. K. Cassava et al., "Myths, presumptions, and facts about obesity," *New England Journal of Medicine* 368, no. 5 (Jan. 31, 2013): 446–54, doi:10.1056/NEJMsa1208051.

Well, the great news is you've found the right plan! In Cycle 1 of the Virgin Diet, you eliminate the 7 foods that most commonly cause food intolerance, which means you can also kiss the weight and symptoms they create good-bye. You replace those highly reactive foods with whole, unprocessed foods that rev fat burning, muscle building, and metabolism.

Many of my clients lose 7 pounds in the first week, and a few have lost up to 12 pounds! In a week! Your mileage will vary, of course, but Cycle 1 puts the *fast* in my fast-and-lasting fat loss promise for even the most weight-loss-resistant people.

Best of all, you get these benefits without starvation, deprivation, or calorie counting. You'll start every day with a shake packed full of protein, good fats, antioxidants, and fiber in a single pour right out of the blender to keep you full, focused, and burning fat all morning. The same goes for your meals, because the Virgin Diet Plate sets you up with the perfect balance of nutritious, whole food to pump your energy and stoke your fat-burning fire. You'll get the hang of my fat-burning formula in no time, and soon it will be second nature whether you're dining out, hanging out with friends, or even traveling.

## STEP IT UP WITH THESE STRATEGIES

1. **Swap starchy carbs for non-starchy veggies.** Slow-release starchy carbs like sweet potatoes and legumes are nutrient-rich powerhouses, but when you want fat loss fast, their higher carb count can hold you back. To crank your fat loss into high gear, keep starches to one serving per meal and swap out the rest for broccoli, asparagus, and other green veggies, which pack the same—and often *better*—fiber and nutrient punch as those starchy carbs.

2. **Limit your fruit.** Most fruits are powerhouses of nutrients, antioxidants, and fiber. But along with all that delicious goodness comes sugar, much of it in the form of fructose that your liver converts to fat. To crank up fat loss, limit fruit to 1 cup total per day and stick with the lower-glycemic rock stars like berries and cherries. If you notice your weight stalling and really want to kick things up, remove fruit altogether till you're near your goal weight.

3. **Stay in Cycle 1 longer.** I'm not joking when I say Cycle 1 puts the "fast" in fast and lasting fat loss; many of my clients lose up to 7 pounds in their first week.

In *The Virgin Diet* I ask you to stay in Cycle 1 for 3 weeks. But here's something I get asked pretty often, and you may be wondering, too: "I feel so good pulling these highly reactive foods, so can I stay on Cycle 1 forever?" Here's the deal: At some point I want you to challenge the four foods in Cycle 2 to pinpoint food intolerances. That said, I pretty much live in Cycle 1 and you can, too—especially for accelerated fat loss. Once you're within 5 pounds of your goal weight, shift into Cycle 2, challenge the four foods to connect the dots between them and your symptoms, and then you can return to Cycle 1 indefinitely.

4. **Have protein smoothies for 2 meals.** You've got less than 2 months until beach season and you want to rock that new swimsuit. The fastest, easiest way to get there is with a yummy protein smoothie for 2 out of 3 meals a day. Blend plant-based (but not soy) protein powder, frozen organic berries, leafy greens (trust me, you won't taste them!), and flax or chia seeds with unsweetened coconut or almond milk. It's a crave-busting blend of protein, good fats, and fiber that keeps you full and burning fat for hours. And again, for even faster weight loss, toss the fruit for a few weeks and burn, baby, burn.

5. **Drink more water.** Studies show that water curbs your appetite. One study reported in the journal *Obesity*[3] found that people who drank 8 ounces of water before meals had greater fat loss than people who didn't drink up. Midnight cravings? A study at the University of Washington[4] showed that one glass of water before bed knocked out hunger for every single one of the study participants. But if your goal is to lose fat, and I am betting it is, then it's important to drink water all day, anyway. Even slight dehydration can crash your metabolic machinery and stall fat loss; so drink up according to my guidelines on pages 50–52. If plain water isn't sassy enough for you, just add lemon or lime for a little zing—whatever works to get it in.

6. **Drink more green tea.** Research is inconclusive about whether it's the epi-gallocatechin gallate (EGCG) or the caffeine in green tea that makes it thermogenic

3. E. A. Dennis et al., "Water consumption increases weight loss during a hypocaloric diet intervention in middle-aged and older adults," *Obesity* (Silver Spring) 18, no. 2 (Feb. 2010): 300–307, doi:10.1038/oby.2009.235. Epub 2009 Aug 6.

4. University of Washington Study, reported in *Integrated and Alternative Medicine Clinical Highlights* 4 (2002): 1(16).

(which means it boosts your metabolism and helps burn fat). As with most things, it's probably a little of both. But it doesn't really matter because what we do know is that green tea can help increase fat loss. The evidence comes from a study covered in the *Journal of the American College of Nutrition*,[5] which found that EGCG could reduce abdominal fat in overweight post-menopausal women when they also exercised. Since you'll need several cups to light the fat-burning fire, consider not only swapping your dark roast for green tea but also adding a green tea EGCG supplement.

**7. Stretch the "fast" between dinner and breakfast.** A study reported in the journal *Cell Metabolism*[6] found that mice restricted to eating during only 8 hours a day burned more fat than mice that grazed whenever they wanted, even though both groups ate the same high-fat diet. In other words, for 16 hours every day, the restricted mice went into a "fasting" fat-burning mode. So what's the takeaway? Close the kitchen after dinner! You can get the same benefits as those mice if you create a 12- to 14-hour fat-burning "fast" (don't worry, you'll be sleeping for most of it!) until your morning protein smoothie begins a new fat-burning day. You can even take it one step further and extend the fast by dropping dinner two nights a week!

**8. Eat a big breakfast.** Ever noticed that on those mornings when you skimp on breakfast (or worse, skip it entirely), you're hungrier throughout the day and craving a blueberry scone with your afternoon green tea? A study in the *American Journal of Clinical Nutrition*[7] found that a higher-protein breakfast shuts down your noisy hunger hormone ghrelin much better than cereal with skim milk or other high-carb eats. Aim for a 400- to 600-calorie breakfast to beat back cravings and stay full for hours. If you're doing a protein smoothie, take it to the next level with a spoonful of almond butter or a scoop of avocado. Otherwise, think outside the breakfast box: Salmon and spinach are the perfect way to rev the fat-burning at the start of your busy day.

5. A. M. Hill et al., "Can EGCG reduce abdominal fat in obese subjects?" *Journal of the American College of Nutrition* 26, no. 4 (Aug. 2007): 396S–402S.

6. M. Hatori et al., "Time-restricted feeding without reducing caloric intake prevents metabolic diseases in mice fed a high-fat diet," *Cell Metabolism* 15, no. 6 (June 2012): 848–60, doi:10.1016/j .cmet.2012.04.019. Epub 2012 May 17.

7. W. A. Blom et al., "Effect of a high-protein breakfast on the postprandial ghrelin response," *American Journal of Clinical Nutrition* 83, no. 2 (Feb. 2006): 211–20.

9. **Burst to blast fat.** Treadmills and overheated aerobics classes can raise your stress hormone cortisol and actually stall fat loss. Besides, who has hours every day to work out? And who wants to? Numerous studies show that burst training, which is high-intensity interval training (alternating periods of 30 to 60 seconds of full-out—full-out!—exercise and active recovery for twice as long), can spike your fat-burning metabolism in just minutes a day. Now you're happy! I go into depth on burst training in Cycle 3 of *The Virgin Diet*. One study, reported in the *Journal of Applied Physiology*,[8] found that moderately active women got impressive fat loss doing burst training for just 2 weeks. For fast fat loss, I like to double the basics: double veggies at meals, double protein smoothies, and double burst training. You'll be down a size in no time!

10. **Curb your appetite with fiber.** It's not sexy and it won't be the hot topic next month on your favorite news blog, but fiber reduces gastric emptying, balances blood sugar levels, and promotes satiety. All you have to do is get more in and let it do its thing. Mix a tablespoon of chia seeds, flaxseeds, or a fiber-blend powder into a glass of water 30 to 60 minutes before your meals, drink it down, and you'll be far less likely to pile the food high or reach for seconds. Bonus points for adding fiber in your water before bed to completely shut down late-night cravings and hunger.

11. **Get your zzz's.** Research at the University of Chicago[9] found that even with the right food and exercise plans, you inhibit fast fat loss when you don't get 8 hours of uninterrupted sleep every night. Even one bad night's sleep can crash your fat-burning hormones, lower your fountain-of-youth growth hormone (GH), raise your stress hormone cortisol, and leave you absentmindedly reaching for a cheese Danish with your vat of morning coffee. Sleep your way lean with 7 to 9 hours of high-quality sleep every night. It sounds elusive, but I know you can do it!

For additional meal plans tailored to specific conditions and lifestyle needs, visit thevirgindietcookbook.com/bonus.

---

8. J. L. Talanian et al., "Two weeks of high-intensity aerobic interval training increases the capacity for fat oxidation during exercise in women," *Journal of Applied Physiology* 102, no. 4 (April 2007): 1439–47.

9. University of Chicago, "Sleep loss limits fat loss, study finds," *UChicagoNews*, Oct. 4, 2010, http://news.uchicago.edu/article/2010/10/03/sleep-loss-limits-fat-loss-study-finds.

## WEEK 1 MEAL PLAN

Feel free to add a mixed green salad, lightly dressed with your choice of vinaigrette, or crudités to any meal (including your shakes!). In this meal plan the types of shakes you make are entirely your choice. Choose from any of the ingredients listed in the weekly shopping lists under "Your Shake Ingredients." Be creative, but be sure each shake includes at least 2 scoops of protein powder per serving.

### Day 1

Breakfast: Shake (pages 92 to 97)

Lunch: Scallion Shrimp Stir-Fry with Snow Peas (page 154), over shirataki noodles

Dinner: Shake (pages 92 to 97)

### Day 2

Breakfast: Shake (pages 92 to 97)

Lunch: Vietnamese Chicken-and-Cabbage Salad (page 109)

Dinner: Shake (pages 92 to 97)

### Day 3

Breakfast: Shake (pages 92 to 97)

Lunch: Pan-Seared Salmon over Tri-Color Salad with Dijon Dressing (page 108)

Dinner: Shake (pages 92 to 97)

### Day 4

Breakfast: Shake (pages 92 to 97)

Lunch: Cilantro Turkey Burger with Chipotle Ketchup (page 150; no wrap), on a bed of mixed greens

Dinner: Shake (pages 92 to 97)

### Day 5

Breakfast: Shake (pages 92 to 97)

Lunch: Seared Ahi Tuna over Asian Slaw (page 107)

Dinner: Shake (pages 92 to 97)

## Day 6

Breakfast: Shake (pages 92 to 97)
Lunch: Shake (pages 92 to 97)
Skip Dinner

## Day 7

Breakfast: Shake (pages 92 to 97)
Lunch: Shake (pages 92 to 97)
Skip Dinner

# WEEK 1 SHOPPING LIST

### Proteins

Ahi tuna steaks
Cooked organic free-range boneless, skinless chicken breast
Natural lean ground turkey
Wild salmon fillets, such as king or sockeye
Wild shrimp

### Vegetables/Fruits/Herbs

| | | |
|---|---|---|
| Avocado | Fresh ginger | Napa cabbage |
| Baby arugula | Garlic cloves | Radicchio |
| Baby spinach | Green onions | Red cabbage |
| Belgian endive | Lemons | Shallots |
| Carrots | Limes | Snow peas |
| Fresh basil | Medium cucumber | Tomatoes |
| Fresh cilantro | Mixed greens for salads | |

### Grains/Nuts/Seeds

Slow-roasted cashews

### Miscellaneous

Shirataki noodles

### Your Shake Ingredients

Your shakes are your choice, so you will need to fill in the quantities to have on hand for this week.

Apple

Avocado

Baby kale

Baby spinach

Cashew butter

Chai vegan protein powder

Chocolate vegan protein powder

Instant espresso/coffee powder

Frozen organic blueberries

Frozen organic dark cherries

Frozen organic mixed berries

Frozen organic peaches

Frozen organic strawberries, unsweetened

Unsweetened coconut milk

Unsweetened almond milk

Vanilla vegan protein powder

# WEEK 2 MEAL PLAN

Feel free to add a mixed green salad, lightly dressed with your choice of vinaigrette, or crudités to any meal (including your shakes!).

### Day 1

Breakfast: Shake (pages 92 to 97)
Lunch: Flank Steak Bistro Chopped Salad (page 105)
Dinner: Shake (pages 92 to 97)

### Day 2

Breakfast: Shake (pages 92 to 97)
Lunch: Seafood Salad with Italian Salsa Verde (page 110)
Dinner: Shake (pages 92 to 97)

### Day 3

Breakfast: Shake (pages 92 to 97)
Lunch: Asian Chicken in Lettuce Cups (page 146)
Dinner: Shake (pages 92 to 97)

### Day 4

Breakfast: Shake (pages 92 to 97)
Lunch: Pan-Seared Scallops with Bacon and Spinach (page 155)
Dinner: Shake (pages 92 to 97)

### Day 5

Breakfast: Shake (pages 92 to 97)
Lunch: Pounded Chicken Paillards Topped with Tomato and Fresh Basil Salad
  (page 147)
Dinner: Shake (pages 92 to 97)

### Day 6

Breakfast: Shake (pages 92 to 97)
Lunch: Shake (pages 92 to 97)
Skip Dinner

### Day 7

Breakfast: Shake (pages 92 to 97)
Lunch: Shake (pages 92 to 97)
Skip Dinner

## WEEK 2 SHOPPING LIST

### Proteins

Grass-fed flank steak
Nitrate-free bacon slices
Organic free-range boneless, skinless chicken breast halves
Organic free-range lean ground chicken
Wild prawns or shrimp
Wild squid
Wild sea scallops

### Vegetables/Fruits/Herbs

Baby spinach or baby arugula

Boston lettuce

Campari or large vine-ripened cherry
tomatoes

Carrots

Celery

Fennel

Fresh basil

Fresh cilantro

Fresh ginger

Fresh parsley

Fresh rosemary

Garlic cloves

Green onions

Lemons

Limes

Medium cucumber

Medium onion

Medium red bell pepper

Medium red onion

Mixed greens for salad

Radishes

Romaine

Shallots

Small red onion

Vegetables for crudités

### Grains/Nuts/Seeds

Slow-roasted cashews

### Frozen

Organic spinach

### Your Shake Ingredients

Your shakes are your choice, so you will need to fill in the quantities to have on
hand for this week.

Apple

Avocado

Baby kale

Baby spinach

Cashew butter

Chai vegan protein powder

Chocolate vegan protein powder

Frozen organic blueberries

Frozen organic dark cherries

Frozen organic mixed berries

Frozen organic peaches

Frozen organic strawberries, unsweetened

Instant espresso/coffee powder

Unsweetened almond milk

Unsweetened coconut milk

Vanilla vegan protein powder

## WEEK 3 MEAL PLAN

Feel free to add a mixed green salad, lightly dressed with your choice of vinaigrette, or crudités to any meal (including your shakes!)

**Day 1**

Breakfast: Shake (pages 92 to 97)

Lunch: Scallion Shrimp Stir-Fry with Snow Peas (page 154), over shirataki noodles

Dinner: Shake (pages 92 to 97)

**Day 2**

Breakfast: Shake (pages 92 to 97)

Lunch: Tex-Mex Burger with Avocado Salsa (page 134), on a bed of greens

Dinner: Shake (pages 92 to 97)

**Day 3**

Breakfast: Shake (pages 92 to 97)

Lunch: Shepherd's Salad with Prawns (page 106)

Dinner: Shake (pages 92 to 97)

**Day 4**

Breakfast: Shake (pages 92 to 97)

Lunch: Grilled Turkey Cutlet with Chimchurri (page 151); Braised Kale (page 205)

Dinner: Shake (pages 92 to 97)

**Day 5**

Breakfast: Shake (pages 92 to 97)

Lunch: Poached Salmon with Rémoulade Sauce,★ (page 160); Roasted Asparagus with Lemon Zest (page 198)

Dinner: Shake (pages 92 to 97)

★ Substitute chicken broth for the white wine.

**Day 6**
Breakfast: Shake (pages 92 to 97)
Lunch: Shake (pages 92 to 97)
Skip Dinner

**Day 7**
Breakfast: Shake (pages 92 to 97)
Lunch: Shake (pages 92 to 97)
Skip Dinner

# WEEK 3 SHOPPING LIST

### Proteins

Grass-fed lean ground beef
Natural turkey breast cutlets
Nitrate-free bacon slices
Shrimp
Wild prawns
Wild salmon fillets, such as king or sockeye

### Vegetables/Fruits/Herbs

Asparagus
Avocado
Boston or romaine
    lettuce leaves
Carrots
Celery
Fresh basil
Fresh cilantro
Fresh ginger
Fresh parsley

Garlic cloves
Green onions
Kale
Lemons
Limes
Medium onions
Medium red bell pepper
Mini or Persian
    cucumbers
Mixed greens for salad

Plum tomatoes
Shallots
Small bunch celery
Small jalapeño pepper
Small onion
Small red bell pepper
Small red onions
Snow peas
Vegetables for crudités

### Miscellaneous

Shirataki noodles

### Your Shake Ingredients

Your shakes are your choice, so you'll need to fill in the quantities to have on hand for this week.

Apple
Avocado
Baby kale
Baby spinach
Cashew butter
Chai vegan protein powder
Chocolate vegan protein powder
Frozen organic blueberries
Frozen organic dark cherries

Frozen organic mixed berries
Frozen organic peaches
Frozen organic strawberries, unsweetened
Instant espresso/coffee powder
Raw or homemade almond butter (see page 128)
Unsweetened almond milk
Unsweetened coconut milk
Vanilla vegan protein powder

## STAPLES LIST

### Oils and Vinegars

Asian sesame oil
Coconut oil
Extra-virgin olive oil
Macadamia nut oil
Malaysian red palm fruit oil

Cider vinegar
Red wine vinegar
White balsamic vinegar
White wine vinegar

### Spices

Cinnamon
Chili powder
Dried oregano
Freshly ground black pepper
Garlic powder

Ground allspice
Ground dried cumin
Onion powder
Sea salt
Smoked paprika

### Extracts

Almond extract
Coconut extract

Monk fruit extract
Vanilla extract

### Grains/Seeds

Chia seeds

Flaxseeds

Gluten-free oats

### Jarred and Canned

Capers

Chili garlic sauce

Chipotle pepper in adobo sauce

Coconut aminos

Dijon mustard

Fish sauce

Organic low-sodium chicken broth

Tabasco sauce

(8-oz) bottle clam juice

(6-oz) cans organic tomato paste

(8-oz) cans organic tomato sauce

### Miscellaneous

Homemade Ketchup (recipe on page 211)

# VEGAN AND VEGETARIAN 14

Most of the world depends on vegetarian foods as a major source of nutrition. There are a lot of variations under the umbrella of plant-based eaters. They include lacto vegetarians, who eat dairy; lacto-ovos, who also eat eggs; and pescetarians, who eat fish. The strictest are vegans; they exclude all animal products (meat, poultry, fish, eggs, milk, cheese, and other dairy products).

If you're a vegan or a vegetarian, this cookbook will offer you incredible choices for delicious, healthy, easy ways to eat according to your bliss. Because no matter why you've decided to be a vegan or a vegetarian—and there are many good reasons—there's no denying the real health benefits that result from a plant-based diet. Generally speaking, vegetarian diets tend to be lower in damaged fats, cholesterol, and, of course, animal protein, and higher in fiber and folate than an omnivore's (a plant-and-animal eater's) diet. As such, many vegetarians are at a lower risk for developing heart disease, some cancers, diabetes, obesity, and high blood pressure.

One of the reasons you may have chosen to give up meat or other animal by-products is the sorry state of animal welfare in this country. Abysmal living conditions, inhumane treatment, and rampant use of hormones and antibiotics are hard to ignore. To make matters worse, these conditions and practices also compromise the quality of meat, eggs, dairy, and other foods animals provide.

That being said, humans developed high-functioning, large brains—which use 20 percent of our energy—directly as a result of including meat in our diet. So going vegetarian or vegan is still not a choice I recommend for most people. In fact, I go even further than not recommending it—I actually try to encourage my vegetarian clients to *reintroduce* lean animal protein into their diets (hey, you have to give me credit for trying!). Why? For two reasons. One, because I believe our bodies and brains still thrive on animal-based protein; and two, there *are* ways to eat meat and make healthy choices that are thoughtful of animals and the conditions they live in.

Don't get me wrong: If your choice is rooted in spiritual beliefs, I respect that. And I want to reiterate that if you're a vegetarian or a vegan, you have my full support through the awesome plant-based recipes in this cookbook! But the advice I'm offering comes from a place of knowledge and experience. I was a vegan and a vegetarian for many years, and during that time I had higher body fat than I do now, had to work out twice as much to maintain that weight, and suffered with chronic cystic acne and cratered energy.

I also know nutrition, and the reason I evangelize animal-based protein for a high-functioning metabolism is that when you eat only plant-based protein, it's more difficult to get the full spectrum of nutrients that the combination of plants and clean, lean animal protein can provide ("clean, lean" being the key). Besides, a plant-based diet, by its very nature, is high in carbohydrates. A high-carb diet can mean a roller-coaster ride of blood sugar spikes and crashes that set you up for insulin resistance and type 2 diabetes.

And—surprise—if you're eating a nutritionally bankrupt, calorie-dense vegetarian diet (there's no meat in French fries!), you can seriously pack on some pounds. And that is not the goal here! An unhealthy vegetarian diet is no better than a diet heavy in corn-fed red meat, which has been linked to atherosclerosis and heart disease.

So as a vegetarian or a vegan, you need to work that much harder to be sure you're getting enough complete quality protein into your diet from the right sources. Make that commitment—it's critical. You'll be happy to know this cookbook has done a lot of the work for you; it has rock-star vegetable recipes to help you get all the nutritional support you can from food, without being overloaded with carbs and sugar.

Vegetarians and vegans also often test low or deficient in essential fatty acids, and a few crucial vitamins and minerals as well. If that's true for you, supplementing can save you. Supplement to ensure you get not only the amino acids you need, but also $B_{12}$ (which you can't get from plants) and possibly iron, vitamin D, and the omega-3s DHA and EPA, as well.

## HOW THE VIRGIN DIET CAN HELP

A vegetarian walks into a restaurant…No, I don't have a joke. But as a vegetarian you probably want to laugh (or cry?) when you open some restaurant menus. They offer you a nice pat on the head with a token vegetarian choice, and I'm going to go out on a limb here and bet it's a grilled vegetable sandwich.

That's not only happening at the delis. You've no doubt had the experience of looking forward to a nice evening out at a posh restaurant only to find yourself blinking vacantly at the meat-heavy fare. Or maybe you've been to a dinner party your friend *swore* was vegetarian-friendly, which turned out to mean there was no bacon in the mashed potatoes.

There's no reason to feel frustrated and defeated just because there are times the world makes eating as a vegetarian harder than it needs to be. You don't have to succumb to bland noodles and marinara or other last-resort, carb-heavy diet wreckers; a meal can be completely satisfying and nutritious without meat.

Here's the thing: Whether you're Paleo or vegan, the Virgin Diet is completely agnostic—its principles complement and even supercharge any eating plan. For example, about a quarter of the Virgin Diet Plate is allocated to clean, lean protein. But *which* protein is entirely up to you. You have the flexibility to choose higher-protein plant-based foods and still easily meet your quota.

One secret we can keep from hard-core carnivores is that everyone is a vegan for breakfast on the Virgin Diet (and that doesn't mean you get to keep your scone!). The Virgin Diet Shake is a fast, easy, fat-burning shake that keeps you full and focused for hours, so get ready to fire up the blender. Toss in some plant-based (but not soy) protein powder, frozen berries, kale or other leafy greens, flaxseeds or chia seeds, and unsweetened coconut or almond milk, then press...Make Delicious!

My vegetarian meals are also a cinch. The Virgin Diet fills your plate with a burst of colorful vegetables, fruits, nuts and seeds, legumes, and other healthy starches. And good fats like avocado, olive and coconut oils, and nut butters. You'll replace the meat portion of the Virgin Diet Plate with protein-rich foods like quinoa, lentils, and non-gluten grains like amaranth. In Cycle 3, once you've passed the soy challenge, you can even enjoy the occasional organic tofu or fermented soy dish. Easy!

Your days will be filled with foods that pack a nutrient and antioxidant wallop. Many are high-fiber, so you won't have any trouble meeting your 50-gram quota. Actually, you'll probably have an easier time meeting that number than your meat-eating friends!

I know vegetarians are also always on the lookout for more creative, delicious, easy-to-make meals that won't leave them feeling deprived. So look no further! This cookbook will become a great weapon in your culinary arsenal.

My recipes incorporate nutrition-savvy strategies to address the concerns I've just laid out, so you can follow them to the letter or use them to guide your inner artist in designing the perfect vegetarian or vegan diet for you. You can become a lean, healthy, energetic force to be reckoned with without going anywhere near a grass-fed steak (assuming I haven't persuaded you!).

## STEP IT UP WITH THESE STRATEGIES

1. **Get optimal protein.** Meeting your protein quota as a vegetarian or vegan becomes easy once you know which foods should be your go-to sources. Combine ½ cup of lentils, ½ cup of quinoa, and 2 tablespoons of walnuts, for instance, and you'll get 17 grams of protein. Homemade vegetable burgers, legumes, nuts and nut butters, and non-gluten grains also make excellent protein sources. Aim for two or three higher-protein foods at every meal, and getting enough will become an afterthought.

2. **Make lateral shifts.** *Deprivation* is not a word I want in your dietary vocabulary. Instead of being preoccupied with what you can't have, turn your attention to the many other choices you have. I guarantee there are lots of substitutes for your favorite foods and they'll make you just as happy, or happier for having made a healthier choice. I call these lateral shifts. Here are a few: Swap nutrient-empty spaghetti for corn-free quinoa pasta or spaghetti squash. Dump the cow's milk (you probably have anyway) for unsweetened coconut or almond milk. Who needs stale chips and salsa when you can enjoy kale chips with hummus or guacamole? Cashew cheese smeared on portobello mushroom caps with tomato sauce is decadent. Once you get the hang of lateral shifts, they become easy, fun, and more satisfying than your old favorites.

3. **Be mindful of food intolerances.** Organic soy, eggs, and grass-fed dairy provide good sources of protein and good fats, but too many vegans and lacto-ovo vegetarians over-rely on these foods, triggering food sensitivities that manifest as weight loss resistance, inflammation, and symptoms like fatigue, bloating, and headaches. Eliminate the 7 highly reactive foods for 3 weeks and then challenge soy, gluten, eggs, and dairy. (Vegans, you're exempt from those last two.) Even if you do okay challenging these foods, they can't become everyday staples again or you'll risk having the food intolerance symptoms return with a vengeance.

**4. Address nutrient deficiencies.** Studies confirm what I often find with testing in my own clients: Vegans and vegetarians can have lower levels of certain nutrients. A study reported in the journal *Nutrition in Clinical Practice*[1] found that vegetarians often show deficiencies in vitamins $B_{12}$ and D, omega-3 fatty acids, calcium, iron, and zinc. Nutrient-rich foods can correct those deficiencies. A simple example is eating more raw nuts and seeds, which are a good source of zinc and calcium. A comprehensive multivitamin/mineral supplement can also be an insurance policy to fill in nutrient gaps. And if you suffer from fatigue, brain fog, or mood imbalances, look for an integrative practitioner who can test and help optimize your nutrient levels.

**5. Swap the processed carbs for high-fiber starches.** Food manufacturers create all kinds of crazy meal-in-a-box vegetarian and vegan-friendly comfort foods produced with unrecognizable ingredients designed to prolong shelf life. They're often loaded with preservatives, added sugars, and an overall carb load that tell your body to raise insulin and store fat. Skip the mac 'n' vegan cheese and other meat-free Frankenfoods for nutrient-rich unprocessed carbs like sweet potatoes, lentils and other legumes, and quinoa.

**6. Don't fall into the sugar trap.** Manufacturers also masquerade sweet treats like agave-sweetened ice cream and organic cane sugar–sweetened cookies as health food to people like you, since you're more health conscious than the average person. But whether it's gluten-free or vegan-friendly, junk food is junk food, and your pancreas isn't going to know the difference between table sugar and whatever sweetener du jour lurks in those vegan muffins. My one exception is locally grown organic raw honey, which offers some homeopathic benefits for allergies. If you have immune responses to bits of mold and dust, local raw organic honey can strengthen your immune system and help you handle those things better. But don't get carried away: ½ to 1 teaspoon a day will do the job.

**7. Make an oil change.** Sure, vegetable oils *sound* healthy, but safflower and other predominantly omega-6 oils can contribute to inflammation and upset the omega-6/omega-3 balance essential for reducing the risk of serious health issues. That's a real concern because current estimates are that the Standard American Diet

1. W. J. Craig, "Nutrition concerns and health effects of vegetarian diets," *Nutrition in Clinical Practice* 25, no. 6 (Dec. 2010): 613–20, doi: 10.1177/0884533610385707.

contains about fourteen to twenty-five times more omega-6 fatty acids than omega-3 fatty acids. For high-heat cooking, choose coconut oil and Malaysian red palm fruit oil, and use extra-virgin olive oil for delicious drizzling. Incorporate healthy fats like avocados and raw almonds to your heart's content. Flaxseeds, chia seeds, and walnuts are good choices for an anti-inflammatory omega-3 wallop. So is fish oil, so if you're unwilling to supplement with fish oil, look for a vegan DHA algae supplement to get these essential fatty acids.

For additional meal plans tailored to specific conditions and lifestyle needs, visit the virgindietcookbook.com/bonus.

## WEEK 1 MEAL PLAN

### Day 1
Breakfast: Mixed Berry and Avocado Protein Shake (page 93)
Lunch: Chocolate-Cherry-Chia Protein Shake (page 94)
Optional Snack: Babaganoush (page 118) with crudités or rice chips
Dinner: Lentil Nut Burger with Cilantro Vinaigrette (page 163); Roasted Cauliflower and Broccoli (page 202)

### Day 2
Breakfast: Green Coconut Protein Shake (page 94)
Lunch: Strawberry "Milkshake" Protein Shake (page 95)
Optional Snack: Roasted Jalapeño Guacamole with Toasted Pumpkin Seeds (page 121) with crudités
Dinner: Mushroom Lentil Loaf with Barbecue Glaze (page 164); mixed green salad with Toasted Macadamia Nut Dressing (page 216)

### Day 3
Breakfast: Nutty Chai Breakfast Blast Shake (page 97)
Lunch: Peach-Berry-Almond Protein Shake (page 95)
Optional Snack: Kale Chips with Cumin and Sea Salt (page 120)
Dinner: Quinoa Fusilli with Cherry Tomatoes, Garlic, Basil, and Olive Oil (page 166); spinach salad with Shallot-Champagne Vinaigrette (page 215)

### Day 4

Breakfast: Rise and Shine Mocha Espresso Protein Shake (page 96)

Lunch: Green Coconut Protein Shake (page 94)

Optional Snack: Cinnamon Roasted Pecans (page 123)

Dinner: Chickpeas with Spinach, Lemon, and Tomatoes (page 191); Confetti Quinoa (page 186); Green Beans with Shiitakes and Shallots (page 199)

### Day 5

Breakfast: Chocolate-Cherry-Chia Protein Shake (page 94)

Lunch: Chickpea Falafel Salad with Tahini Dressing (page 112)

Optional Snack: Sea Salt and Black Pepper Cashew Cheese (page 125) with crudités

Dinner: Mixed Berry and Avocado Protein Shake (page 93)

### Day 6

Breakfast: Rise and Shine Mocha Espresso Protein Shake (page 96)

Lunch: Peach-Berry-Almond Protein Shake (page 95)

Optional Snack: Smoked Paprika and Cayenne Roasted Almonds (page 124)

Dinner: Quinoa and Chickpea Tabbouleh with Mint, Parsley, and Lemon Dressing (page 167); Cauliflower and Nut Stir-Fry (page 206)

### Day 7

Breakfast: Nutty Chai Breakfast Blast Shake (page 97)

Lunch: Strawberry "Milkshake" Protein Shake (page 95)

Optional Snack: Roasted Red Pepper Hummus (page 118) with crudités

Dinner: Vegetarian Chili (page 166); mixed green salad with Toasted Macadamia Nut Dressing (page 216)

## WEEK 1 SHOPPING LIST

### Vegetables/Fruits/Herbs

| | | |
|---|---|---|
| Apples | Broccoli | Eggplants |
| Avocados | Cauliflower | Fresh basil |
| Baby kale | Celery | Fresh cilantro |
| Baby spinach | Cremini mushrooms | Fresh mint |

Fresh parsley
Fresh thyme
Garlic cloves
Grape tomatoes
Green beans
Green onions
Kale
Large cucumber
Large shallot
Lemons
Limes
Medium cucumber

Medium green bell pepper
Medium jalapeño peppers
Medium onion
Medium orange bell pepper
Medium plum tomatoes
Medium red bell peppers
Medium red onion
Medium yellow bell pepper

Mixed greens for salads
Mixed spring greens
Orange
Shiitake mushrooms
Small onions
Small plum tomato
Small red bell pepper
Small red onion
Small shallots
Vegetables for crudités
White mushrooms

### Grains/Nuts/Seeds

Pine nuts
Raw cashews
Raw macadamia nuts
Raw pumpkin seeds

Raw sunflower seeds
Raw walnuts
Slow-roasted almonds
Slow-roasted pecans

### Milks

Cultured coconut milk
Unsweetened almond milk
Unsweetened coconut milk

## WEEK 2 MEAL PLAN

### Day 1

Breakfast: Blueberry Power Muffin (page 87)
Lunch: Mixed Berry and Avocado Protein Shake (page 93)
Optional Snack: Classic Tapenade on Endive (page 122)
Dinner: Kale and Bean Soup* (page 174); Spaghetti Squash Arrabbiata
  (page 203)

*Replace the chicken broth with organic vegetable broth.

**Day 2**

Breakfast: Chocolate-Cherry-Chia Protein Shake (page 94)

Lunch: Quinoa and Chickpea Tabbouleh with Mint, Parsley, and Lemon Dressing (page 167), on a bed of arugula

Optional Snack: Kale Chips with Cumin and Sea Salt (page 120)

Dinner: Red Quinoa with Kale, Onions, and Pine Nuts (page 190); Tuscan White Beans with Sage* (page 193)

**Day 3**

Breakfast: Hot Quinoa Flake Cereal with Warm Berry Compote (page 90)

Lunch: Peach-Berry-Almond Protein Shake (page 95)

Optional Snack: Freeze-Dried Fruit, Nut, and Seed Mix (page 127)

Dinner: Black Bean Soup (page 171); Roasted Brussels Sprouts with Hazelnuts (page 194)

**Day 4**

Breakfast: Nutty Chai Breakfast Blast Shake (page 97)

Lunch: Chickpea Falafel Salad with Tahini Dressing (page 112)

Optional Snack: Romesco Dip (page 126) with rice chips

Dinner: Quinoa Fusilli with Cherry Tomatoes, Garlic, Basil, and Olive Oil (page 166); Easy Spinach-and-Garlic Sauté (page 195)

**Day 5**

Breakfast: Swedish-Style Pecan Pancakes with Orange and Strawberries (page 89)

Lunch: Kale and Bean Soup** (page 174); mixed green salad with sliced avocado and Shallot-Champagne Vinaigrette (page 215)

Optional Snack: Homemade Almond Butter (page 128) with apple slices

Dinner: Green Coconut Protein Shake (page 94)

**Day 6**

Breakfast: Rise and Shine Mocha Espresso Protein Shake (page 96)

Lunch: Cucumber and Radish Salad with Arugula, Nuts, and Seeds (page 113)

*Replace the chicken broth with organic vegetable broth.

**Replace the chicken broth with organic vegetable broth.

Optional Snack: Avocado-Lime Black Bean Salsa (page 120) with crudités

Dinner: Mushroom Lentil Loaf with Barbecue Glaze (page 164); Roasted Cauliflower and Broccoli (page 202)

### Day 7

Breakfast: Strawberry "Milkshake" Protein Shake (page 95)

Lunch: Lentil Nut Burger with Cilantro Vinaigrette (page 163), on a bed of spinach and arugula

Optional Snack: Roasted Red Pepper Hummus (page 118) with crudités

Dinner: Red Quinoa with Kale, Onions, and Pine Nuts (page 190); Tuscan White Beans with Sage (page 193)

## WEEK 2 SHOPPING LIST

### Vegetables/Fruits/Herbs

Apples

Avocados

Baby arugula

Baby kale

Baby spinach

Belgian endive

Broccoli

Brussels sprouts

Cauliflower

Celery

Cremini mushrooms

Extra-large onions

Fresh basil

Fresh blueberries (or use frozen)

Fresh cilantro

Fresh mint

Fresh parsley

Fresh rosemary

Fresh sage

Fresh spinach

Fresh strawberries

Fresh thyme

Garlic cloves

Grape tomatoes

Green onions

Kale

Large cucumber

Large jalapeño pepper

Large shallots

Lemons

Limes

Medium cucumber

Medium onions

Medium plum tomatoes

Medium red bell peppers

Medium spaghetti squash

Mini or Persian cucumbers

Mixed greens and arugula for salad

Mixed spring greens

Radishes

Small jalapeño pepper

Small onions

Small oranges

Small red bell pepper

Small red onion

Small shallots

Vegetables for crudites

White mushrooms

### Grains/Nuts/Seeds

Pine nuts

Raw almonds

Raw hazelnuts

Raw pecans

Raw pumpkin seeds

Raw sunflower seeds

Raw walnuts

Sliced raw almonds

Slow-roasted almonds

Slow-roasted cashews

Slow-roasted pecans

### Milks

Cultured coconut milk

Unsweetened almond milk

Unsweetened coconut milk

## WEEK 3 MEAL PLAN

### Day 1

Breakfast: Chocolate-Cherry-Chia Protein Shake (page 94)

Lunch: Cauliflower and Nut Stir-Fry (page 206); Curried Lentils (page 190)

Optional Snack: Sea Salt and Black Pepper Cashew Cheese (page 125) with crudités

Dinner: Chickpeas with Spinach, Lemon, and Tomatoes (page 191); Confetti Quinoa (page 186); Swiss Chard with Olives (page 200)

### Day 2

Breakfast: Nutty Chai Breakfast Blast Shake (page 97)

Lunch: Minestrone Soup (page 172); mixed green salad with Shallot-Champagne Vinaigrette (page 215)

Optional Snack: Avocado-Lime Black Bean Salsa (page 120) with crudités

Dinner: Spaghetti Squash Arrabbiata (page 203); Tuscan White Beans with Sage (page 193)

### Day 3

Breakfast: Blueberry Power Muffin (page 87)

Lunch: Chickpea Falafel Salad with Tahini Dressing (page 112)

Optional Snack: Smoky Black Bean Hummus (page 119) with crudités

Dinner: Green Coconut Protein Shake (page 94)

## Day 4

Breakfast: Mixed Berry and Avocado Protein Shake (page 93)

Lunch: Quinoa and Chickpea Tabbouleh with Mint, Parsley, and Lemon Dressing (page 167), on a bed of arugula

Optional Snack: Roasted Artichoke Dip (page 123) with crudités

Dinner: Mushroom Lentil Loaf with Barbecue Glaze (page 164); Jicama, Apple, and Pear Slaw (page 114)

## Day 5

Breakfast: Hot Quinoa Flake Cereal with Warm Berry Compote (page 90)

Lunch: Kale and Bean Soup* (page 174); mixed green salad with Toasted Macadamia Nut Dressing (page 216)

Optional Snack: Roasted Jalapeño Guacamole with Toasted Pumpkin Seeds (page 121), with crudités

Dinner: Peach-Berry-Almond Protein Shake (page 95)

## Day 6

Breakfast: Rise and Shine Mocha Espresso Protein Shake (page 96)

Lunch: Lentil Nut Burger with Cilantro Vinaigrette (page 163), over Cauliflower Puree (page 196)

Optional Snack: Classic Tapenade on Endive (page 122)

Dinner: Kale and Bean Soup** (page 174); Spaghetti Squash Arrabbiata (page 203)

## Day 7

Breakfast: Swedish-Style Pecan Pancakes with Orange and Strawberries (page 89)

Lunch: Strawberry "Milkshake" Protein Shake (page 95)

Optional Snack: Babaganoush (page 118) with bean chips

Dinner: Vegetarian Chili (page 166) with mixed green salad and your choice of vinaigrette

*Replace the chicken broth with organic vegetable broth.

**Replace the chicken broth with organic vegetable broth.

# WEEK 3 SHOPPING LIST

## Vegetables/Fruits/Herbs

Apples
Avocados
Baby kale
Baby spinach
Belgian endive
Carrots
Cauliflower
Celery
Cremini mushrooms
Eggplants
Fennel
Fresh basil
Fresh blueberries (or use frozen)
Fresh cilantro
Fresh mint
Fresh parsley
Fresh sage
Fresh strawberries
Fresh thyme

Garlic cloves
Grape tomatoes
Green cabbage
Green onions
Kale
Large cucumber
Large shallots
Lemons
Limes
Medium cucumber
Medium green bell pepper
Medium jalapeño peppers
Medium onions
Medium orange bell pepper
Medium plum tomatoes
Medium red bell peppers
Medium red onions

Medium spaghetti squash
Medium Vidalia or other sweet onion
Medium yellow bell pepper
Medium zucchini
Mixed greens and arugula for salads
Mixed spring greens
Pear
Red cabbage
Small jalapeño pepper
Small jicama
Small onions
Small orange
Small red bell pepper
Small shallots
Swiss chard
Vegetables for crudités
White mushrooms

## Grains/Nuts/Seeds

Pine nuts
Raw almonds
Raw cashews
Raw macadamia nuts
Raw pecans

Raw pumpkin seeds
Raw sunflower seeds
Raw walnuts
Slow-roasted pecans

## Milks

Cultured coconut milk
Unsweetened almond milk

Unsweetened coconut milk

## STAPLES LIST

### Protein Powders

Chai vegan protein powder

Chocolate vegan protein powder

Vanilla vegan protein powder

### Oils and Vinegars

Coconut oil

Extra-virgin olive oil

Macadamia nut oil

Malaysian red palm fruit oil

Champagne vinegar

Cider vinegar

Sherry vinegar

White wine vinegar

### Spices

Arrowroot

Bay leaf

Cayenne pepper

Chili powder

Cinnamon

Coriander

Crushed red pepper flakes

Curry powder

Dried basil

Dried oregano

Freshly ground black pepper

Garlic powder

Ground allspice

Ground ancho chili pepper

Ground chipotle pepper

Ground cumin

Sea salt

Smoked paprika

### Extracts

Almond extract

Coconut extract

Monk fruit extract

Stevia extract

Vanilla extract

### Grains/Seeds/Legumes

Bean chips

Bob's Red Mill Gluten-Free All-
Purpose Baking Flour

Brown rice

Chia seeds

Dry quinoa

Dry red quinoa
Dry, sprouted lentils
Fennel seeds
Flaxseeds
Gluten-free oats

Quinoa flakes cereal
Quinoa fusilli pasta
Quinoa pasta shells
Rice chips
Sesame seeds

## Jarred and Canned

Anchovies in oil
Capers
Cashew butter
Coconut aminos
Dijon mustard
Kalamata olives
Organic low-sodium vegetable broth
Organic tahini paste
Picholine olives
Roasted red peppers
Tabasco sauce
(6-oz) cans organic tomato paste

(14.5-oz) cans fire-roasted diced tomatoes
(14.5-oz) cans organic diced tomatoes
(15-oz) cans organic black lentils
(15-oz) cans organic no-salt-added black beans
(15-oz) cans organic no-salt-added cannellini beans
(15-oz) cans organic no-salt-added chickpeas (garbanzo beans)
(15-oz) cans organic no-salt-added red kidney beans
(28-oz) cans organic crushed tomatoes
(28-oz) cans organic diced tomatoes

## Frozen

Artichoke hearts
Organic blueberries
Organic dark cherries

Organic mixed berries
Organic peaches
Organic strawberries, unsweetened

## Miscellaneous

Aluminum-free baking powder
Baking soda
Instant espresso/coffee powder

Organic freeze-dried blueberries
Organic freeze-dried raspberries
Organic freeze-dried strawberries

# DIABETES AND PRE-DIABETES 15

High blood sugar creates a perfect metabolic storm.

When you eat, your blood sugar goes up. All foods raise blood sugar, but refined carbohydrates and sugary foods make your blood sugar go *way* up. High blood sugar is toxic, so your pancreas produces a hormone called insulin that gets that sugar (glucose) out of your bloodstream and shuttles it to your cells to use for energy. What your cells can't use, your liver and muscles can store in the form of glycogen to be used for energy later.

At least that's what should happen. If your metabolic machinery is broken, your cells stop responding to insulin and your liver and muscles don't effectively store that sugar as glycogen. That's when the trouble starts.

Excess glucose gets stored as fat, especially when your glycogen stores are overloaded or you eat foods high in fructose, an especially damaging sugar that goes straight to the liver and starts *making* fat.

Remember that insulin's job involves getting sugar out of your blood. But insulin sometimes overcompensates and pulls your blood sugar down *too* low, leading to a crash-and-burn roller coaster of hunger and cravings.

When you pummel your bloodstream with high doses of sugar and carbohydrates on a regular basis, you're forcing your pancreas to work overtime, cranking out heaps of insulin to remove that sugar. Your liver repackages that excess sugar as triglycerides (a type of fat found in the blood), and your cells eventually get burned out from the insulin barrage and stop responding, leading to a condition called insulin resistance.

Inflammation is closely linked to insulin resistance. Insulin resistance by itself increases chronic inflammation, and it leads to weight gain. To add insult to injury, fat cells further increase inflammation. Inflammation is guaranteed to stall fat loss, damage your organs, and contribute to nearly every illness from heart disease to cancer.

My good friend Dr. Mark Hyman writes in his book *The Blood Sugar Solution* that more than 100 million Americans have insulin resistance, also called metabolic syndrome, a collection of symptoms that increases the risk of serious disease. That's 1 in 3 people! People with metabolic syndrome usually have high triglycerides, which raise the risk of heart disease. People who have metabolic syndrome are also at a higher risk of getting diabetes. That's especially frightening since total deaths from diabetes are projected to increase by more than 50 percent in the next 10 years.

So why does blood sugar matter? When you have high blood sugar for too long, you're also heading down a dangerous road not just to significant weight gain but also to high insulin levels (hyperinsulinemia), inflammation, high triglycerides, metabolic syndrome, diabetes, heart disease, hypertension, and illness.

People with blood sugar problems come in all shapes and sizes. Symptoms often develop slowly, and many people who have had type 2 diabetes for years don't even know it. But most are dealing with the same issues. If you have blood sugar imbalances, you probably struggle with your weight, brain fog, and irritating mood swings that make you miserable. You're tired, you're stressed, you have no sex drive, and you can't find the energy or motivation to tackle your ballooning to-do list. So before you convince yourself that you're one of the other two people in Dr. Hyman's statistic, see if any of this sounds familiar:

- Feeling lousy after meals
- Fuzzy thinking
- Stressed out
- Discolored skin on the back of the neck and underarms
- A waist circumference of greater than 34 inches for a woman or 40 inches for a man
- High blood pressure
- High blood sugar (pre-diabetes)
- High triglycerides
- Low HDL cholesterol
- Women: irregular periods, acne, and facial hair

Any one of those conditions puts your health at risk, but having more than one means you might need to balance your blood sugar.

So how did you get here? It could be that you have been following the wrong set of rules: wasting years of your life counting calories and eating low-fat diets.

Maybe you start your day at your favorite coffee spot, ordering a soy latte and a low-fat muffin, feeling good that you stayed on track with your weight-loss point system. But by midmorning you're famished, your fuse is short, and you're craving something sweet.

You just need a little something to get you through. Thank goodness your favorite coworker brought homemade biscotti. They're low-fat and low-calorie, right? So you grab one and get a sugar hit that *almost* carries you to lunch. Except that within an hour or two you feel like you've wilted; you're light-headed, sleepy, and worst of all, really craving another biscotto.

Those spikes and crashes punish you throughout the day—you swing between bursts of energy and crushing exhaustion. You're up; you're down. Even though you're diligently counting points and eating everything in moderation, you can't shake those unsightly extra pounds you carry around your middle.

Sound familiar? It's time to get the right information and stop the cycle. Because what you're experiencing can be far more detrimental than some unflattering extra weight, and how you address it can literally save your life.

The good news is that if you have high blood sugar, you're not doomed to bad health. You can make some simple, easy, delicious changes that balance your blood sugar and put you in charge of how you feel.

## HOW THE VIRGIN DIET CAN HELP

On the Virgin Diet, you're not only losing fat fast, you're healing your body. That's because the basic tenets of the diet are designed to target food intolerance, reduce inflammation, and normalize your immune response (which is kicked into high gear as a result of food intolerance). By homing in on these conditions, the Virgin Diet also addresses the dangerous issues they cause, including blood sugar imbalance.

Simply put, the Virgin Diet pulls you off the blood sugar spike-and-crash roller coaster that sucks your energy, ages you, and intensifies your hunger and cravings (inexplicably, for the same foods that got you into this mess!).

Both the Virgin Diet Shake and the Virgin Diet Plate make for a blood sugar–balancing blend of clean, lean protein; good fats; high-fiber slow-release carbs; leafy greens; and cruciferous vegetables. And they leave out higher-sugar fruits and other high-glycemic foods that provoke blood sugar imbalance.

The fiber I just mentioned is especially key here. Fiber is a blood sugar–balancing rock star, and I want you to be its groupie! Aim for 50 grams of fiber a day—entirely possible with all the Virgin Diet's recommended high-fiber foods, including avocados, berries (raspberries are highest), lentils and other legumes, and leafy greens. But if getting that amount from food seems daunting, opt for a multifiber supplement powder to meet your quota.

The good news is that in a matter of weeks, most people will become more insulin sensitive. That means their bodies have recalibrated their response to sugar and they can occasionally enjoy something sweet without enduring the subsequent sugar crash. Sweets can't ever become an everyday thing again, though. To keep your blood sugar stable and cravings a thing of the past, you'll start most mornings with the Virgin Diet Shake and then eat by the Plate for your meals.

Staying in control of your health is easy with *The Virgin Diet Cookbook*, because it's filled with recipes designed to help you do just that!

## STEP IT UP WITH THESE STRATEGIES

1. **Up your omega-3s.** High blood pressure, triglycerides, and inflammation are the nasty trifecta that leads to insulin resistance and diabetes. Omega-3 fatty acids can lower all three and help offset the massive amounts of pro-inflammatory omega-6s most people get in their diets. Omega-3 fats can also help your insulin receptors work better. Wild fish is your best source for omega-3s. I also love tossing flaxseeds or chia seeds into my morning shake for an omega-3 boost. If you're not eating wild fish at least three or four times each week, supplement with a high-quality essential fatty acid formula.

2. **Increase your vitamin D.** Research reported and in the *Journal of Biomedicine and Biotechnology*[1] connects the dots between vitamin D deficiencies and insulin resistance! Even if you're lucky enough to live in a sunnier climate (and most of us *aren't*), your body might not be making enough vitamin D. Some foods like wild fish are a good source of vitamin D, but you'll also want to take a supplement to make sure you

1. C. C. Sung et al., "Role of vitamin D in insulin resistance," *Journal of Biomedicine and Biotechnology* (2012): 1–11, 634195, doi: 10.1155/2012/634195. Epub 2012 Sep 3.

get the therapeutic dose you need. Take a 25-hydroxy vitamin D test and work with an integrative practitioner until you reach 60 to 80 ng/ml. Once you've reached those levels, you will probably need 2,000 to 5,000 IUs per day to maintain your D levels. This will vary based on your genetics, biochemistry, and environment.

3. **Nix the sugar.** The glycemic index measures how quickly your blood sugar increases after you eat. Sugar, processed carbs, and other high-glycemic foods create blood sugar spikes and crashes that trigger even more cravings for problem foods. Opt instead for blood sugar–balancing foods like protein, good fats, and high-fiber starchy carbs. One study reported in the *American Journal of Clinical Nutrition*[2] found that increasing protein helped people with diabetes have better control over their blood sugar levels. Other studies, reported in the *Asia Pacific Journal of Clinical Nutrition*,[3] show that good fats like raw nuts also help even out sugar for people with diabetes.

4. **Burst.** Burst training, or high-intensity interval training (HIIT), is the most efficient, effective exercise for balancing blood sugar levels. One study discussed in the journal *BMC Endocrine Disorders*[4] even showed that burst training could reduce diabetes risks for young people. Another, in the *Journal of Applied Physiology*,[5] showed that bursting could improve blood sugar levels and reduce complications for people who already have diabetes. No time for exercise? Sorry, nice try—time is no excuse, since you can do burst training in just 15 minutes a day (actually, it's only 4 minutes of bursting…the rest of the time you're warming up, cooling down, or in active recovery!). If you don't own an X-iser (my favorite burst training machine), your nearest park, hill, or stairwell can provide all the "equipment" you need to get your burst on. I go into how to burst train in depth in Cycle 3 in *The Virgin Diet Book*.

2. M. C. Gannon et al., "An increase in dietary protein improves the blood glucose response in persons with type 2 diabetes," *American Journal of Clinical Nutrition* 78, no. 4. (Oct. 2003): 734–41.

3. C. W. Kendall et al., "Health benefits of nuts in prevention and management of diabetes," *Asia Pacific Journal of Clinical Nutrition* 19, no. 1 (2010): 110–16.

4. J. A. Babraj et al., "Extremely short duration high intensity interval training substantially improves insulin action in young healthy males," *BMC Endocrine Disorders* 9, no. 3 (Jan. 2009), doi: 10.1186/1472-6823-9-3.

5. J. P Little et al., "Low-volume high-intensity interval training reduces hyperglycemia and increases muscle mitochondrial capacity in patients with type 2 diabetes," *Journal of Applied Physiology* 111, no. 6 (Dec. 2011): 1554–60, doi: 10.1152/japplphysiol.00921.2011. Epub 2011 Aug 25.

**5. Get enough sleep.** Just one night of poor sleep can knock insulin and other blood sugar–related hormones out of whack. And that can have serious consequences. One study, reported in the *Journal of Applied Physiology*,[6] made it clear that chronic sleep loss could lead to fat gain, insulin resistance, and diabetes! That's all I needed to hear (good night!). Aim for 7 to 9 hours of quality, uninterrupted sleep every night to optimize insulin and other hormone levels.

**6. Reduce your stress.** You can't avoid stress, but there are lots of things you can do to control it—and they're more than worth it. Constant anxiety, worry, and fear keep the pedal to the floor on your adrenal glands, and they flood your system with the stress hormone cortisol. A study reported in the journal *Diabetes Care* determined that "the degree of cortisol secretion is directly associated with the presence and the number of diabetes complications."[7] Meditation, yoga, deep breathing, or even walking your dog around the block—find out what works for *you* to de-stress.

For additional meal plans tailored to specific conditions and lifestyle needs, visit thevirgindietcookbook.com/bonus.

## WEEK 1 MEAL PLAN

**Day 1**
Breakfast: Mixed Berry and Avocado Protein Shake (page 93)
Lunch: Green Coconut Protein Shake (page 94)
Optional Snack: Roasted Red Pepper Hummus (page 118) with crudités
Dinner: Salmon Puttanesca (page 161); Braised Kale (page 205)

**Day 2**
Breakfast: Rise and Shine Mocha Espresso Protein Shake (page 96)
Lunch: Strawberry "Milkshake" Protein Shake (page 95)
Optional Snack: Smoked Paprika and Cayenne Roasted Almonds (page 124)

---

6. K. Spiegel et al., "Sleep loss: A novel risk factor for insulin resistance and Type 2 diabetes," *Journal of Applied Physiology* 99, no. 5 (Nov. 2005) 2008–19.

7. I. Chiodini et al., "Cortisol secretion in patients with type 2 diabetes: Relationship with chronic complications," *Diabetes Care* 30, no. 1 (Jan. 2007): 83–88.

Dinner: Quinoa Fusilli with Cherry Tomatoes, Garlic, Basil, and Olive Oil (page 166); Balsamic Roasted Vegetables (page 205)

## Day 3

Breakfast: Nutty Chai Breakfast Blast Shake (page 97)

Lunch: Chocolate-Cherry-Chia Protein Shake (page 94)

Optional Snack: Classic Tapenade on Endive (page 122)

Dinner: Pounded Chicken Paillards Topped with Tomato and Fresh Basil Salad (page 147); French Beans with Macadamia Nuts (page 203)

## Day 4

Breakfast: Rise and Shine Mocha Espresso Protein Shake (page 96)

Lunch: Green Coconut Protein Shake (page 94)

Optional Snack: Smoky Black Bean Hummus (page 119) with crudités

Dinner: Halibut en Papillote (page 158); Roasted Acorn Squash Puree (page 192); mixed green salad with Shallot-Champagne Vinaigrette (page 215)

## Day 5

Breakfast: Nutty Chai Breakfast Blast Shake (page 97)

Lunch: Strawberry "Milkshake" Protein Shake (page 95)

Optional Snack: Cinnamon Roasted Pecans (page 123)

Dinner: Broiled Rosemary-and-Fennel Lamb Chops (page 140); Roasted Root Vegetables with Thyme (page 193); simple mixed green salad with Toasted Macadamia Nut Dressing (page 216)

## Day 6

Breakfast: Peach-Berry-Almond Protein Shake (page 95)

Lunch: Mixed Berry and Avocado Protein Shake (page 93)

Optional Snack: Sea Salt and Black Pepper Cashew Cheese (page 125) with crudités

Dinner: Mediterranean Turkey-and-Peppers Skillet (page 149); Chickpeas with Spinach, Lemon, and Tomatoes (page 191)

## Day 7

Breakfast: Peach-Berry-Almond Protein Shake (page 95)

Lunch: Chocolate-Cherry-Chia Protein Shake (page 94)

Optional Snack: Avocado-Lime Black Bean Salsa (page 120) with crudités
Dinner: Minestrone Soup (page 172); Chicken with 40 Cloves of Garlic (page 145)

# WEEK 1 SHOPPING LIST

### Proteins

Grass-fed lean bone-in loin lamb chops
Natural turkey breast cutlets
Organic free-range boneless, skinless chicken breast halves
Whole organic free-range chicken
Wild halibut fillets
Wild salmon fillets, such as king or sockeye

### Vegetables/Fruits/Herbs

Acorn squash
Apples
Asparagus
Avocados
Baby kale
Baby spinach
Belgian endive
Butternut squash
Campari or large vine-ripened cherry tomatoes
Carrots
Celery
Fresh basil

Fresh cilantro
Fresh parsley
Fresh rosemary
Fresh thyme
Garlic cloves
Grape tomatoes
Haricots verts
Japanese eggplants
Kale
Large red bell pepper
Limes
Lemons
Medium fennel bulbs
Medium green bell pepper

Medium onions
Medium red bell pepper
Medium red onions
Medium yellow squash
Medium zucchini
Mixed greens for salad
Plum tomato
Small jalapeño pepper
Small onions
Small red onion
Small shallots
Small sweet potato
Vegetables for crudités
White turnip

### Grains/Nuts/Seeds

Raw cashews
Raw macadamia nuts
Slow-roasted almonds
Slow-roasted pecans

**Milks**

Unsweetened almond milk

Unsweetened coconut milk

## WEEK 2 MEAL PLAN

### Day 1

Breakfast: Green Coconut Protein Shake (page 94)

Lunch: Shepherd's Salad with Prawns (page 106)

Optional Snack: Smoky Black Bean Hummus (page 119) with crudités

Dinner: Slow Cooker Coq au Vin (page 180)

### Day 2

Breakfast: Strawberry "Milkshake" Protein Shake (page 95)

Lunch: Vegetarian Chili (page 166); mixed green salad with olive oil and fresh-squeezed lemon juice

Optional Snack: Classic Tapenade on Endive (page 122)

Dinner: Kale and Bean Soup (page 174); Blackened Salmon (page 159); Cauliflower Puree (page 196)

### Day 3

Breakfast: Mixed Berry and Avocado Protein Shake (page 93)

Lunch: Flank Steak Bistro Chopped Salad (page 105)

Optional Snack: Roasted Red Pepper Hummus (page 118) with crudités

Dinner: Turkey Meat Loaf with Kale (page 148); Orange-Scented Mashed Sweet Potatoes with Coconut (page 188); Roasted Cauliflower and Broccoli (page 202)

### Day 4

Breakfast: Chocolate-Cherry-Chia Protein Shake (page 94)

Lunch: Hearty Chicken Soup (page 169); mixed green salad with Toasted Macadamia Nut Dressing (page 216)

Optional Snack: Cinnamon Roasted Pecans (page 123)

Dinner: Mushroom Lentil Loaf with Barbecue Glaze (page 164); Jicama, Apple, and Pear Slaw (page 114)

### Day 5

Breakfast: Rise and Shine Mocha Espresso Protein Shake (page 96)

Lunch: Cilantro Turkey Burger with Chipotle Ketchup (page 150), on a bed of greens

Optional Snack: Sea Salt and Black Pepper Cashew Cheese (page 125) with crudités

Dinner: Mushroom Bisque (page 178); Dijon-and-Almond-Crusted Halibut with Lemon and Parsley (page 156); Roasted Asparagus with Lemon Zest (page 198)

### Day 6

Breakfast: Nutty Chai Breakfast Blast Shake (page 97)

Lunch: Vietnamese Chicken-and-Cabbage Salad (page 109)

Optional Snack: Smoked Paprika and Cayenne Roasted Almonds (page 124)

Dinner: Chicken with 40 Cloves of Garlic (page 145); Roasted Root Vegetables with Thyme (page 193); mixed green salad with Shallot-Champagne Vinaigrette (page 215)

### Day 7

Breakfast: Peach-Berry-Almond Protein Shake (page 95)

Lunch: Grilled Pesto Chicken Wrap (page 100) with crudités

Optional Snack: Avocado-Lime Black Bean Salsa (page 120) with rice chips

Dinner: Weeknight Cioppino (page 181); Cucumber and Radish Salad with Arugula, Nuts, and Seeds (page 113; reduce nuts and seeds by half)

## WEEK 2 SHOPPING LIST

### Proteins

Cooked organic free-range boneless, skinless chicken breast

Grass-fed flank steak

Littleneck clams

Natural lean ground turkey

Nitrate-free bacon slices

Organic free-range bone-in chicken thighs

Organic free-range bone-in, skinless chicken breast halves

Organic free-range whole chicken

Wild halibut fillet

Wild prawns

Wild salmon fillets, such as king or sockeye

## Vegetables/Fruits/Herbs

Apples
Asparagus
Assorted wild
  mushrooms
Avocados
Baby arugula
Baby kale
Baby spinach
Belgian endive
Broccoli
Butternut squash
Carrots
Cauliflower
Celery
Cremini mushrooms
Fresh basil
Fresh cilantro
Fresh parsley
Fresh rosemary
Fresh sage

Fresh thyme
Garlic cloves
Green cabbage
Green onions
Jicama
Kale
Large shallot
Leeks
Lemons
Limes
Medium cucumbers
Medium green bell
  peppers
Medium onions
Medium red bell peppers
Medium red onions
Medium sweet potatoes
Mini or Persian
  cucumbers
Mixed greens for salad

Orange
Parsnip
Pear
Plum tomatoes
Radishes
Red cabbage
Romaine lettuce
Shallot
Small fennel bulb
Small jalapeño pepper
Small jicama
Small onions
Small red bell peppers
Small red onions
Small shallots
Small sweet potato
Tomato
Vegetables for crudités
White mushrooms
White turnip

## Grains/Nuts/Seeds

Brown rice tortillas
Pine nuts
Raw almonds
Raw cashews
Raw macadamia nuts
Raw pecans

Raw walnuts
Slow-roasted almonds
Slow-roasted cashews
Slow-roasted pecans
Unsweetened shredded coconut

## Milks

Unsweetened almond milk
Unsweetened coconut milk

## WEEK 3 MEAL PLAN

### Day 1

Breakfast: Nutty Chai Breakfast Blast Shake (page 97)

Lunch: Seafood Salad with Italian Salsa Verde (page 110)

Optional Snack: Smoky Black Bean Hummus (page 119) with crudités

Dinner: Kale and Bean Soup (page 174); Grass-Fed Beef Tenderloin Steaks with Sautéed Shiitakes (page 131); Roasted Fennel and Onions (page 201)

### Day 2

Breakfast: Mixed Berry and Avocado Protein Shake (page 93)

Lunch: Lentil Nut Burger with Cilantro Vinaigrette (page 163), with sliced avocado on a bed of spinach leaves

Optional Snack: Classic Tapenade on Endive (page 122)

Dinner: Coconut Red Curry Chicken (page 144); Vegetable Fried Rice (page 187); mixed green lettuce and shredded cabbage salad with Sesame-Ginger Vinaigrette (page 216)

### Day 3

Breakfast: Rise and Shine Mocha Espresso Protein Shake (page 96)

Lunch: Pan-Seared Salmon over Tri-Color Salad with Dijon Dressing (page 108)

Optional Snack: Cinnamon Roasted Pecans (page 123)

Dinner: Grilled Turkey Cutlet with Chimichurri (page 151); Cuban-Style Black Beans (page 189); Easy Spinach-and-Garlic Sauté (page 195)

### Day 4

Breakfast: Strawberry "Milkshake" Protein Shake (page 95)

Lunch: Tex-Mex Turkey Wrap with Salsa, Avocado, and Arugula (page 104)

Optional Snack: Roasted Red Pepper Hummus (page 118) with crudités

Dinner: Scallion Shrimp Stir-Fry with Snow Peas (page 154); Sesame Spinach with Scallions (page 200); Vegetable Fried Rice (page 187)

### Day 5

Breakfast: Chocolate-Cherry-Chia Protein Shake (page 94)

Lunch: Kale and Bean Soup (page 174; double portion)

Optional Snack: Sea Salt and Black Pepper Cashew Cheese (page 125) with crudités

Dinner: Lemon and Herb Broiled Sole (page 158); Confetti Quinoa (page 186); Roasted Asparagus with Lemon Zest (page 198)

## Day 6

Breakfast: Green Coconut Protein Shake (page 94)

Lunch: Asian Chicken in Lettuce Cups (page 146)

Optional Snack: Smoked Paprika and Cayenne Roasted Almonds (page 124)

Dinner: Easy Pasta Bolognese (page 135; Balsamic Roasted Vegetables (page 205)

## Day 7

Breakfast: Peach-Berry-Almond Protein Shake (page 95)

Lunch: Chicken Salad Wrap (page 101) with crudités

Optional Snack: Avocado-Lime Black Bean Salsa (page 120) with rice chips

Dinner: Chicken Sloppy Joes over Brown Rice (page 144); Roasted Cauliflower and Broccoli (page 202)

## WEEK 3 SHOPPING LIST

### Proteins

Deli-sliced nitrate-free turkey breast

Grass-fed beef tenderloin steaks

Grass-fed lean ground beef

Natural turkey breast cutlets

Organic free-range boneless, skinless chicken breast halves

Organic free-range lean ground chicken

Wild prawns or shrimp

Wild salmon fillets, such as king or sockeye

Wild sea scallops

Wild sole fillets

Wild squid

### Vegetables/Fruits/Herbs

Apples

Asparagus

Avocados

Baby arugula

Baby kale

Baby spinach

Belgian endive
Boston lettuce
Carrots
Cauliflower
Celery
Fresh basil
Fresh cilantro
Fresh ginger
Fresh parsley
Fresh sage
Fresh spinach
Fresh tarragon
Fresh thyme
Garlic cloves
Green cabbage

Green onions
Japanese eggplants
Kale
Large red bell pepper
Large shallots
Lemons
Limes
Medium fennel bulbs
Medium green bell
  peppers
Medium head broccoli
Medium onions
Medium orange bell
  pepper
Medium red bell
  peppers

Medium red onions
Medium yellow bell
  pepper
Medium yellow squash
Medium zucchini
Orange
Plum tomatoes
Shiitake mushrooms
Small head radicchio
Small jalapeño peppers
Small onions
Snow peas
Spinach and mixed
  greens for salads
Vegetables for crudités
White mushrooms

### Grains/Nuts/Seeds

Brown rice tortillas
Raw cashews
Raw walnuts
Slow-roasted almonds

Slow-roasted cashews
Slow-roasted pecans
Sunflower seeds

### Milks

Unsweetened almond milk
Unsweetened coconut milk

## STAPLES LIST

### Protein Powders

Chai vegan protein powder
Chocolate vegan protein powder
Vanilla vegan protein powder

## Oils and Vinegars

Asian sesame oil

Coconut butter

Coconut oil

Extra-virgin olive oil

Macadamia nut oil

Malaysian red palm fruit oil

Balsamic vinegar

Champagne vinegar

Cider vinegar

Red wine vinegar

Rice vinegar

Sherry vinegar

White balsamic vinegar

White wine vinegar

## Spices

Arrowroot

Bay leaves

Cayenne pepper

Chili powder

Cinnamon

Coriander

Crushed red pepper flakes

Curry powder

Dried oregano

Dried thyme

Fennel seeds

Freshly ground black pepper

Garlic powder

Ground allspice

Ground ancho chile pepper

Ground chipotle pepper

Ground cumin

Nutmeg

Onion powder

Saffron threads

Sea salt

Smoked paprika

Sweet paprika

## Extracts

Almond extract

Coconut extract

Monk fruit extract

Vanilla extract

## Grains/Seeds/Legumes

Brown rice

Chia seeds

Dry quinoa

Dry, sprouted lentils

Gluten-free oats

Quinoa fusilli pasta

Quinoa linguine pasta

Quinoa pasta shells

Rice chips

Sesame seeds

## Jarred and Canned

Anchovies in oil

Capers

Cashew butter

Chili garlic sauce

Coconut aminos

Dijon mustard

Fish sauce

Kalamata olives

Oil-packed sun-dried tomatoes

Organic low-sodium beef broth

Organic low-sodium chicken broth

Organic low-sodium vegetable broth

Organic tahini paste

Picholine olives

Red curry paste (such as Thai Kitchen)

Roasted red peppers

Tabasco sauce

(6-oz) cans organic tomato paste

(8-oz) bottle clam juice

(8-oz) cans organic tomato sauce

(14.5-oz) cans fire-roasted diced tomatoes

(14.5-oz) cans organic diced tomatoes

(15-oz) cans organic black lentils

(15-oz) cans organic no-salt-added black beans

(15-oz) cans organic no-salt-added cannellini beans

(15-oz) cans organic no-salt-added chickpeas (garbanzo beans)

(15-oz) cans organic no-salt-added red kidney beans

(28-oz) cans organic diced tomatoes

### Frozen

Organic blueberries

Organic dark cherries

Organic mixed berries

Organic peaches

Organic strawberries, unsweetened

Pearl onions

### Miscellaneous

Instant espresso/coffee powder

# PALEO/LOW CARB 16

We know we're in a battle with an enemy. An invisible enemy. But invisible or not, we have to know our enemy to defeat it. For many years, health-care professionals and nutritionists believed the biggest evildoer preventing fat loss was fat. It sounded right: Fat makes you fat. But over the past decade there's been a gradual shift to understanding that carbohydrates are the real adversary fat loss faces. Doctors once vilified low-carb diets as unsafe and even dangerous, but studies continue to confirm that for fat loss and overall health, eating low-carb works as well as (and often better than) a low-fat diet.

One such study, reported in the journal *Nutrition in Clinical Practice*,[1] declared it was "time to embrace [low-carb] diets as a viable option to aid in reversing diabetes mellitus, risk factors for heart disease, and the epidemic of obesity." That's because a low-carb diet consistently delivers impressive results without the oppressive hunger or feelings of deprivation low-fat and low-calorie diets can create.

Low-carb diets vary, but overall they reduce carbohydrate count anywhere from 20 to 100 grams a day. Despite popular lore, low-carb diets are *not* meat-only diets. Even the strictest among them can include leafy greens and cruciferous veggies, nuts and seeds, and even low-glycemic fruits like berries.

The popular Paleo diet shares a lot of traits with most low-carb diets. Followers debate an official definition, but they agree it revolves around high protein, high fiber, and lots of good fats. Its focus is the nutrient-rich whole, unprocessed foods our ancestors (from the Paleolithic era, naturally) thrived on thousands of years ago. It's not a style of eating that requires "net carb" counting. If you can gather, hunt, fish, or pluck

1. A. H. Hite et al., "Low-carbohydrate diet review: Shifting the paradigm," *Nutrition in Clinical Practice* 26, no. 3 (June 2011): 300–308, doi: 10.1177/0884533611405791.

it, chances are it qualifies as Paleo. Lean meats, leafy green veggies, berries, insects, and nuts and seeds are all staples of the Paleo diet.

Sure, Paleolithic humans didn't live as long as modern-day humans, but I bet they were more likely to die from old age (unless a saber-toothed tiger *had them* for dinner). They likely weren't plagued with cancer, diabetes, obesity, or other modern-day ills.

## HOW THE VIRGIN DIET CAN HELP

Is it any coincidence that most highly reactive foods didn't exist for Paleo humans? Dairy, soy, gluten, corn, peanuts, and added sugar are relatively new to our diet, and the result in our daily lives is weight gain, fatigue, inflammation, gut issues, diabetes, and obesity. When people stop eating these foods, they become lean and healthy, their energy soars, they look and feel younger, and those frustrating symptoms disappear.

I call the Virgin Diet "Paleo with benefits." That's because I include nutrient- and fiber-rich slow-release carbs for a little variety. Okay, so maybe your Paleo ancestors didn't have legumes growing in their backyards. But you do! You're the big winner! Allow yourself a little leeway and edge in some nutrient-dense foods even if they aren't strictly Paleo or low-carb. A sweet potato is higher in carbs, but it's a great source of fiber and beta-carotene, and it can inject much-needed pizzazz into what can become a monotonous diet. To honor those of you who land on the hard-core side of Paleo, I've left legumes and grains out of this meal plan. But you can always reincorporate them.

And you'll start every morning with the Virgin Diet Shake—a fast, easy infusion of protein, good fats, fiber, and antioxidants. If you're committed to Paleo principles of whole foods, you can simply eat a Virgin Diet lunch or dinner recommendation for breakfast. To make it simple, I've given you both options in the meal plan.

What's out? Vegetable oils, grain-fed beef, and the processed foods we can be sure our ancestors didn't eat. Inflammation plays a part in nearly every modern disease, from obesity to diabetes to cancer. Our Paleo ancestors got about a 4:1 ratio of omega-6s to omega-3s, but today we're more like 20:1 in favor of pro-inflammatory fats.

On the Virgin Diet you'll rebalance that ratio by focusing on good fats like coconut oil, olives, avocados, and raw almonds. Flaxseeds or chia seeds and walnuts are great sources of the omega-3 fatty acid alpha-linolenic acid (ALA), which is theoretically a precursor to the longer-chain eicosapentaenoic acid (EPA) and docosahexaenoic acid (DHA). And if you're not eating wild fish three times a week, you should also supplement with an essential fatty acids formula.

## STEP IT UP WITH THESE STRATEGIES

**1. Low-carb doesn't mean all-you-can-eat.** Too much of even the healthiest foods can stall fat loss, since those excess calories have to go somewhere. Most Paleo and low-carb plans don't shine a spotlight on calories, but they still matter. Thanks to a hormone called cholecystokinin (CCK), when you eat protein and good fats your brain gets the message to put your fork down, so you're less likely to overeat. We can agree you're probably not going to eat six chicken breasts, but overdoing nuts and avocados (staples on many low-carb diets) can derail your hard work and create fat-loss plateaus.

**2. Stay away from the processed stuff.** Looking at *you*, Paleo bread, low-carb granola bars, and "low-net-carb" chocolate chip cookies. Manufacturers know you're craving "legal" versions of ice cream, candy bars, and other junk foods, so they've concocted a low-carb or Paleo version of just about every comfort food imaginable. Watch out: They frequently come loaded with whey protein isolate, gluten, preservatives, artificial sweeteners, trans fats, and lots of other stuff your Paleo ancestors wouldn't recognize. Steer clear of the middle aisles at the grocery store and of most foods with a bar code on the package. If you're craving something sweet, have a few squares of low-sugar dark chocolate, with 80 percent or higher cacao. But if a few squares become the whole bar, back away from the chocolate quickly!

**3. Choose the best-quality meats.** Chicken, beef, and fish provide excellent amounts of protein, fats, and nutrients like zinc and carnitine. Unfortunately, most commercial meat also comes from antibiotic-injected animals subjected to wretched living conditions and other atrocities our Paleo ancestors didn't have to confront. Skip the feedlot steaks and hormone-injected chicken breasts and look for the best-quality meats you can afford, ideally from farmers who humanely raise their own cows and chickens. Grass-fed meat provides higher amounts of anti-inflammatory omega-3 fatty acids and the fat-burning fatty acid conjugated linoleic acid (CLA).

Likewise, choose free-range poultry and wild fish rather than the farm-raised fish and chicken-on-steroids most grocery stores sell.

**4. Stay hydrated.** Among its many benefits, your kidneys need extra water to filter the higher amounts of protein you're getting on a low-carb or Paleo diet. Even slight dehydration can stall your metabolic machinery, so if you're plateauing, stepping up your water intake might be the needle mover for you. Start with a glass of water when you get up, and drink throughout your day. The only time I don't want you drinking is *during* meals, when too much liquid can dilute the stomach enzymes that break down protein.

**5. Increase your fiber.** Researchers estimate Paleo humans got 100 grams of fiber every day. We pale in comparison, with a paltry 5 to 14 grams a day. If meat is the centerpiece of your meals, you could be shortchanging the nutrients in leafy greens and other high-fiber foods. A study in the journal *Nutrition*[2] found that while most people consume less than half of the recommended fiber allowance in their diets, low-carb dieters get even less than that. I'll meet you halfway: On the Virgin Diet, I want you to get 50 grams a day. You can meet that quota with high-fiber avocados, lentils and other legumes, quinoa, nuts, and seeds. You'll also nudge up your fiber intake when you throw freshly ground flaxseeds or chia seeds into your Virgin Diet Shake. Even with the best intentions, though, we can't always get there. So I recommend a professional-quality fiber supplement to hit your 50 grams.

For additional meal plans tailored to specific conditions and lifestyle needs, visit thevirgindietcookbook.com/bonus.

## MEAL PLANS

If you're 100 percent Paleo and won't do the protein shakes, you can substitute any other meal for breakfast, as I have here. I understand there are varying degrees of Paleo "adherence," so you may have to adjust these meal plans slightly if you're more hard-core!

So you have two meal plans below—one with protein shakes and one without. Each has its own Shopping List and Staples Shopping List.

2. J. L. Slavin, "Dietary fiber and body weight," *Nutrition* 21, no. 3 (March 2005): 411–18.

## *Week 1 Meal Plan (no shakes)*

### Day 1

Breakfast: Bacon-and-Mushroom Sweet Potato Hash (page 91)

Lunch: Flank Steak Bistro Chopped Salad (page 105)

Optional Snack: Homemade Almond Butter (page 128) on apple slices

Dinner: Weeknight Cioppino (page 181); mixed green salad with Shallot-Champagne Vinaigrette (page 215)

### Day 2

Breakfast: Cilantro Turkey Burger with Chipotle Ketchup (page 150; no wrap), on a bed of salad greens

Lunch: Seafood Salad with Italian Salsa Verde (page 110)

Optional Snack: Roasted Jalapeño Guacamole with Toasted Pumpkin Seeds (page 121) and crudités

Dinner: Grilled Marinated Duck Breasts (page 153; no sherry); Roasted Brussels Sprouts with Hazelnuts (page 194)

### Day 3

Breakfast: Salmon Puttanesca (page 161); Balsamic Roasted Vegetables (page 205)

Lunch: Flank Steak Bistro Chopped Salad (page 105)

Optional Snack: Cinnamon Roasted Pecans (page 123)

Dinner: Chicken with 40 Cloves of Garlic (page 145); Italian-Style Escarole (page 208)

### Day 4

Breakfast: Grilled Fresh Sardines (page 162); Grilled Marinated Portobello Mushrooms (page 207)

Lunch: Vietnamese Chicken-and-Cabbage Salad (page 109)

Optional Snack: Roasted Artichoke Dip (page 123) with crudités

Dinner: Mushroom Beef Stew (page 179)

### Day 5

Breakfast: Tex-Mex Burger with Avocado Salsa (page 134), on a bed of mixed greens

Lunch: Pounded Chicken Paillards Topped with Tomato and Fresh Basil Salad (page 147)

Optional Snack: Kale Chips with Cumin and Sea Salt (page 120)

Dinner: Pork Souvlaki Kabobs with Tzatziki (page 139); Roasted Fennel and Onions (page 201)

## Day 6

Breakfast: Bacon-and-Mushroom Sweet Potato Hash (page 91)

Lunch: Seared Ahi Tuna over Asian Slaw (page 107)

Optional Snack: Sea Salt and Black Pepper Cashew Cheese (page 125) with crudités

Dinner: BBQ Glazed Chicken (page 143); Easy Spinach-and-Garlic Sauté (page 195)

## Day 7

Breakfast: Turkey Meat Loaf with Kale (page 148)

Lunch: Thai Coconut Shrimp Soup (page 175)

Optional Snack: Homemade Almond Butter (page 128) on celery sticks

Dinner: Grass-Fed Beef Tenderloin Steaks with Sautéed Shiitakes (page 131); Wild Mushrooms and Onions (page 197)

## Week 1 Shopping List (no shakes)

### Proteins

Ahi tuna steaks

Boneless duck breasts

Cooked organic free-range boneless, skinless chicken breast

Fresh sardines

Grass-fed beef round roast

Grass-fed beef tenderloin steaks

Grass-fed flank steak

Grass-fed lean ground beef

Littleneck clams

Natural lean ground turkey

Natural lean pork loin

Nitrate-free bacon slices

Organic free-range bone-in, skinless chicken breast halves

Organic free-range whole chicken

Wild halibut fillet

Wild prawns or shrimp

Wild salmon fillets, such as king or sockeye

Wild sea scallops

Wild squid

## Vegetables/Fruits/Herbs

Apples

Avocados

Baby arugula

Baby spinach

Boston or romaine
lettuce leaves

Brussels sprouts

Campari or large vine-
ripened cherry
tomatoes

Carrots

Celery

Cremini mushrooms

Escarole

Fresh basil

Fresh cilantro

Fresh ginger

Fresh parsley

Fresh rosemary

Fresh spinach

Fresh tarragon

Fresh thyme

Garlic cloves

Grape tomatoes

Green onions

Japanese eggplants

Kale

Large onion

Large portobello
mushrooms

Large red bell pepper

Large shallots

Large Vidalia or other
sweet onion

Lemongrass

Lemons

Limes

Medium cucumbers

Medium fennel bulbs

Medium jalapeño
peppers

Medium onions

Medium red bell peppers

Medium red onion

Medium Vidalia or other
sweet onion

Medium yellow squash

Medium zucchini

Mixed greens
for salads

Napa cabbage

Orange

Oyster mushrooms

Plum tomatoes

Radishes

Red cabbage

Shiitake mushrooms

Small cucumber

Small fennel bulbs

Small green bell pepper

Small head romaine

Small jalapeño pepper

Small onions

Small red bell pepper

Small red onions

Small shallots

Small sweet potatoes

Snow peas

Tomatoes

Vegetables for crudités

White mushrooms

## Grains/Nuts/Seeds

Raw cashews

Raw hazelnuts

Raw pumpkin seeds

Slow-roasted almonds

Slow-roasted cashews

Slow-roasted pecans

## Milks

Plain cultured coconut milk

Unsweetened coconut milk

## *Week 1 Meal Plan (with shakes)*

### Day 1

Breakfast: Mixed Berry and Avocado Protein Shake (page 93)

Lunch: Nutty Chai Breakfast Blast Shake (page 97)

Optional Snack: Homemade Almond Butter (page 128) on apple slices

Dinner: Weeknight Cioppino (page 181); mixed green salad with Shallot–Champagne Vinaigrette (page 215)

### Day 2

Breakfast: Peach-Berry-Almond Protein Shake (page 95)

Lunch: Seafood Salad with Italian Salsa Verde (page 110)

Optional Snack: Roasted Jalapeño Guacamole with Toasted Pumpkin Seeds (page 121) and crudités

Dinner: Green Coconut Protein Shake (page 94)

### Day 3

Breakfast: Nutty Chai Breakfast Blast Shake (page 97)

Lunch: Chocolate-Cherry-Chia Protein Shake (page 94)

Optional Snack: Cinnamon Roasted Pecans (page 123)

Dinner: Chicken with 40 Cloves of Garlic (page 145); Italian-Style Escarole (page 208)

### Day 4

Breakfast: Rise and Shine Mocha Espresso Protein Shake (page 96)

Lunch: Chocolate-Cherry-Chia Protein Shake (page 94)

Optional Snack: Roasted Artichoke Dip (page 123) with crudités

Dinner: Mushroom Beef Stew★ (page 179)

### Day 5

Breakfast: Rise and Shine Mocha Espresso Protein Shake (page 96)

Lunch: Pounded Chicken Paillards Topped with Tomato and Fresh Basil Salad (page 147)

★Substitute additional beef broth for the red wine.

Optional Snack: Kale Chips with Cumin and Sea Salt (page 120)
Dinner: Green Coconut Protein Shake (page 94)

## Day 6

Breakfast: Bacon-and-Mushroom Sweet Potato Hash (page 91)
Lunch: Mixed Berry and Avocado Protein Shake (page 93)
Optional Snack: Sea Salt and Black Pepper Cashew Cheese (page 125) with crudités
Dinner: Strawberry "Milkshake" Protein Shake (page 95)

## Day 7

Breakfast: Peach-Berry-Almond Protein Shake (page 95)
Lunch: Green Coconut Protein Shake (page 94)
Optional Snack: Homemade Almond Butter (page 128) on celery sticks
Dinner: Grass-Fed Beef Tenderloin Steaks with Sautéed Shiitakes (page 131);
    Wild Mushrooms and Onions (page 197)

### *Week 1 Shopping List (with shakes)*

#### Proteins

Grass-fed beef round roast

Grass-fed beef tenderloin steaks

Littleneck clams

Nitrate-free bacon slices

Organic free-range boneless, skinless
    chicken breast halves

Organic free-range whole chicken

Wild halibut fillet

Wild prawns or shrimp

Wild sea scallops

Wild squid

#### Vegetables/Fruits/Herbs

Apples

Avocado

Baby arugula

Baby kale

Baby spinach

Campari or large vine-ripened cherry
    tomatoes

Carrots

Celery

Cremini mushrooms

Escarole

Fresh basil

Fresh cilantro

Fresh parsley

Fresh rosemary

Fresh tarragon

Fresh thyme

Garlic cloves

Kale

Large onion

Large shallot

Large Vidalia or other sweet onion

Lemons

Lime

Medium jalapeño peppers

Medium onions

Medium red bell pepper

Medium red onions

Medium Vidalia or other sweet onion

Mixed greens for salads

Oyster mushrooms

Shiitake mushrooms

Small fennel bulbs

Small plum tomato

Small red onions

Small shallots

Small sweet potatoes

Vegetables for crudités

White mushrooms

### Grains/Nuts/Seeds

Raw cashews

Raw pumpkin seeds

Slow-roasted almonds

Slow-roasted pecans

### Milks

Unsweetened almond milk

Unsweetened coconut milk

## Week 2 Meal Plan (no shakes)

### Day 1

Breakfast: Cilantro Turkey Burger with Chipotle Ketchup (page 150)

Lunch: Flank Steak Bistro Chopped Salad (page 105)

Optional Snack: Roasted Artichoke Dip (page 123) with crudités

Dinner: Dijon-and-Almond-Crusted Halibut with Lemon and Parsley (page 156); Cauliflower Puree (page 196)

### Day 2

Breakfast: Bacon-and-Mushroom Sweet Potato Hash (page 91)

Lunch: Asian Chicken in Lettuce Cups (page 146)

Optional Snack: Freeze-Dried Fruit, Nut, and Seed Mix (page 127)

Dinner: Pounded Chicken Paillards Topped with Tomato and Fresh Basil Salad (page 147)

## Day 3

Breakfast: Pan-Seared Scallops with Bacon and Spinach (page 155)

Lunch: Hearty Chicken Soup (page 169); mixed green salad with Toasted Macadamia Nut Dressing (page 216)

Optional Snack: Roasted Jalapeño Guacamole with Toasted Pumpkin Seeds (page 121) and crudités

Dinner: Meatballs in Tomato Sauce (page 133); Easy Spinach-and-Garlic Sauté (page 195)

## Day 4

Breakfast: Tex-Mex Burger with Avocado Salsa (page 134)

Lunch: Mediterranean Turkey-and-Peppers Skillet (page 149)

Optional Snack: Homemade Almond Butter (page 128) on celery sticks

Dinner: Blackened Salmon (page 159); Swiss Chard with Olives (page 200)

## Day 5

Breakfast: Grilled Dijon-Lemon Lamb Kabobs (page 140); Roasted Asparagus with Lemon Zest (page 198)

Lunch: Vietnamese Chicken-and-Cabbage Salad (page 109)

Optional Snack: Cinnamon Roasted Pecans (page 123)

Dinner: Halibut en Papillote (page 158); Cauliflower and Nut Stir-Fry (page 206)

## Day 6

Breakfast: Bacon-and-Mushroom Sweet Potato Hash (page 91)

Lunch: Gazpacho with Lump Crab (page 177)

Optional Snack: Classic Tapenade on Endive (page 122)

Dinner: BBQ Glazed Chicken (page 143); Roasted Cauliflower and Broccoli (page 202)

### Day 7

Breakfast: Cilantro Turkey Burger with Chipotle Ketchup (page 150; wrapped in lettuce)

Lunch: Poached Salmon with Rémoulade Sauce (page 160); Braised Kale (page 205)

Optional Snack: Babaganoush (page 118) with crudités

Dinner: Herb-Marinated Pork Chop with Balsamic Drizzle (page 138); Balsamic Roasted Vegetables (page 205)

## Week 2 Shopping List (no shakes)

### Proteins

Cooked organic free-range boneless, skinless chicken breast

Grass-fed flank steak

Grass-fed lean boneless leg of lamb

Grass-fed lean ground beef

Lump crabmeat

Natural lean boneless center-cut pork chops

Natural lean ground turkey

Natural turkey breast cutlets

Nitrate-free bacon slices

Organic free-range bone-in, skinless chicken thighs

Organic free-range bone-in, skinless chicken breast halves

Organic free-range boneless, skinless chicken breast halves

Organic free-range lean ground chicken

Wild halibut fillets

Wild sea scallops

Wild salmon fillets, such as king or sockeye

### Vegetables/Fruits/Herbs

Avocados

Asparagus

Baby arugula

Baby spinach

Belgian endive

Boston lettuce

Broccoli

Campari or large vine-ripened cherry tomatoes

Carrots

Cauliflower

Celery

Eggplants

Fresh basil

Fresh cilantro

Fresh ginger

Fresh marjoram

Fresh parsley

Fresh rosemary

Fresh sage

Fresh spinach

Fresh thyme

Garlic cloves

Grape tomatoes

Green onions

Jalapeño pepper

Japanese eggplants

Kale

Large red bell pepper

Leeks

Lemons

Limes

Medium cucumbers

Medium fennel bulb

Medium green bell pepper

Medium jalapeño peppers

Medium onions

Medium red bell peppers

Medium red onions

Medium Vidalia or other sweet onion

Medium yellow squash

Medium zucchini

Mixed greens for salads

Orange

Parsnip

Plum tomatoes

Radishes

Red cabbage

Romaine lettuce

Seedless cucumber

Shallots

Small jalapeño pepper

Small red onions

Small sweet potatoes

Swiss chard

Tomatoes

Vegetables for crudités

White mushrooms

### Grains/Nuts/Seeds

Pine nuts

Raw almonds

Raw macadamia nuts

Raw pumpkin seeds

Raw sunflower seeds

Slow-roasted almonds

Slow-roasted cashews

Slow-roasted pecans

### Milks

Unsweetened coconut milk

## Week 2 Meal Plan (with shakes)

### Day 1

Breakfast: Mixed Berry and Avocado Protein Shake (page 93)

Lunch: Flank Steak Bistro Chopped Salad (page 105)

Optional Snack: Roasted Artichoke Dip (page 123) with crudités

Dinner: Dijon-and-Almond-Crusted Halibut with Lemon and Parsley (page 156); Cauliflower Puree (page 196)

### Day 2

Breakfast: Bacon-and-Mushroom Sweet Potato Hash (page 91)

Lunch: Chocolate-Cherry-Chia Protein Shake (page 94)

Optional Snack: Freeze-Dried Fruit, Nut, and Seed Mix (page 127)

Dinner: Pounded Chicken Paillards Topped with Tomato and Fresh Basil Salad (page 147)

### Day 3

Breakfast: Nutty Chai Breakfast Blast Shake (page 97)

Lunch: Hearty Chicken Soup (page 169); mixed green salad with Toasted Macadamia Nut Dressing (page 216)

Optional Snack: Roasted Jalapeño Guacamole with Toasted Pumpkin Seeds (page 121) and crudités

Dinner: Meatballs in Tomato Sauce (page 133); Easy Spinach-and-Garlic Sauté (page 195)

### Day 4

Breakfast: Green Coconut Protein Shake (page 94)

Lunch: Mediterranean Turkey-and-Peppers Skillet (page 149)

Optional Snack: Homemade Almond Butter (page 128) on celery sticks

Dinner: Blackened Salmon (page 159); Swiss Chard with Olives (page 200)

### Day 5

Breakfast: Peach-Berry-Almond Protein Shake (page 95)

Lunch: Vietnamese Chicken-and-Cabbage Salad (page 109)

Optional Snack: Cinnamon Roasted Pecans (page 123)

Dinner: Halibut en Papillote (page 158); Cauliflower and Nut Stir-Fry (page 206)

### Day 6

Breakfast: Bacon-and-Mushroom Sweet Potato Hash (page 91)

Lunch: Strawberry "Milkshake" Protein Shake (page 95)

Optional Snack: Classic Tapenade on Endive (page 122)

Dinner: BBQ Glazed Chicken (page 143); Roasted Cauliflower and Broccoli (page 202)

## Day 7

Breakfast: Rise and Shine Mocha Espresso Protein Shake (page 96)

Lunch: Poached Salmon with Rémoulade Sauce (page 160); Braised Kale (page 205)

Optional Snack: Babaganoush (page 118) with crudités

Dinner: Herb-Marinated Pork Chop with Balsamic Drizzle (page 138); Balsamic Roasted Vegetables (page 205)

## Week 2 Shopping List (with shakes)

### Proteins

Cooked organic free-range boneless, skinless chicken breast

Grass-fed flank steak

Grass-fed lean ground beef

Natural lean boneless center-cut pork chops

Natural turkey breast cutlets

Nitrate-free bacon slices

Organic free-range bone-in, skinless chicken breast halves

Organic free-range bone-in, skinless chicken thighs

Organic free-range boneless, skinless chicken breast halves

Wild halibut fillets

Wild salmon fillets, such as king or sockeye

### Vegetables/Fruits/Herbs

Apples

Asparagus

Avocados

Baby arugula

Baby kale

Baby spinach

Belgian endive

Broccoli

Campari or large vine-ripened cherry tomatoes

Carrot

Cauliflower

Celery

Eggplant

Fresh basil

Fresh cilantro

Fresh parsley

Fresh rosemary

Fresh sage

Fresh spinach

Fresh thyme

Garlic cloves

Grape tomatoes

Green onions

Japanese eggplants

Kale

Large red bell pepper

Leeks

Lemons

Limes

Medium cucumbers

Medium fennel bulb

Medium green bell pepper

Medium jalapeño peppers

Medium onions

Medium red bell pepper

Medium red onions

Medium Vidalia or other sweet onion

Medium yellow squash

Medium zucchini

Mixed greens for salads

Orange

Parsnip

Radishes

Red cabbage

Romaine lettuce

Shallots

Small plum tomato

Small red onions

Small sweet potatoes

Swiss chard

Vegetables for crudités

White mushrooms

### Grains/Nuts/Seeds

Pine nuts

Raw almonds

Raw macadamia nuts

Raw pumpkin seeds

Raw sunflower seeds

Slow-roasted almonds

Slow-roasted cashews

Slow-roasted pecans

### Milks

Unsweetened almond milk

Unsweetened coconut milk

## Week 3 Meal Plan (no shakes)

### Day 1

Breakfast: Salmon Puttanesca (page 161)

Lunch: Shepherd's Salad with Prawns (page 106)

Optional Snack: Sea Salt and Black Pepper Cashew Cheese (page 125) with crudités

Dinner: Grilled Turkey Cutlet with Chimichurri (page 151); Cauliflower Puree (page 196)

### Day 2

Breakfast: Bacon-and-Mushroom Sweet Potato Hash (page 91)

Lunch: Seafood Salad with Italian Salsa Verde (page 110)

Optional Snack: Smoked Paprika and Cayenne Roasted Almonds (page 124)

Dinner: Coconut Red Curry Chicken (page 144); Braised Kale (page 205)

### Day 3

Breakfast: Turkey Meat Loaf with Kale (page 148); Cauliflower Puree (page 196)

Lunch: Scallion Shrimp Stir-Fry with Snow Peas (page 154; no brown rice)

Optional Snack: Homemade Almond Butter (page 128) on celery sticks

Dinner: Broiled Rosemary-and-Fennel Lamb Chop (page 140); Wild Mushrooms and Onions (page 197)

### Day 4

Breakfast: Grilled Fresh Sardines (page 162)

Lunch: Pork Tenderloin Fajitas* (page 136)

Optional Snack: Cinnamon Roasted Pecans (page 123)

Dinner: Slow Cooker Coq au Vin** (page 180)

### Day 5

Breakfast: Bacon-and-Mushroom Sweet Potato Hash (page 91)

Lunch: Seared Ahi Tuna over Asian Slaw (page 107)

Optional Snack: Kale Chips with Cumin and Sea Salt (page 120)

Dinner: Shallot-Thyme Marinated Flank Steak (page 132); Braised Kale (page 205)

### Day 6

Breakfast: Pan-Seared Scallops with Bacon and Spinach (page 155)

Lunch: Gazpacho with Lump Crab (page 177)

Optional Snack: Freeze-Dried Fruit, Nut, and Seed Mix (page 127)

Dinner: Grilled Dijon-Lemon Lamb Kabobs (page 140); Swiss Chard with Olives (page 200)

### Day 7

Breakfast: Tex-Mex Burger with Avocado Salsa (page 134), on a bed of mixed greens

Lunch: Spice-Rubbed Pulled Pork (page 137); Roasted Fennel and Onions (page 201)

*Use lettuce leaves to wrap.

**Replace the wine with chicken broth.

Optional Snack: Classic Tapenade on Endive (page 122)

Dinner: Lemon and Herb Broiled Sole (page 158); Cauliflower and Nut Stir-Fry (page 206)

## Week 3 Shopping List (no shakes)

### Proteins

Ahi tuna steaks

Fresh sardines

Grass-fed flank steak

Grass-fed lean bone-in loin lamb chops

Grass-fed lean boneless leg of lamb

Grass-fed lean ground beef

Lump crabmeat

Natural lean ground turkey

Natural lean pork loin

Natural lean pork tenderloin

Natural turkey breast cutlets

Nitrate-free bacon slices

Organic free-range bone-in, skinless chicken thighs

Organic free-range boneless, skinless chicken breast halves

Shrimp

Wild prawns

Wild salmon fillets, such as king or sockeye

Wild sea scallops

Wild sole fillets

Wild squid

### Vegetables/Fruits/Herbs

Avocado

Belgian endive

Boston or romaine lettuce leaves

Carrots

Cauliflower

Celery

Cremini mushrooms

Fresh basil

Fresh cilantro

Fresh ginger

Fresh marjoram

Fresh parsley

Fresh rosemary

Fresh thyme

Garlic cloves

Grape tomatoes

Green onions

Jalapeño pepper

Kale

Medium fennel bulbs

Large Vidalia or other sweet onion

Lemons

Limes

Medium green bell pepper

Medium onions

Medium red bell peppers

Medium red onions

Mini or Persian cucumbers

Mixed greens for salads

Napa cabbage

Oyster mushrooms

Plum tomatoes

Seedless cucumber

Shallots

Shiitake mushrooms

Small fennel bulb

Small jalapeño pepper

Small onions

Small red bell peppers

Small red onions

Small sweet potatoes

Snow peas

Swiss chard

Vegetables for crudités

White mushrooms

### Grains/Nuts/Seeds

Pine nuts

Raw cashews

Raw pumpkin seeds

Raw sunflower seeds

Slow-roasted almonds

Slow-roasted cashews

Slow-roasted pecans

### Milks

Plain cultured coconut milk

Unsweetened coconut milk

## Week 3 Meal Plan (with shakes)

### Day 1

Breakfast: Mixed Berry and Avocado Protein Shake (page 93)

Lunch: Shepherd's Salad with Prawns (page 106)

Optional Snack: Sea Salt and Black Pepper Cashew Cheese (page 125) with crudités

Dinner: Grilled Turkey Cutlet with Chimichurri (page 151); Cauliflower Puree (page 196)

### Day 2

Breakfast: Bacon-and-Mushroom Sweet Potato Hash (page 91)

Lunch: Chocolate-Cherry-Chia Protein Shake (page 94)

Optional Snack: Smoked Paprika and Cayenne Roasted Almonds (page 124)

Dinner: Coconut Red Curry Chicken (page 144); Braised Kale (page 205)

### Day 3

Breakfast: Green Coconut Protein Shake (page 94)

Lunch: Scallion Shrimp Stir-Fry with Snow Peas★ (page 154)

Optional Snack: Homemade Almond Butter (page 128) on celery sticks

Dinner: Broiled Rosemary-and-Fennel Lamb Chops (page 140); Wild Mushrooms and Onions (page 197)

### Day 4

Breakfast: Peach-Berry-Almond Protein Shake (page 95)

Lunch: Pork Tenderloin Fajitas★★ (page 136)

Optional Snack: Cinnamon Roasted Pecans (page 123)

Dinner: Slow Cooker Coq au Vin★★★ (page 180)

### Day 5

Breakfast: Bacon-and-Mushroom Sweet Potato Hash (page 91)

Lunch: Strawberry "Milkshake" Protein Shake (page 95)

Optional Snack: Kale Chips with Cumin and Sea Salt (page 120)

Dinner: Shallot-Thyme Marinated Grilled Flank Steak (page 132); Braised Kale (page 205)

### Day 6

Breakfast: Nutty Chai Breakfast Blast Shake (page 97)

Lunch: Gazpacho with Lump Crab (page 177)

Optional Snack: Freeze-Dried Fruit, Nut, and Seed Mix (page 127)

Dinner: Grilled Dijon-Lemon Lamb Kabobs (page 140); Swiss Chard with Olives (page 200)

### Day 7

Breakfast: Rise and Shine Mocha Espresso Protein Shake (page 96)

Lunch: Spice-Rubbed Pulled Pork (page 137); Roasted Fennel and Onions (page 201)

★No brown rice.

★★Use lettuce leaves to wrap.

★★★Replace wine with chicken broth.

Optional Snack: Classic Tapenade on Endive (page 122)

Dinner: Lemon and Herb Broiled Sole (page 158); Cauliflower and Nut Stir-Fry (page 206)

## Week 3 Shopping List (with shakes)

### Proteins

Grass-fed flank steak

Grass-fed lean bone-in loin lamb chops

Grass-fed lean boneless leg of lamb

Lump crabmeat

Natural lean pork loin

Natural lean pork tenderloin

Natural turkey breast cutlets

Nitrate-free bacon slices

Organic free-range bone-in, skinless chicken thighs

Organic free-range boneless, skinless chicken breast halves

Wild prawns

Wild shrimp

Wild sole fillets

### Vegetables/Fruits/Herbs

Apples

Avocado

Baby kale

Baby spinach

Belgian endive

Carrots

Cauliflower

Celery

Cremini mushrooms

Fresh basil

Fresh cilantro

Fresh ginger

Fresh marjoram

Fresh parsley

Fresh rosemary

Fresh thyme

Garlic cloves

Green onions

Jalapeño peppers

Kale

Large Vidalia or other sweet onion

Lemons

Lime

Medium fennel bulbs

Medium green bell pepper

Medium onions

Medium plum tomatoes

Medium red bell peppers

Medium red onions

Mini or Persian cucumbers

Mixed greens for salads

Oyster mushrooms

Peaches

Seedless cucumber

Shallots

Shiitake mushrooms

Small onion
Small red bell pepper
Small red onions
Small sweet potatoes

Snow peas
Swiss chard
Vegetables for crudités
White mushrooms

### Grains/Nuts/Seeds

Pine nuts
Raw cashews
Raw pumpkin seeds
Raw sunflower seeds

Slow-roasted almonds
Slow-roasted cashews
Slow-roasted pecans

### Milks

Plain cultured coconut milk
Unsweetened almond milk
Unsweetened coconut milk

## Staples List (no shakes)

### Oils and Vinegars

Asian sesame oil
Coconut oil
Extra-virgin olive oil
Macadamia nut oil
Malaysian red palm fruit oil
Balsamic vinegar

Champagne vinegar
Cider vinegar
Red wine vinegar
White balsamic vinegar
White wine vinegar

### Spices

Arrowroot
Bay leaf
Cayenne pepper
Chili powder
Cinnamon
Coriander
Crushed red pepper flakes
Dried basil

Dried oregano
Dried thyme
Freshly ground black pepper
Garlic powder
Ground allspice
Ground chipotle pepper
Ground cumin
Onion powder

Saffron threads

Sea salt

Smoked paprika

Sweet paprika

### Extracts

Monk fruit extract

### Grains/Seeds

Fennel seeds

Gluten-free oats

Quinoa linguine

### Jarred and Canned

Anchovies in oil

Canned organic, non-GMO
    unsweetened coconut milk

Capers

Chili garlic sauce

Chipotle peppers in adobo sauce

Coconut aminos

Dijon mustard

Fish sauce

Green curry paste

Kalamata olives

Low-sodium vegetable juice

Organic low-sodium beef broth

Organic low-sodium chicken broth

Organic tahini paste

Picholine olives

Red curry paste (such as Thai Kitchen)

Tabasco sauce

(6-oz) cans organic tomato paste

(8-oz) bottle clam juice

(8-oz) cans organic tomato sauce

(14.5-oz) cans organic diced tomatoes

(28-oz) cans organic crushed tomatoes

### Frozen

Artichoke hearts

Organic spinach

Pearl onions

### Miscellaneous

Organic freeze-dried blueberries

Organic freeze-dried raspberries

Organic freeze-dried strawberries

## *Staples List (with shakes)*

### Protein Powders

Chai vegan protein powder

Chocolate vegan protein powder

Vanilla vegan protein powder

### Oils and Vinegars

Coconut oil

Extra-virgin olive oil

Macadamia nut oil

Malaysian red palm fruit oil

Balsamic vinegar

Champagne vinegar

Cider vinegar

Red wine vinegar

White balsamic vinegar

White wine vinegar

### Spices

Arrowroot

Cayenne pepper

Chili powder

Cinnamon

Coriander

Crushed red pepper
flakes

Dried basil

Dried oregano

Dried thyme

Freshly ground black
pepper

Garlic powder

Ground allspice

Ground chipotle pepper

Ground cumin

Saffron threads

Sea salt

Smoked paprika

Sweet paprika

### Extracts

Almond extract

Coconut extract

Monk fruit extract

Vanilla extract

### Grains/Seeds

Chia seeds

Fennel seeds

Flaxseeds

Quinoa linguine

## Jarred and Canned

Anchovies in oil

Capers

Cashew butter

Chili garlic sauce

Coconut aminos

Dijon mustard

Fish sauce

Kalamata olives

Low-sodium vegetable juice

Organic low-sodium beef broth

Organic low-sodium chicken broth

Organic tahini paste

Picholine olives

Red curry paste (such as Thai Kitchen)

Tabasco sauce

(6-oz) cans organic tomato paste

(8-oz) bottle clam juice

(14.5-oz) cans organic diced tomatoes

(28-oz) cans organic crushed tomatoes

## Frozen

Artichoke hearts

Organic blueberries

Organic dark cherries

Organic mixed berries

Organic peaches

Organic strawberries, unsweetened

Pearl onions

## Miscellaneous

Instant espresso/coffee powder

Organic freeze-dried blueberries

Organic freeze-dried raspberries

Organic freeze-dried strawberries

I know this drill well. You spend most of your days feeling as if you've been shot out of a cannon. As you race from a crazy afternoon at the office to grab your son at soccer practice and then pick up your daughter from her track meet, it dawns on you that you have no idea what's for dinner. It's after five and you're approaching famished. At this point, a drive-thru burger sounds awfully tempting, and you know your kids would love you for it.

Stay strong! As a single mom with two teenage boys, I know what it's like to feel overwhelmed. As priorities go, dinner often gets short shrift. But when that happens, so does your family's health.

I know every night can't be a Rockwellian family dinner, but I'm sure you can set aside a few nights—okay, even *one night*—a week to eat together. Whether you're laughing or bickering around the table, you'll be strengthening the bonds that make you a family. In today's fast-faster frenzy, family dinner may be the only time you really hear and see each other.

The meal is just as important as your time together. On those harried days (*every day?*), it can feel as though the only path is the one of least resistance and that a pepperoni deep dish is your salvation. But you're making choices that impact your family's health, and every one counts. Give them the fuel they need to build strong, healthy bodies. Besides, your kids follow your example, and there will be a big payoff for you down the road when you see them modeling your stellar food choices.

Trust me: There's nothing much more important than feeding your family well. Researchers at the American Society for Nutrition looked at sixty-eight studies about family mealtime and children's health. Among their findings, which they presented at Scientific Sessions in San Diego, California: Kids who have more family meals get more fruits, vegetables, fiber, calcium-rich foods, and vitamins. They are less likely to reach for junk food than their friends. Researchers even found family mealtime helped reduce obesity![1]

So now that we agree that feeding your family nutritious meals is worth investing in, I'm going to walk it back a little. Don't feel like it has to be an all-or-nothing descent into battle every day. If you get some push-back when you try to pull the family together for dinner, or even over the meals themselves, there's no need for a meltdown. You'll win some and you'll lose some. Do your best and don't sweat it if it doesn't go your way.

## HOW THE VIRGIN DIET CAN HELP

I designed the Virgin Diet for fast and lasting fat loss. But I've also made the guidelines flexible so they work with any eating plan, in any situation. Which is just what a crazy-busy family like yours needs! I've chosen the most nutrient-rich, whole, delicious foods to help you burn fat and discover (and *maintain*) the vibrant health you and your family deserve.

One mom recently told me her kids weren't overweight and that they were actually really athletic. Was she trying to tell me she didn't think they'd benefit from the Virgin Diet? Not exactly. She said what she loves about the Virgin Diet is that *she* can eat delicious food for fat loss and also give it to her kids so they stay lean and healthy and well fueled for sports. She said the diet also sets a great example and is helping her kids learn good habits for life. Well, that's it in a nutshell, isn't it? That mom nailed the Virgin Diet's versatility and flexibility.

Breakfast can feel overwhelming when you're running against the clock and kids are flying out the door. So I totally get why many families resort to sugary cereals and other easy-access foods. Unfortunately, those foods spike and crash blood sugar, and the results of that reveal themselves midmorning at school, when your kids become lethargic, mentally foggy, and start clawing for the birthday cupcakes their classmate brought in.

In about the time it takes to pour cereal and milk, you can whip up a fast, filling Virgin Diet Shake. Kids love the sweetness of frozen berries, raw cacao nibs, and almond butter. You can even slip some kale into the mix and they'll never know! The nutrient-rich protein/good fats/fiber combo steadies blood sugar so they're focused

1. http://www.eurekalert.org/pub releases/2012-04/foas-rfa041812.php.

and not craving whatever sweet treats their classmates snuck in (no promise their grades will improve, but it's a possibility!).

Family meals are also a cinch. The Virgin Diet Plate takes the guesswork out of planning and preparing healthy, delicious food. Simply follow my Plate formula with clean protein, good fats, low-glycemic veggies, and slow-release high-fiber carbs. With a little creativity and a few lateral shifts, you can checkerboard the plate with different choices to your heart's content, knowing you can never get the "tasty" and "healthy" parts of the equation wrong.

Let's say your child wants burgers and fries. Upgrade to grass-fed beef in gluten-free wraps with sweet potato fries. Chicken fingers? Buy free-range chicken and "bread" them with almond or coconut flour. If your kid has a hankering for pasta, try spaghetti squash or corn-free quinoa pasta instead. Not every swap will slip by them unnoticed, but you'll hit healthy home runs that your child won't turn their nose up at, and you'll have peace of mind knowing you're giving them the foundation for a strong, healthy life.

## STEP IT UP WITH THESE STRATEGIES

1. **Involve your kids.** Relieve yourself of top-chef duties with your kids' help. Assigning them tasks—chopping, slicing, or, for the littlest ones, setting the table—makes them feel important and reduces your burden. Be patient, allow a wide margin for error, and provide praise for a job well done.

2. **Plan ahead.** Mealtime stress often comes from a lack of preparation. Eliminate that sinking *What's for dinner?* feeling by creating a meal plan. On Saturday or Sunday, make a list of your grocery essentials, buy everything in one fell swoop (bulk purchases save you time and money), and begin prep work on Sunday night. When you have organic chicken and garlic green beans planned for Tuesday night, you're less likely to stress or succumb to takeout on the way home.

3. **Don't be perfect.** In an ideal world, each meal would have you serving up plated perfection, like fresh, organic vegetables and wild salmon, seasoned to please even your pickiest eater. Of course, your kids would also praise your culinary efforts, devour their broccoli, and joyfully clean their rooms to repay your herculean efforts. Reality check: Your world is not perfect, kids will occasionally resist healthy

foods, and some nights you'll stop by Whole Foods for a rotisserie chicken and vegetables. Do your best and you'll probably find that "good enough" is better than it sounds.

4. **Make a no-media rule.** Endless distractions and the white noise of the TV and video games can make family time seem more like just people in the same room. I get it: Sometimes merely being together is enough. But trust me, your son's soccer game is more interesting than a stock market crash or your best friend's text dishing about a bad date. Be present and make a no-gadgets rule at the dinner table.

5. **Make it fun.** If you're a drill sergeant, your kids will greet dinner with the same enthusiasm as a visit to the dentist. Instead, create a fun, relaxed environment that combines kid-friendly (animal shapes!), healthy favorites. Try broccoli trees and hummus sharks (hummus with kale chips), or make an apple butter wheel (almond butter between apple slices).

6. **Double up.** Planning dinner can be hassle enough. Afterward, the last thought on your mind is what to make for tomorrow's lunch. Make it easy and create extras for the next day's lunchboxes. The grilled chicken you made for dinner goes easily in a gluten-free wrap with some guacamole. Add some raw almonds and fresh blueberries for a simple, healthy, kid-friendly lunch.

7. **Rinse and repeat.** As you well know from your own successful New Year's resolutions, creating a new habit takes daily consistency and persistence. Likewise, repeated exposure can turn your kids on to broccoli or kimchi. (Okay, maybe not kimchi!) Experts estimate it may take twelve times of eating a particular food for your kids to like it. I take the middle ground here: While I don't want to turn the dinner table into a battleground, my kids must try a bite of everything before they leave the table. You may have more misses than hits, but if you turn them on to quinoa or a new vegetable, you've hit a home run.

8. **Exploit their tastes.** Kids gravitate to sweet and salty foods. Try drizzling marinara on their cauliflower or sprinkling goat cheese (if they're not dairy sensitive) on their broccoli. A little olive or coconut oil gives rich flavor to spinach and other veggies. Ever tried faux-tatoes (pureed cauliflower) as a nutrient-rich mashed potato alternative? Kids also love the natural sweetness of sweet potatoes sprinkled with cinnamon.

**9. Keep it at eye level.** The journal *Environment and Behavior*[2] reported a study, involving 96 college kids, where fruits and veggies in clear or opaque bowls were placed either nearby or about 7 feet away from students. No surprise: The closer bowls got more action. Trust me, if researchers could get college students to eat healthier, there's hope for your finicky kids. For snacking, keep fresh fruit, hummus and kale chips, and veggies with guacamole on your coffee table or another accessible area, and you'll likely find they reach for healthy foods more often.

For additional meal plans tailored to specific conditions and lifestyle needs, visit thevirgindietcookbook.com/bonus.

## WEEK 1 MEAL PLAN

### Day 1

Breakfast: Green Coconut Protein Shake (page 94)—make double and take in thermos for lunch

Lunch: Green Coconut Protein Shake

Optional Snack: Freeze-Dried Fruit, Nut, and Seed Mix (page 127)

Dinner: Grilled Dijon-Lemon Lamb Kabobs (page 140); Roasted Sweet Potato Salad (page 114); Roasted Cauliflower and Broccoli (page 202)

### Day 2

Breakfast: Mixed Berry and Avocado Protein Shake (page 93)—make double and take in thermos for lunch

Lunch: Mixed Berry and Avocado Protein Shake

Optional Snack: Kale Chips with Cumin and Sea Salt (page 120)

Dinner: Chicken Sloppy Joes over Brown Rice (page 144); Braised Kale (page 205)

### Day 3

Breakfast: Peach-Berry-Almond Protein Shake (page 95)—make double and take in thermos for lunch

Lunch: Peach-Berry-Almond Protein Shake

2. G. J. Privitera et al., "Proximity and visibility of fruits and vegetables influence intake in a kitchen setting among college students," *Environment and Behavior* 45, no. 7 (Oct. 2013): 876–86.

Optional Snack: Freeze-Dried Fruit, Nut, and Seed Mix (page 127)

Dinner: Easy Pasta Bolognese (page 135); mixed green salad with Toasted Macadamia Nut Dressing (page 216)

## Day 4

Breakfast: Nutty Chai Breakfast Blast Shake (page 97)—make double and take in thermos for lunch

Lunch: Nutty Chai Breakfast Blast Shake

Optional Snack: Cinnamon Roasted Pecans (page 123)

Dinner: Pan-Seared Scallops with Bacon and Spinach (page 155); Confetti Quinoa (page 186)

## Day 5

Breakfast: Chocolate-Cherry-Chia Protein Shake (page 94)—make double and take in thermos for lunch

Lunch: Chocolate-Cherry-Chia Protein Shake

Optional Snack: Homemade Almond Butter (page 128) on apple slices

Dinner: Minestrone Soup (page 172); Salmon Puttanesca (page 161) over spaghetti squash

## Day 6

Breakfast: Strawberry "Milkshake" Protein Shake (page 95)—make double and take in thermos for lunch

Lunch: Strawberry "Milkshake" Protein Shake

Optional Snack: Babaganoush (page 118) with rice crackers

Dinner: Turkey Meat Loaf with Kale (page 148); Roasted Acorn Squash Puree (page 192); Balsamic Roasted Vegetables (page 205)

## Day 7

Breakfast: Mixed Berry and Avocado Protein Shake (page 93)—make double and take in thermos for lunch

Lunch: Mixed Berry and Avocado Protein Shake

Optional Snack: Cinnamon Roasted Pecans (page 123)

Dinner: Mushroom Bisque (page 178); Mushroom Lentil Loaf with Barbecue Glaze (page 164)

# WEEK 1 SHOPPING LIST

### Proteins

Grass-fed lean boneless leg of lamb

Grass-fed lean ground beef

Natural lean ground turkey

Nitrate-free bacon slices

Organic free-range lean ground chicken

Wild salmon fillets, such as king or sockeye

Wild sea scallops

### Vegetables/Fruits/Herbs

Acorn squash

Apples

Assorted wild mushrooms

Avocados

Baby kale

Baby spinach

Carrots

Cauliflower

Celery

Cremini mushrooms

Eggplants

Fennel

Fresh marjoram

Fresh parsley

Fresh thyme

Garlic cloves

Grape tomatoes

Japanese eggplants

Kale

Large red bell pepper

Large shallot

Lemons

Medium green bell pepper

Medium head broccoli

Medium onions

Medium orange bell pepper

Medium red bell peppers

Medium red onions

Medium sweet potatoes

Medium yellow bell pepper

Medium yellow squash

Medium zucchini

Mixed greens for salads

Orange

Shallots

Small onions

Small red bell pepper

Spaghetti squash

Veggies for crudités

White mushrooms

### Grains/Nuts/Seeds

Raw macadamia nuts

Raw pumpkin seeds

Raw sunflower seeds

Slow-roasted almonds

Slow-roasted cashews

Slow-roasted pecans

Milks

Unsweetened almond milk

Unsweetened coconut milk

# WEEK 2 MEAL PLAN

### Day 1

Breakfast: Blueberry Power Muffin (page 87) with a side of nitrate-free chicken breakfast sausage

Lunch: Mixed Berry and Avocado Protein Shake (page 93)—take in thermos

Optional Snack: Kale Chips with Cumin and Sea Salt (page 120)

Dinner: Creamy Sweet Potato Soup (page 173); Blackened Salmon (page 159); Braised Kale (page 205)

### Day 2

Breakfast: Peach-Berry-Almond Protein Shake (page 95)

Lunch: Chicken Caesar Salad Wrap (page 100) and crudités

Optional Snack: Roasted Red Pepper Hummus (page 118) with crudités or rice crackers

Dinner: Cilantro Turkey Burger with Chipotle Ketchup (page 150); Butternut Squash "Fries" (page 185); mixed green salad with Toasted Macadamia Nut Dressing (page 216)

### Day 3

Breakfast: Bacon-and-Mushroom Sweet Potato Hash (page 91)

Lunch: Green Coconut Protein Shake (page 94)—take in thermos

Optional Snack: Homemade Almond Butter (page 128) with apple slices

Dinner: Slow Cooker Coq au Vin (page 180); Red Quinoa with Kale, Onions, and Pine Nuts (page 190)

### Day 4

Breakfast: Nutty Chai Breakfast Blast Shake (page 97)

Lunch: Chicken Salad Wrap (page 101) with crudités

Optional Snack: Freeze-Dried Fruit, Nut, and Seed Mix (page 127)

Dinner: Easy Pasta Bolognese (page 135); mixed green salad with Shallot-Champagne Vinaigrette (page 215)

## Day 5

Breakfast: Swedish-Style Pecan Pancakes with Orange and Strawberries (page 89), with a side of nitrate-free chicken breakfast sausage

Lunch: Strawberry "Milkshake" Protein Shake (page 95)—take in thermos

Optional Snack: Cinnamon Roasted Pecans (page 123)

Dinner: Broiled Rosemary-and-Fennel Lamb Chops (page 140); Roasted Root Vegetables with Thyme (page 193); Cauliflower Puree (page 196)

## Day 6

Breakfast: Chocolate-Cherry-Chia Protein Shake (page 94)

Lunch: Vegetarian Chili (page 166); mixed green salad with Shallot-Champagne Vinaigrette (page 215)

Optional Snack: Homemade Almond Butter (page 128) with apple slices

Dinner: Minestrone Soup (page 172); Chicken with 40 Cloves of Garlic (page 145); Cauliflower and Nut Stir-Fry (page 206)

## Day 7

Breakfast: Hot Quinoa Flake Cereal with Warm Berry Compote (page 90), with a side of nitrate-free bacon

Lunch: Mixed Berry and Avocado Protein Shake (page 93)—take in thermos

Optional Snack: Sea Salt and Black Pepper Cashew Cheese (page 125) with rice crackers

Dinner: Grilled Marinated Duck Breasts (page 153); Orange-Scented Mashed Sweet Potatoes with Coconut (page 188); Roasted Brussels Sprouts with Hazelnuts (page 194)

## WEEK 2 SHOPPING LIST

### Proteins

Boneless duck breasts

Grass-fed lean bone-in loin lamb chops

Grass-fed lean ground beef

Natural lean ground turkey

Nitrate-free bacon slices

Nitrate-free chicken breakfast sausages

Organic free-range bone-in, skinless chicken thighs

Organic free-range boneless, skinless chicken breast halves

Organic free-range whole chicken

Wild salmon fillets, such as king or sockeye

### Vegetables/Fruits/Herbs

Apples

Avocados

Baby kale

Baby spinach

Brussels sprouts

Butternut squash

Carrots

Cauliflower

Celery

Extra-large onion

Fresh basil

Fresh blueberries (or use frozen)

Fresh cilantro

Fresh ginger

Fresh rosemary

Fresh strawberries

Fresh thyme

Garlic cloves

Green onions

Kale

Lemons

Medium green bell pepper

Medium onions

Medium red bell pepper

Medium red onions

Medium sweet potatoes

Medium zucchini

Mixed greens for salads

Oranges

Romaine lettuce

Small fennel bulb

Small shallots

Small sweet potatoes

Tomatoes

Vegetables for crudités

White mushrooms

White turnip

### Grains/Nuts/Seeds

Brown rice tortillas

Pine nuts

Raw cashews

Raw hazelnuts

Raw macadamia nuts

Raw pecans

Raw pumpkin seeds

Raw sunflower seeds

Raw walnuts

Slow-roasted almonds

Slow-roasted cashews

Slow-roasted pecans

### Milks

Unsweetened almond milk

Unsweetened coconut milk

## WEEK 3 MEAL PLAN

**Day 1**

Breakfast: Bacon-and-Mushroom Sweet Potato Hash (page 91)

Lunch: Green Coconut Protein Shake (page 94)—take in thermos

Optional Snack: Kale Chips with Cumin and Sea Salt (page 120)

Dinner: Lemon and Herb Broiled Sole (page 158); Roasted Asparagus with Lemon Zest (page 198); Confetti Quinoa (page 186)

**Day 2**

Breakfast: Nutty Chai Breakfast Blast Shake (page 97)

Lunch: Tex-Mex Turkey Wrap with Salsa, Avocado, and Arugula (page 104), with crudités

Optional Snack: Cinnamon Roasted Pecans (page 123)

Dinner: Meatballs in Tomato Sauce (page 133) on quinoa pasta; Italian-Style Escarole (page 208)

**Day 3**

Breakfast: Blueberry Power Muffin (page 87) with a side of nitrate-free chicken breakfast sausage

Lunch: Mixed Berry and Avocado Protein Shake (page 93)—take in thermos

Optional Snack: Freeze-Dried Fruit, Nut, and Seed Mix (page 127)

Dinner: Mushroom Beef Stew (page 179); mixed green salad with Toasted Macadamia Nut Dressing (page 216)

**Day 4**

Breakfast: Peach-Berry-Almond Protein Shake (page 95)

Lunch: Vegetarian Chili (page 166); mixed green salad with Toasted Macadamia Nut Dressing (page 216)

Optional Snack: Homemade Almond Butter (page 128) with apple slices

Dinner: Turkey Meat Loaf with Kale (page 148); Butternut Squash "Fries" (page 185); Cauliflower Puree (page 196)

Day 5

Breakfast: Swedish-Style Pecan Pancakes with Orange and Strawberries
(page 89), with a side of nitrate-free chicken breakfast sausage

Lunch: Strawberry "Milkshake" Protein Shake (page 95)—take in thermos

Optional Snack: Roasted Red Pepper Hummus (page 118) with crudités

Dinner: Stir-Fried Shrimp with Ginger, Black Beans, and Cashews (page 157);
Vegetable Fried Rice (page 187)

Day 6

Breakfast: Chocolate-Cherry-Chia Protein Shake (page 94)

Lunch: Chicken Caesar Salad Wrap (page 100) with crudités

Optional Snack: Babaganoush (page 118) with rice crackers

Dinner: Herb-Marinated Pork Chop with Balsamic Drizzle (page 138);
Roasted Sweet Potato Salad (page 114); Balsamic Roasted Vegetables
(page 205)

Day 7

Breakfast: Hot Quinoa Flake Cereal with Warm Berry Compote (page 90)

Lunch: Strawberry "Milkshake" Protein Shake (page 95)

Optional Snack: Roasted Jalapeño Guacamole with Toasted Pumpkin Seeds
(page 121), with rice chips

Dinner: Chicken Sloppy Joes over Brown Rice (page 144); Roasted Cauliflower
and Broccoli (page 202)

## WEEK 3 SHOPPING LIST

### Proteins

Deli-sliced nitrate-free turkey breast

Grass-fed beef round roast

Grass-fed lean ground beef

Natural lean boneless center-cut pork
chops

Natural lean ground turkey

Nitrate-free bacon slices

Nitrate-free chicken breakfast sausage

Organic free-range boneless, skinless
chicken breast halves

Organic free-range lean ground
chicken

Wild shrimp

Wild sole fillets

## Vegetables/Fruits/Herbs

Asparagus

Apples

Avocados

Baby arugula

Baby kale

Baby spinach

Broccoli

Butternut squash

Cauliflower

Celery

Eggplants

Escarole

Fresh blueberries (can use frozen)

Fresh cilantro

Fresh ginger

Fresh parsley

Fresh sage

Fresh strawberries

Fresh thyme

Garlic cloves

Green onions

Japanese eggplants

Kale

Large onion

Large red bell pepper

Large shallot

Lemons

Limes

Medium green bell peppers

Medium jalapeño peppers

Medium onions

Medium orange bell pepper

Medium plum tomatoes

Medium red bell peppers

Medium red onions

Medium sweet potatoes

Medium yellow bell pepper

Medium yellow squash

Medium zucchini

Mixed greens for salads

Napa cabbage

Shiitake mushrooms

Small onions

Small oranges

Small plum tomato

Small sweet potato

Vegetables for crudités

White mushrooms

## Grains/Nuts/Seeds

Brown rice tortillas

Raw almonds

Raw macadamia nuts

Raw pecans

Raw pumpkin seeds

Raw sunflower seeds

Slow-roasted almonds

Slow-roasted cashews

Slow-roasted pecans

## Milks

Unsweetened almond milk

Unsweetened coconut milk

## STAPLES LIST

### Protein Powders

Chai vegan protein powder

Chocolate vegan protein powder

Vanilla vegan protein powder

### Oils and Vinegars

Asian sesame oil

Coconut butter

Coconut oil

Extra-virgin olive oil

Macadamia nut oil

Malaysian red palm fruit oil

Balsamic vinegar

Champagne vinegar

Cider vinegar

Sherry vinegar

White wine vinegar

### Spices

Allspice

Arrowroot

Bay leaves

Cayenne pepper

Chili powder

Cinnamon

Crushed red pepper flakes

Dried basil

Dried oregano

Dried thyme

Freshly ground black pepper

Garlic powder

Ground ancho chile pepper

Ground chipotle pepper

Ground coriander

Ground cumin

Ground nutmeg

Onion powder

Sea salt

Smoked paprika

Sweet paprika

### Extracts

Almond extract

Coconut extract

Monk fruit extract

Stevia extract

Vanilla extract

### Grains/Seeds

Bob's Red Mill Gluten-Free All-Purpose Baking Flour

Brown rice

Chia seeds

Dry quinoa

Flaxseeds

Fennel seeds
Gluten-free oats
Quinoa flakes cereal
Quinoa linguine pasta

Quinoa pasta of choice
Quinoa pasta shells
Red quinoa
Rice crackers

## Jarred and Canned

Canned chipotle pepper in adobo sauce
Capers
Cashew butter
Coconut aminos
Dijon mustard
Kalamata olives
Oil-packed anchovies
Organic low-sodium beef broth
Organic low-sodium chicken broth
Organic low-sodium vegetable broth
Organic tahini paste
Roasted red peppers
Tabasco sauce

(4.5-oz) cans organic diced tomatoes
(6-oz) cans organic tomato paste
(8-oz) cans organic tomato sauce
(14.5-oz) cans organic fire-roasted diced tomatoes
(15-oz) cans organic no-salt-added black beans
(15-oz) cans organic no-salt-added cannellini beans
(15-oz) cans organic no-salt-added chickpeas (garbanzo beans)
(15-oz) cans organic no-salt-added red kidney beans
(28-oz) cans organic diced tomatoes

## Frozen

Organic blueberries
Organic dark cherries
Organic mixed berries
Organic peaches

Organic spinach
Organic strawberries, unsweetened
Pearl onions

## Miscellaneous

Aluminum-free baking powder
Baking soda
Organic freeze-dried blueberries
Organic freeze-dried raspberries
Organic freeze-dried strawberries

# ON THE GO 18

If you're like me, "on the road" doesn't bring Jack Kerouac to mind; it stirs up premature anxiety about how I'm going to survive a gauntlet of airport pubs without packing on pounds and slogging through sugar crashes. If I were queen of the world, road-trip calories wouldn't count. But, sigh, they do.

Whether I'm doing a cross-country book tour or taking a rare vacation, I'm away from home a lot. I also know what it means to be scheduled wall-to-wall (anyone?), and to hear the siren call of the drive-thru during a long commute. That means there's probably not a dietary disaster you can come up with that I haven't faced. And you know from your own experience that eating well when you're crazy busy or when you travel can be a major challenge (yes, I also have relatives who think a healthy breakfast consists of low-fat pancakes drowned in "lite" syrup with bananas).

So let's tackle this head-on. Finding grass-fed beef or quinoa pasta or wild salmon at even the best hotel or airport restaurant isn't always easy—okay, sometimes it's almost *impossible*. To make matters worse, restaurant fare is filled with food-intolerance land mines. News flash—chefs don't always play by the Virgin Diet rules! They liberally infuse food with ingredients that may trigger a reaction...and stick to your hips.

But over the years I've learned how to navigate everything from hole-in-the-wall diners, where the menus themselves are dripping with grease, to airport kiosks where pesticide-ridden iceberg lettuce is the only green vegetable. And I'm going to help you do the same.

With the strategies I've developed, you'll always have a way to dodge diet-busting calorie grenades like a food superhero, even in the face of a double bacon cheeseburger and greasy fries during a 3-hour airport delay, or fettuccine Alfredo at your carb-loving in-laws'. While you can't control a delayed flight or mysteriously canceled hotel reservation, you do have the means to make wise decisions about what you eat, no matter where you are. And with a little creativity and know-how, even a fast-food restaurant can become a relatively healthy haven.

A little planning before you hit the road (or before a hectic week with little time to prepare meals every night) can also save you major hassles and potential dietary disaster. I scope out the locations of my favorites like Whole Foods or Chipotle because I know I can get consistent, fast, healthy meals there, no matter what city I'm in. When I don't have those options, I travel armed with nutrient-dense portable foods that keep me full and focused so food doesn't become a hassle or a preoccupation.

Along the way, I've racked up millions of frequent-flier miles and some effective strategies to help navigate the worst culinary travel nightmare with ease and, dare I say, pleasure.

## HOW THE VIRGIN DIET CAN HELP

I designed the Virgin Diet with the most challenging situations in mind, and traveling tops that list. I mean, why is breakfast on the road so frustrating when all you want is a healthy protein source that hasn't been sitting under a heat lamp for hours and doesn't cost more than your last grocery bill? Is that too much to ask? Not anymore! The Virgin Diet Shake is your answer.

I always travel with plant-based (but not soy) all-in-one protein powder, little cartons of unsweetened coconut milk, and my favorite travel accessory, the Magic Bullet blender. I skip the $18 continental breakfasts and the morning coffee shop lines for a fast, filling breakfast in minutes and for less money than a bottle of designer water.

Whether you're dining out or eating at your long-lost cousin's family reunion, you'll follow that same strategy for your meals, using the Virgin Diet Plate to help you plot a route through the road-food obstacle course. Look at menus as suggestions, not absolutes. Maybe the filet mignon comes with spinach and mashed potatoes. Easy: Swap the starch for a second green vegetable.

Gargantuan restaurant salads notoriously come loaded with crunchy, creamy, sweet toppings that make them more like desserts. Switch the candied bits for avocado and walnuts, and ask for your dressing on the side. I love salads customized with grilled chicken, avocado, salsa, and black beans.

You'll quickly get the hang of this formula, and even fast-food and hotel-pub ventures will become Virgin Diet–friendly encounters. With a little improvisation, you can make even the most diet-hostile situation work in your favor.

## STEP IT UP WITH THESE STRATEGIES

1. **Do your research.** An Internet search followed by a phone call can eliminate on-the-road culinary confusion and frustration. If you're dining with high-end clients in a new city, research the restaurant ahead of time and figure out your healthiest choice. A quick call to the restaurant will let you know whether they'll make accommodations for food intolerances or make substitutions. That way you can focus on your clients while everyone else is studying the menu.

2. **Don't dashboard-dine.** Racing to the airport for a 6 a.m. flight provides little time for a sit-down breakfast, but resist the temptation to devour a biscuit sandwich or low-fat muffin while you're multitasking on your drive. You're only inviting indigestion and other gut-related issues, not to mention the catastrophic ride you're sending your blood sugar on. A meta-analysis in the *American Journal of Clinical Nutrition*[1] showed that mindfulness when you eat helps you burn more fat. Crowded airports and other on-the-go conveniences almost encourage eat-and-run situations, but you'll benefit if you slow down and give your food the attention it deserves.

3. **Ask your server questions.** I've been there, and so have you: You order an innocuous-sounding chicken breast and it arrives breaded or drowning in a syrupy sweet sauce. Questioning your server might seem impolitic, but it's far less hassle and embarrassing than sending a dish back. Be nice but firm, not interrogating (think Sally, in *When Harry Met Sally*), and remember that what you put in your mouth is *your* responsibility regardless of whether what's on your plate is or isn't what you ordered.

4. **Keep emergency food nearby.** You're stuck at a conference where the speaker drones into the lunch hour, or maybe your pilot alerts passengers you'll be sitting on the tarmac for 45 minutes. Hunger crashes your blood sugar and makes hectic

1. E. Robinson et al., "Eating attentively: A systematic review and meta-analysis of the effect of food intake memory and awareness on eating," *American Journal of Clinical Nutrition* 97, no. 4 (Apr. 2013): 728–42, doi: 10.3945/ajcn.112.045245. Epub 2013 Feb 27.

travel situations even more miserable. Not to mention you're vulnerable and more likely to grab the nearest stale pastry to tide you over until your meal. Don't even put yourself in that position. Keep healthy snacks in your bag or car. Some of my favorite on-the-go munchies include raw nuts and seeds, nitrate-free jerky, almond butter in individual packets with apple slices or celery, and, if you won't eat for several hours, aseptic-packed wild salmon.

**5. Stay hydrated.** Coffee is often synonymous with travel and chances are that even when you're well rested, you stay amped up on caffeine to keep you moving. Airplanes, hotels, and new climates create dehydration, which your morning dark roast, coupled with last night's pinot noir, only exacerbates. Keep purified water with you and sip it throughout the day so you're not suffering brain fog and other miseries of dehydration. Many hotel gyms provide filtered water, so I travel with a water bottle and refill there.

**6. Get enough sleep.** Noisy, uncomfortable hotel rooms, changing time zones, and red-eyes with screaming toddlers are three of the many reasons restful sleep becomes challenging and sometimes downright impossible on the road. Even one night's poor sleep can knock your fat-burning hormones out of whack, leaving you irritable and hyper-caffeinated the following morning. Turn off your laptop and use the hour before bed to relax with a hot bath, chamomile tea, and deep breathing or meditation. Earplugs, an eye mask, and even a noise machine can become the best friends that help you get steady, optimal slumber in less-than-conducive travel environments.

**7. Don't neglect exercise.** Ditching your workout is all too easy when you have a jam-packed travel schedule, whether you're sightseeing or stuck in hotel meetings. But being on the road *isn't an excuse to blow off* exercise—you need it to handle the stress, keep your energy up, and ensure you don't curse the scales once you get home. If you don't have an hour to spend at your hotel gym, you can do burst training in the stairwell or my travel *4x4 Workout* in your hotel room. (Find it at JJVirgin.com/4x4workout.) And wear a pedometer and take every opportunity to move more. Manage your time well so exercise becomes a top priority, no matter how hectic your schedule.

For additional meal plans tailored to specific conditions and lifestyle needs, visit thevirgindietcookbook.com/bonus.

## WEEK 1 MEAL PLAN

**Day 1**

Breakfast: Green Coconut Protein Shake (page 94)—make double and take in
thermos

Lunch: Green Coconut Protein Shake

Optional Snack: Cinnamon Roasted Pecans (page 123)

Dinner: Weeknight Cioppino (page 181)—make extra for tomorrow's dinner;
serve with mixed green salad and Shallot-Champagne Vinaigrette (page 215)

**Day 2**

Breakfast: Rise and Shine Mocha Espresso Protein Shake (page 96)—make
double and take in thermos

Lunch: Rise and Shine Mocha Espresso Protein Shake

Optional Snack: Freeze-Dried Fruit, Nut, and Seed Mix (page 127)

Dinner: Weeknight Cioppino (from last night); with mixed green salad and
Shallot-Champagne Vinaigrette (page 215)

**Day 3**

Breakfast: Peach-Berry-Almond Protein Shake (page 95)—make double and take
in thermos

Lunch: Peach-Berry-Almond Protein Shake

Optional Snack: Smoked Paprika and Cayenne Roasted Almonds (page 124)

Dinner: Chicken with 40 Cloves of Garlic (page 145)—make extra for Hearty
Chicken Soup (page 169); Easy Spinach-and-Garlic Sauté (page 195)—make
extra for tomorrow's dinner; Curried Lentils (page 190)—make extra for
tomorrow's dinner

**Day 4**

Breakfast: Nutty Chai Breakfast Blast Shake (page 97)—make double and take in
thermos

Lunch: Nutty Chai Breakfast Blast Shake

Optional Snack: Freeze-Dried Fruit, Nut, and Seed Mix (page 127)

Dinner: Hearty Chicken Soup (page 169)—freeze extra for next week's lunch; serve
with Easy Spinach-and-Garlic Sauté and Curried Lentils (both from last night)

### Day 5

Breakfast: Chocolate-Cherry-Chia Protein Shake (page 94)—make double and take in thermos

Lunch: Chocolate-Cherry-Chia Protein Shake

Optional Snack: Cinnamon Roasted Pecans (page 123)

Dinner: Mushroom Beef Stew (page 179)—make extra and freeze for next week

### Day 6

Breakfast: Strawberry "Milkshake" Protein Shake (page 95)—make double and take in thermos

Lunch: Strawberry "Milkshake" Protein Shake

Optional Snack: Freeze-Dried Fruit, Nut, and Seed Mix (page 127)

Dinner: Coconut Red Curry Chicken (page 144)—make extra and freeze for next week; Vegetable Fried Rice (page 187)—make extra and freeze for next week; serve with a mixed green salad with Toasted Macadamia Nut Dressing (page 216)

### Day 7

Breakfast: Mixed Berry and Avocado Protein Shake (page 93)—make double and take in thermos

Lunch: Mixed Berry and Avocado Protein Shake

Optional Snack: Freeze-Dried Fruit, Nut, and Seed Mix (page 127)

Dinner: Turkey Chili (page 182)—make extra and freeze for next week; serve with mixed green salad and Toasted Macadamia Nut Dressing (page 216)

## WEEK 1 SHOPPING LIST

### Proteins

Grass-fed beef round roast

Littleneck clams

Natural lean ground turkey

Organic free-range bone-in, skinless chicken thighs

Organic free-range boneless, skinless chicken breast halves

Organic free-range whole chicken

Wild halibut fillet

Wild prawns

### Vegetables/Fruits/Herbs

| | | |
|---|---|---|
| Apples | Fresh thyme | Mixed greens for salad |
| Avocados | Fresh rosemary | Parsnip |
| Baby kale | Garlic cloves | Shiitake mushrooms |
| Baby spinach | Green onions | Small fennel bulb |
| Carrot | Large green bell pepper | Small shallots |
| Celery | Large onion | Small onions |
| Fresh basil | Leeks | Small sweet potato |
| Fresh cilantro | Medium onions | Snow peas |
| Fresh ginger | Medium plum tomatoes | Vegetables for crudités |
| Fresh spinach | Medium red bell peppers | White mushrooms |

### Grains/Nuts/Seeds

| | |
|---|---|
| Raw macadamia nuts | Slow-roasted almonds |
| Raw pumpkin seeds | Slow-roasted cashews |
| Raw sunflower seeds | Slow-roasted pecans |

### Milks

Unsweetened almond milk
Unsweetened coconut milk

## WEEK 2 MEAL PLAN

### Day 1

Breakfast: Blueberry Power Muffin (page 87) with a side of nitrate-free chicken breakfast sausage

Lunch: Mixed Berry and Avocado Protein Shake (page 93)

Optional Snack: Cinnamon Roasted Pecans (page 123)

Dinner: Easy Pasta Bolognese (page 135)—double recipe; pack for tomorrow's lunch; serve with Balsamic Roasted Vegetables (page 205)—double recipe; add to pasta for tomorrow's lunch

### Day 2

Breakfast: Nutty Chai Breakfast Blast Shake (page 97)

Lunch: Easy Pasta Bolognese with Balsamic Roasted Vegetables (from last night)

Optional Snack: Freeze-Dried Fruit, Nut, and Seed Mix (page 127)—double recipe for 3 days of snacks

Dinner: Poached Salmon with Rémoulade Sauce (page 160)—double recipe for tomorrow's lunch; Roasted Fennel and Onions (page 201); Confetti Quinoa (page 186)

### Day 3

Breakfast: Rise and Shine Mocha Espresso Protein Shake (page 96)

Lunch: Poached Salmon with Rémoulade Sauce, on a bed of greens

Optional Snack: Freeze-Dried Fruit, Nut, and Seed Mix (page 127)

Dinner: Mushroom Beef Stew (in freezer from Week 1); mixed green salad with Toasted Macadamia Nut Dressing (page 216)

### Day 4

Breakfast: Blueberry Power Muffin (page 87) with a side of nitrate-free chicken breakfast sausage

Lunch: Hearty Chicken Soup (in freezer from Week 1) with crudités

Optional Snack: Cinnamon Roasted Pecans (page 123)

Dinner: Green Coconut Protein Shake (page 94)

### Day 5

Breakfast: Chocolate-Cherry-Chia Protein Shake (page 94)

Lunch: Turkey Chili (in freezer from Week 1) with crudités

Optional Snack: Smoked Paprika and Cayenne Roasted Almonds (page 124)

Dinner: Coconut Red Curry Chicken and Vegetable Fried Rice (both in freezer from Week 1); mixed green salad with Toasted Macadamia Nut Dressing (page 216)

### Day 6

Breakfast: Peach-Berry-Almond Protein Shake (page 95)

Lunch: Chicken Salad Wrap (page 101) with crudités

Optional Snack: Freeze-Dried Fruit, Nut, and Seed Mix (page 127)

Dinner: Cilantro Turkey Burger with Chipotle Ketchup (page 150)—double burgers and freeze extra patties for next week; Butternut Squash "Fries" (page 185); Cauliflower Puree (page 196)

### Day 7

Breakfast: Blueberry Power Muffin (page 87) with a side of nitrate-free chicken breakfast sausage
Lunch: Strawberry "Milkshake" Protein Shake (page 95)
Optional Snack: Smoked Paprika and Cayenne Roasted Almonds (page 124)
Dinner: Pan-Seared Scallops with Bacon and Spinach (page 155); Vegetable Fried Rice (page 187)—double recipe for tomorrow's dinner

## WEEK 2 SHOPPING LIST

### Proteins

Grass-fed beef round roast

Grass-fed lean ground beef

Natural lean ground turkey

Nitrate-free bacon slices

Nitrate-free chicken breakfast sausages

Organic free-range boneless, skinless chicken breast halves

Wild salmon fillets, such as king or sockeye

Wild sea scallops

### Vegetables/Fruits/Herbs

Apples

Avocados

Baby kale

Baby spinach

Butternut squash

Carrot

Cauliflower

Celery

Fresh basil

Fresh blueberries (or use frozen)

Fresh cilantro

Fresh ginger

Fresh parsley

Fresh thyme

Garlic cloves

Green onions

Japanese eggplants

Large onion

Large red bell pepper

Large shallots

Lemons

Medium fennel bulbs

Medium onions

Medium orange bell pepper

Medium plum tomatoes

Medium red bell peppers

Medium red onion

Medium yellow bell pepper

Medium yellow squash

Medium zucchini

Mixed greens for salad

Shallots

Shiitake mushrooms

Small onions

Small sweet potato

Snow peas

Tomatoes

Vegetables for crudités

White mushrooms

### Grains/Nuts/Seeds

Brown rice tortillas

Raw almonds

Raw macadamia nuts

Raw pumpkin seeds

Raw sunflower seeds

Raw walnuts

Slow–roasted almonds

Slow-roasted cashews

Slow-roasted pecans

### Milks

Unsweetened almond milk

Unsweetened coconut milk

## WEEK 3 MEAL PLAN

### Day 1

Breakfast: Nutty Chai Breakfast Blast Shake (page 97)

Lunch: Hearty Chicken Soup (page 169)

Optional Snack: Freeze-Dried Fruit, Nut, and Seed Mix (page 127)

Dinner: Coconut Red Curry Chicken (page 144); Vegetable Fried Rice (left over from last night)

### Day 2

Breakfast: Chocolate-Cherry-Chia Protein Shake (page 94)

Lunch: Cilantro Turkey Burger with Chipotle Ketchup (in freezer from Week 2), with crudités

Optional Snack: Cinnamon Roasted Pecans (page 123)

Dinner: Mushroom Beef Stew (page 179)

### Day 3

Breakfast: Rise and Shine Mocha Espresso Protein Shake (page 96)

Lunch: Turkey Chili (page 182) with crudités

Optional Snack: Smoked Paprika and Cayenne Roasted Almonds (page 124)

Dinner: Scallion Shrimp Stir-Fry with Snow Peas (page 154); Vegetable Fried Rice (page 187)—double rice recipe for next 2 days

## Day 4

Breakfast: Blueberry Power Muffin (page 87) with a side of nitrate-free chicken breakfast sausage

Lunch: Green Coconut Protein Shake (page 94)

Optional Snack: Cinnamon Roasted Pecans (page 123)

Dinner: Thai Coconut Shrimp Soup (page 175)—double recipe for tomorrow's lunch; Vegetable Fried Rice (from yesterday); mixed greens and cabbage with Sesame-Ginger Vinaigrette (page 216)

## Day 5

Breakfast: Peach-Berry-Almond Protein Shake (page 95)

Lunch: Thai Coconut Shrimp Soup (from yesterday); Vegetable Fried Rice (from Day 3)

Optional Snack: Freeze-Dried Fruit, Nut, and Seed Mix (page 127)

Dinner: Shallot-Thyme Marinated Flank Steak (page 132); Wild Mushrooms and Onions (page 197)—double recipe and add to tomorrow's salad; Spice Roasted Sweet Potatoes (page 187)

## Day 6

Breakfast: Strawberry "Milkshake" Protein Shake (page 95)

Lunch: Flank Steak Bistro Chopped Salad (page 105) with Wild Mushrooms and Onions (from yesterday)

Optional Snack: Smoked Paprika and Cayenne Roasted Almonds (page 124)

Dinner: Slow Cooker Coq au Vin (page 180)—double recipe for tomorrow night's dinner

## Day 7

Breakfast: Blueberry Power Muffin (page 87) with a side of nitrate-free chicken breakfast sausage

Lunch: Mixed Berry and Avocado Protein Shake (page 93)

Optional Snack: Cinnamon Roasted Pecans (page 123)

Dinner: Coq au Vin (from last night)

## WEEK 3 SHOPPING LIST

### Proteins

Grass-fed beef round roast

Grass-fed flank steak

Natural lean ground turkey

Nitrate-free bacon slices

Nitrate-free chicken breakfast sausages

Organic free-range bone-in, skinless chicken thighs

Organic free-range boneless, skinless chicken breast halves

Wild shrimp

### Vegetables/Fruits/Herbs

Apple

Avocado

Baby kale

Baby spinach

Carrots

Celery

Cremini mushrooms

Fresh basil

Fresh blueberries (or use frozen)

Fresh cilantro

Fresh ginger

Fresh rosemary

Fresh thyme

Garlic cloves

Green onions

Large green bell pepper

Large onion

Large Vidalia onions (or other sweet onion)

Leeks

Lemongrass

Lime

Medium cucumber

Medium onions

Medium plum tomatoes

Medium red bell peppers

Medium shallot

Medium sweet potatoes

Mixed greens for salad

Oyster mushrooms

Parsnip

Radishes

Romaine lettuce

Shiitake mushrooms

Small onions

Small red onion

Small sweet potato

Snow peas

Vegetables for crudités

White mushrooms

### Grains/Nuts/Seeds

Raw almonds

Raw pumpkin seeds

Raw sunflower seeds

Slow-roasted almonds

Slow-roasted cashews

Slow-roasted pecans

### Milks

Unsweetened almond milk

Unsweetened coconut milk

## STAPLES LIST

### Protein Powders

Chai vegan protein powder

Chocolate vegan protein powder

Vanilla vegan protein powder

### Oils and Vinegars

Asian sesame oil

Coconut butter

Coconut oil

Extra-virgin olive oil

Macadamia nut oil

Malaysian red palm fruit oil

Balsamic vinegar

Champagne vinegar

Cider vinegar

Rice vinegar

Sherry vinegar

White balsamic vinegar

White wine vinegar

### Spices

Allspice

Arrowroot

Bay leaves

Cayenne pepper

Chili powder

Cinnamon

Coriander

Crushed red pepper flakes

Curry powder

Dried basil

Dried oregano

Freshly ground black pepper

Garlic powder

Ground cumin

Onion powder

Saffron threads

Sea salt

Smoked paprika

### Extracts

Almond extract

Coconut extract

Monk fruit extract

Vanilla extract

### Grains/Seeds/Legumes

Bob's Red Mill Gluten-Free All-Purpose Flour

Brown rice

Chia seeds

Dry quinoa

Dry, sprouted lentils

Flaxseeds

Gluten-free oats

Quinoa linguine pasta

Sesame seeds

### Jarred and Canned

Canned chipotle peppers in adobo
sauce

Capers

Cashew butter

Chile garlic sauce

Coconut aminos

Dijon mustard

Fish sauce

Green curry paste

Organic low-sodium beef broth

Organic low-sodium chicken broth

Red curry paste (such as Thai Kitchen)

Tabasco sauce

Unsweetened organic, non-GMO
coconut milk

(6-oz) cans organic tomato paste

(8-oz) bottles clam juice

(8-oz) cans organic tomato sauce

(14.5-oz) cans fire-roasted diced
tomatoes

(14.5-oz) cans organic diced tomatoes

(15-oz) cans organic no-salt-added red
kidney beans

(28-oz) cans organic diced tomatoes

### Frozen

Organic blueberries

Organic dark cherries

Organic mixed berries

Organic peaches

Organic strawberries, unsweetened

White pearl onions

(10-oz) packages frozen organic
spinach

### Miscellaneous

Aluminum-free baking powder

Instant espresso/coffee powder

Organic freeze-dried blueberries

Organic freeze-dried raspberries

Organic freeze-dried strawberries

# ON A BUDGET  19

You know that putting yourself in the best possible position to achieve your weight loss and health goals comes down to a very simple idea: choosing some foods over others. The right food will propel you to health greatness; it will heal your food intolerances, launch your fat-burning machinery, steady your blood sugar, and combat disease.

But there's no getting around it: That food can be more expensive. And if your paycheck isn't keeping pace with climbing food costs, it can be easy to get discouraged. Many of my clients feel the same squeeze. When you're struggling to pay bills, put gas in the car, and still put a meal on the table every night, organic broccoli and grass-fed beef can feel out of reach.

But my clients are making it work. So how are they doing it? With the strategies I'm going to give you here.

## HOW THE VIRGIN DIET CAN HELP

I designed the Virgin Diet to be practical, easy, and, yes, affordable. I'm going to go out on a limb and suggest *you may even save money* doing the Virgin Diet because you'll no longer be stuffing your cart with overpriced processed foods. Or stocking up on over-the-counter anti-inflammatories and digestive aids. And let's be honest, do you have any idea how much you really spend on those Danish-y add-ons at the coffee shop? The steady drip of those mindless purchases adds up to a big leak from your wallet when all is said and done. On the other side of the ledger, you're getting lean and healthy, which is priceless.

Let's start with breakfast. This one could not be easier or more economical: the

Virgin Diet Shake. For less than a venti dark roast and about the same amount of time you'd stand in line for one, you can make a delicious, filling, fat-burning protein shake. Park the blender on the counter so it's always ready for plant-based (but not soy) protein powder with frozen berries, kale, and chia seeds or flaxseeds in unsweetened coconut or almond milk. Whir away!

For other meals, the geometry of the Virgin Diet Plate guides you through the ideal amounts of clean, lean protein; good fats; low-glycemic veggies; and slow-release high-fiber carbs. Some foods—say, grass-fed beef or wild salmon—might be more expensive in isolation, but on the whole I bet your grocery bill will be roughly the same or even lower.

Another way to ease the strain on your piggy bank is to get some mileage out of your leftovers. We often toss extra food without a second thought, but it can really add up. What you don't eat today can carry you through another meal or two tomorrow and save you time and money in the bargain. That goes for eating out, too. Don't feel pressure to join the clean plate club! Take a doggie bag and enjoy that delicious dinner for lunch the next day. You can also plan for leftovers: Buy in bulk to get the best price, make extra when you cook, then freeze and applaud yourself for being frugal while not giving up a thing in taste or nutrition.

Sugary sodas, individually packaged snacks, and most "convenience" foods in the center aisles have an astronomical markup and deliver little economic value (and certainly no nutritional value). They empty your wallet, balloon your waistline, and set you up for big bills at the doctor's office down the road.

Here's another thing. Many foods on the Virgin Diet are high in fiber, which delays gastric emptying, balances blood sugar, and curbs your appetite. When you eat less, you buy less! Opt for inexpensive fiber-full foods that fill you up faster, like beans, lentils, nuts and seeds, and leafy greens, to meet your 50-gram daily quota. And here's one of my little fat-loss, penny-pinching secrets: 30 to 60 minutes before your meal, stir chia seeds or a fiber powder into a glass of water and drink it. You'll eat less and stretch your food budget!

There's a bigger picture here, too. Eating with "cheap" as your guiding principle in grocery shopping allows toxins and inflammatory foods to sneak into your diet and slowly take a toll on your weight and health over time. Even if healthy food initially seems more expensive, think of it as *buying you health*—which, as you know, is true wealth. When you invest in better food, you invest in you; you'll have a better quality of life (if not a longer one) with fewer health issues, which is money in the bank and peace of mind in the long run.

So let's agree that the extra-value meal hardly provides value when you evaluate its impact on your weight, health, and energy. Making smart choices doesn't demand half your paycheck or that you shop at arcane, expensive health food stores. With the right strategies, you can downsize your food budget while you supersize your health.

## STEP IT UP WITH THESE STRATEGIES

1. **Start your day with a protein shake.** It's quick, cheap, and easy to make, so enjoy a filling, yummy, fat-burning protein shake every morning. Blend plant-based (but not soy) protein powder with frozen berries, kale, and chia seeds or flaxseeds in unsweetened coconut or almond milk.

2. **Eat seasonally and local.** Besides being fresher, locally grown, and more nutrient-rich, seasonal produce usually costs less. Learn your food seasons: Asparagus peaks in spring, while blueberries are best in summer and apples are tastiest in the fall.

3. **Stock up on frozen.** Even though manufacturers have stepped up quality from the soggy, grayish spinach that might haunt you from childhood, frozen produce still gets a bad rap. Unlike fresh produce that goes bad quickly (talk about throwing money away!), you can visit your nearby warehouse store or supermarket during a sale to stock (preferably organic) frozen foods that keep in your freezer for months.

4. **Join a farmers' collective or co-op.** If you have a few hours to spare each month, volunteer at a food co-op. They usually compensate with discounts; you'll have first dibs on fresh, locally grown foods; and you'll probably make a few like-minded friends in the bargain. During warmer weather, stock up on barnyard-raised eggs, grass-fed beef, and fresh produce while getting to know the folks who grow and raise your food.

5. **Make your own.** Salad dressings, spices, and other condiments often contain hidden gluten, soy, dairy, and other ingredients that could sabotage fat loss and your health. You can easily make many of them on your own, saving you time and providing peace of mind that you aren't getting any additives, preservatives, or highly reactive ingredients.

**6. Get a slow cooker.** Especially in cold weather, stews, soups, and other all-in-one-pot meals make easy, inexpensive, satisfying options for your whole family. Be creative and load them with green vegetables and starchy carbs. I have a hybrid of stew and soup that I call "stoup"; you can prepare it in a slow cooker, portion and refrigerate it, and *voilà*! You've got several days' worth of satisfying, money-saving, healthy meals.

**7. Bypass the fancy coffee stores.** People-watching and custom-crafted drinks can make loitering at the coffee shop stimulating (pun!), but a daily habit can take a major hit on your finances. Just one venti green tea daily could tally up to over $100 a month! Brewing your own coffee or tea provides better quality control and environmental friendliness (no paper cups!) for far less money. Opt for organic and switch to decaf if that second cup of breakfast blend keeps you wired at night.

**8. Dine and split.** Cooking your own food saves money and keeps dubious ingredients from slipping into your meals. Still, even the most budget-conscious person needs to splurge occasionally. Restaurants notoriously serve gargantuan portions, so splitting an entrée saves you money and calories. You can always ask your server to divide that filet mignon and sautéed spinach between two plates. If you're dining alone, ask for a doggie bag and portion half for your dinner the next day. Who says there's no such thing as a free lunch?

**9. Less meat, more plant-based foods.** In the Virgin Diet, I encourage you to choose only the best-quality meats and fish, like grass-fed beef and wild salmon. But they can add up, especially if you're trying to feed a family. Rather than buy lower-quality, conventionally produced meats or fish, pile more green veggies, good fats (like avocados), and starchy high-fiber carbs on your plate.

**10. Don't snack.** I have clients tally the money they spend on snacks and they're often shocked at the total. Don't snack unless you absolutely must. You'll save calories and money.

**11. Shop warehouse stores for bulk buys.** Make a list and stick to it; don't be lured in by other "bargains."

**12. Learn when organic is optional and when it isn't.** The Environmental Working Group (ewg.org) has done us all a great service by identifying what they call the "Dirty Dozen" and the "Clean Fifteen." The Dirty Dozen are foods that you absolutely must buy organic because they're more likely to be genetically modified or heavily sprayed. You can also grab a great non-GMO shopping guide through the Institute for Responsible Technology at instituteforresponsibletechnology.org. And of course, when you get to know your local farmers and ranchers, you'll know firsthand how your food is grown.

For additional meal plans tailored to specific conditions and lifestyle needs, visit thevirgindietcookbook.com/bonus.

## WEEK 1 MEAL PLAN

### Day 1
Breakfast: Mixed Berry and Avocado Protein Shake (page 93)
Lunch: Green Coconut Protein Shake (page 94)
Optional Snack: Kale Chips with Cumin and Sea Salt (page 120)
Dinner: Lentil Nut Burger with Cilantro Vinaigrette (page 163); mixed green salad

### Day 2
Breakfast: Rise and Shine Mocha Espresso Protein Shake (page 96)
Lunch: Chocolate-Cherry-Chia Protein Shake (page 94)
Optional Snack: Homemade Almond Butter (page 128) on apple slices
Dinner: Turkey Meat Loaf with Kale (page 148); Cauliflower Puree (page 196); Butternut Squash "Fries" (page 185)

### Day 3
Breakfast: Strawberry "Milkshake" Protein Shake (page 95)
Lunch: Mixed Berry and Avocado Protein Shake (page 93)
Optional Snack: Babaganoush (page 118) with rice crackers
Dinner: Easy Pasta Bolognese (page 135); Italian-Style Escarole (page 208)

### Day 4
Breakfast: Nutty Chai Breakfast Blast Shake (page 97)
Lunch: Peach-Berry-Almond Protein Shake (page 95)

Optional Snack: Roasted Red Pepper Hummus (page 118) with crudités

Dinner: Chicken Sloppy Joes over Brown Rice (page 144); Roasted Cauliflower and Broccoli★ (page 202)

## Day 5

Breakfast: Rise and Shine Mocha Espresso Protein Shake (page 96)

Lunch: Green Coconut Protein Shake (page 94)

Optional Snack: Smoked Paprika and Cayenne Roasted Almonds (page 124)

Dinner: Lemon and Herb Broiled Sole (page 158); Chickpeas with Spinach, Lemon, and Tomatoes (page 191)

## Day 6

Breakfast: Peach-Berry-Almond Protein Shake (page 95)

Lunch: Chocolate-Cherry-Chia Protein Shake (page 94)

Optional Snack: Kale Chips with Cumin and Sea Salt (page 120)

Dinner: BBQ Glazed Chicken (page 143); Braised Kale (page 205); Jicama, Apple, and Pear Slaw★★ (page 114)

## Day 7

Breakfast: Nutty Chai Breakfast Blast Shake (page 97)

Lunch: Strawberry "Milkshake" Protein Shake (page 95)

Optional Snack: Smoky Black Bean Hummus (page 119) with crudités

Dinner: Scallion Shrimp Stir-Fry with Snow Peas (page 154); Vegetable Fried Rice (page 187)

# WEEK 1 SHOPPING LIST

### Proteins

Grass-fed lean ground beef

Natural lean ground turkey

---

★Swap out the macadamia nut oil for palm fruit oil or coconut oil, whichever you can find on sale!

★★Swap out the macadamia nut oil for palm fruit oil or coconut oil, whichever you can find on sale!

Nitrate-free bacon slices
Organic free-range bone-in, skinless chicken breast halves
Organic free-range lean ground chicken
Wild shrimp
Wild sole fillets

### Vegetables/Fruits/Herbs

Apples
Avocados
Baby kale
Baby spinach
Butternut squash
Carrots
Cauliflower
Celery
Eggplants
Escarole
Fresh cilantro
Fresh ginger
Fresh parsley
Garlic cloves
Grape tomatoes
Green cabbage
Green onions

Jicama
Kale
Lemons
Limes
Medium green bell pepper
Medium head broccoli
Medium onions
Medium plum tomato
Mixed greens for salads
Orange
Pear
Red cabbage
Small onions
Snow peas
Vegetables for crudités
White mushrooms

### Grains/Nuts/Seeds

Raw walnuts
Slow-roasted almonds

### Milks

Unsweetened almond milk
Unsweetened coconut milk

## WEEK 2 MEAL PLAN

### Day 1

Breakfast: Chocolate-Cherry-Chia Protein Shake (page 94)

Lunch: Flank Steak Bistro Chopped Salad (page 105)

Optional Snack: Homemade Almond Butter (page 128) with apple slices

Dinner: Chicken with 40 Cloves of Garlic (page 145); Roasted Root Vegetables with Thyme (page 193); mixed green salad with olive oil and fresh-squeezed lemon juice

### Day 2

Breakfast: Blueberry Power Muffin (page 87) with a side of nitrate-free chicken breakfast sausage

Lunch: Peach-Berry-Almond Protein Shake (page 95)

Optional Snack: Smoked Paprika and Cayenne Roasted Almonds (page 124)

Dinner: Mushroom Bisque (page 178); Mushroom Lentil Loaf with Barbecue Glaze (page 164)

### Day 3

Breakfast: Hot Quinoa Flake Cereal with Warm Berry Compote (page 90)

Lunch: Green Coconut Protein Shake (page 94)

Optional Snack: Kale Chips with Cumin and Sea Salt (page 120)

Dinner: Mushroom Beef Stew (page 179)

### Day 4

Breakfast: Swedish-Style Pecan Pancakes with Orange and Strawberries (page 89), with a side of nitrate-free chicken breakfast sausage

Lunch: Strawberry "Milkshake" Protein Shake (page 95)

Optional Snack: Roasted Red Pepper Hummus (page 118) with crudités

Dinner: Creamy Sweet Potato Soup (page 173); Blackened Salmon (page 159); Roasted Cauliflower and Broccoli (page 202)

### Day 5

Breakfast: Rise and Shine Mocha Espresso Protein Shake (page 96)

Lunch: Vietnamese Chicken-and-Cabbage Salad (page 109)

Optional Snack: Smoked Paprika and Cayenne Roasted Almonds (page 124)

Dinner: Pork Tenderloin Fajitas (page 136)

## Day 6

Breakfast: Nutty Chai Breakfast Blast Shake (page 97)

Lunch: Chickpea Falafel Salad with Tahini Dressing (page 112)

Optional Snack: Homemade Almond Butter (page 128) with apple slices

Dinner: Turkey Meat Loaf with Kale (page 148); Cauliflower Puree (page 196); Spice Roasted Sweet Potatoes (page 187)

## Day 7

Breakfast: Mixed Berry and Avocado Protein Shake (page 93)

Lunch: Turkey Chili (page 182); mixed green salad with olive oil and fresh-squeezed lemon juice

Optional Snack: Smoky Black Bean Hummus (page 119) with crudités

Dinner: Scallion Shrimp Stir-Fry with Snow Peas (page 154); Vegetable Fried Rice (page 187)

## WEEK 2 SHOPPING LIST

### Proteins

Cooked organic free-range boneless, skinless chicken breast

Grass-fed beef round roast

Grass-fed flank steak

Natural lean ground turkey

Natural lean pork tenderloin

Nitrate-free chicken breakfast sausages

Whole organic free-range chicken

Wild salmon fillets, such as king or sockeye

Wild shrimp

### Vegetables/Fruits/Herbs

Apples

Assorted wild mushrooms

Avocados

Baby arugula

Baby kale

Baby spinach

Broccoli

Butternut squash

Carrots

Cauliflower

Celery

Cremini mushrooms

Fresh basil

Fresh blueberries (or use frozen)

| | | |
|---|---|---|
| Fresh cilantro | Lemons | Red cabbage |
| Fresh ginger | Limes | Romaine lettuce |
| Fresh parsley | Medium cucumbers | Shallot |
| Fresh rosemary | Medium green bell pepper | Shiitake mushrooms |
| Fresh strawberries | Medium onions | Small onions |
| Fresh thyme | Medium red bell peppers | Small orange |
| Garlic cloves | Medium red onion | Small red bell pepper |
| Grape tomatoes | Medium sweet potatoes | Small red onions |
| Green onions | Mixed greens for salad | Small sweet potatoes |
| Kale | Mixed spring greens | Snow peas |
| Large cucumber | Orange | Vegetables for crudités |
| Large green bell pepper | Plum tomatoes | White mushrooms |
| Large onion | Radishes | White turnip |

### Grains/Nuts/Seeds

Brown rice tortillas
Raw pecans
Slow-roasted almonds
Slow-roasted cashews
Slow-roasted pecans

### Milks

Plain cultured coconut milk
Unsweetened almond milk
Unsweetened coconut milk

## WEEK 3 MEAL PLAN

### Day 1

Breakfast: Blueberry Power Muffin (page 87) with a side of nitrate-free chicken breakfast sausage

Lunch: Green Coconut Protein Shake (page 94)

Optional Snack: Sea Salt and Black Pepper Cashew Cheese (page 125) with rice crackers

Dinner: Hearty Chicken Soup (page 169); Jicama, Apple, and Pear Slaw (page 114)

**Day 2**

Breakfast: Rise and Shine Mocha Espresso Protein Shake (page 96)

Lunch: Chicken Salad Wrap (page 101) with crudités

Optional Snack: Homemade Almond Butter (page 128) on apple slices

Dinner: Easy Pasta Bolognese (page 135); Balsamic Roasted Vegetables (page 205)

**Day 3**

Breakfast: Nutty Chai Breakfast Blast Shake (page 97)

Lunch: Vegetarian Chili (page 166) with crudités

Optional Snack: Avocado-Lime Black Bean Salsa (page 120) with rice chips

Dinner: SlowCooker Coq au Vin (page 180); Tuscan White Beans with Sage (page 193); mixed greens with olive oil and fresh-squeezed lemon juice

**Day 4**

Breakfast: Swedish-Style Pecan Pancakes with Orange and Strawberries (page 89), with a side of nitrate-free chicken breakfast sausage

Lunch: Mixed Berry and Avocado Protein Shake (page 93)

Optional Snack: Roasted Red Pepper Hummus (page 118) with crudités

Dinner: Pork Souvlaki Kabobs with Tzatziki (page 139); Curried Lentils (page 190); Swiss Chard with Olives (page 200)

**Day 5**

Breakfast: Hot Quinoa Flake Cereal with Warm Berry Compote (page 90)

Lunch: Strawberry "Milkshake" Protein Shake (page 95)

Optional Snack: Roasted Jalapeño Guacamole with Toasted Pumpkin Seeds (page 121), with crudités

Dinner: Kale and Bean Soup (page 174); Halibut en Papillote (page 158)

**Day 6**

Breakfast: Peach-Berry-Almond Protein Shake (page 95)

Lunch: Quinoa and Chickpea Tabbouleh with Mint, Parsley, and Lemon Dressing (page 167)

Optional Snack: Sea Salt and Black Pepper Cashew Cheese (page 125) with rice crackers

Dinner: Minestrone Soup (page 172); Meatballs in Tomato Sauce (page 133) over Easy Spinach-and-Garlic Sauté (page 195)

### Day 7

Breakfast: Chocolate-Cherry-Chia Protein Shake (page 94)

Lunch: Lentil, Kale, and Sausage Stew (page 183)

Optional Snack: Cinnamon Roasted Pecans (page 123)

Dinner: Salmon Puttanesca (page 161); Cauliflower Puree (page 196)

## WEEK 3 SHOPPING LIST

### Proteins

Grass-fed lean ground beef

Organic free-range bone-in, skinless chicken breast half

Organic free-range bone-in, skinless chicken thighs

Organic free-range boneless, skinless chicken breast halves

Natural lean pork loin

Nitrate-free bacon slices

Nitrate-free chicken breakfast sausages

Nitrate-free fully cooked organic sweet Italian sausages

Wild halibut fillets

Wild salmon fillets, such as king or sockeye

### Vegetables/Fruits/Herbs

Apples
Asparagus
Avocados
Baby kale
Baby spinach
Carrots
Cauliflower
Celery
Fresh basil

Fresh blueberries (or use frozen)
Fresh cilantro
Fresh mint
Fresh parsley
Fresh sage
Fresh spinach
Fresh strawberries
Fresh thyme

Garlic cloves
Grape tomatoes
Green cabbage
Green onions
Japanese eggplants
Jicama
Kale
Leeks
Large red bell pepper

Large shallot
Lemons
Limes
Medium cucumber
Medium fennel bulb
Medium green bell pepper
Medium jalapeño peppers
Medium onions
Medium red bell peppers

Medium red onions
Medium yellow squash
Medium zucchini
Mixed greens for salad
Parsnip
Pear
Plum tomatoes
Red cabbage
Red or green kale

Small cucumber
Small green bell pepper
Small jalapeño pepper
Small onions
Small orange
Small red bell pepper
Swiss chard
Vegetables for crudités
White mushrooms

### Grains/Nuts/Seeds

Brown rice tortillas
Raw cashews
Raw pumpkin seeds

Raw walnuts
Slow-roasted almonds
Slow-roasted pecans

### Milks

Cultured plain coconut milk
Unsweetened almond milk
Unsweetened coconut milk

# STAPLES LIST

### Protein Powders

Chai vegan protein powder
Chocolate vegan protein powder
Vanilla vegan protein powder

### Oils and Vinegars

Asian sesame oil
Coconut butter
Coconut oil
Extra-virgin olive oil
Macadamia nut oil★

Malaysian red palm fruit oil★
Balsamic vinegar
Cider vinegar
White balsamic vinegar

★You can substitute coconut oil for these—or look for them on sale!

## Spices

Allspice

Arrowroot

Bay leaves

Cayenne pepper

Cinnamon

Coriander

Curry powder

Dried basil

Dried oregano

Freshly ground black pepper

Garlic powder

Ground ancho chile pepper

Ground chipotle pepper

Ground cumin

Onion powder

Red pepper flakes

Sea salt

Smoked paprika

Sweet paprika

## Extracts

Almond extract

Coconut extract

Monk fruit extract

Stevia extract

Vanilla extract

## Grains/Seeds/Legumes

Brown rice

Bob's Red Mill Gluten-Free All-
    Purpose Baking Flour

Chia seeds

Dry, sprouted lentils

Fennel seeds

Flaxseeds

Quinoa

Quinoa linguine pasta

Quinoa pasta of choice

Quinoa pasta shells

Rice chips

Rice crackers

## Jarred and Canned

Capers

Cashew butter

Chili garlic sauce

Coconut aminos

Dijon mustard

Kalamata olives

Organic low-sodium chicken broth

Organic low-sodium vegetable
    broth

Organic tahini paste

Roasted red peppers

Tabasco sauce

(6-oz) cans organic tomato paste

(8-oz) cans organic tomato sauce

(14.5-oz) cans organic fire-roasted
diced tomatoes

(14.5-oz) cans organic diced tomatoes

(15-oz) cans organic black lentils

(15-oz) cans organic no-salt-added
black beans

(15-oz) cans organic no-salt-added
cannellini beans

(15-oz) cans organic no-salt-added
chickpeas (garbanzo beans)

(15-oz) cans organic no-salt-added red
kidney beans

(28-oz) cans organic crushed tomatoes

(28-oz) cans organic diced tomatoes

## Frozen

Organic blueberries

Organic dark cherries

Organic mixed berries

Organic peaches

Organic strawberries, unsweetened

Pearl onions

## Miscellaneous

Aluminum-free baking powder

Baking soda

Instant espresso/coffee powder

# RESTAURANT GUIDE: TRAVEL AND DINING OUT

You have complete control over what you eat, but it's easier if you're prepared. I travel a *lot*. I'm very familiar with navigating carb-heavy continental breakfasts and airline food (I use the word *food* loosely here!).

It also stands to reason that, being on the road, I also eat at restaurants more than I'd care to (okay, sometimes it's fun!).

I'm going to walk you through my top strategies and tips for fast fat loss and making smart choices, whether you're jet-lagged after a 12-hour flight, driving cross-country to visit your family, or just don't feel like cooking one more meal. Hotel buffets, airport fast food, roadside diners where the only vegetables are deep-fried...you name it, I've been there countless times, and I know just how to handle those situations. Most of the time it comes back to that old saw about being prepared: When you package your own meals and snacks, and carry the tools for your success with you, you're making sure you never get backed into a sugar-craving corner. You're making your weight loss and health goals a priority.

But sometimes you have to make do with what's in front of you, or you just can't resist the call of that voice in your head that says you can't go another day without Thai food. All is not lost! I'm going to give you specific ways to get your fix and still come out feeling Virgin Diet–strong on those days when you have to have your favorite ethnic foods.

## General Travel Strategies

1. **Carry a water bottle with filter.** Staying buzzed on caffeine can certainly help you remain alert all morning during that excruciatingly boring meeting, but it

also raises stress hormones and dehydrates you. Keep purified water to sip throughout the day so you're not suffering brain fog and other dehydration miseries.

**2. The Magic Bullet or Blender Bottle.** I want you to eat a protein-rich breakfast within an hour of waking up. Ever tried to do that at a three-star hotel or when racing to the airport to catch your 7:30 a.m. flight? Even if you're a morning person, it's not easy. Fast-food sandwich options don't cut it, what passes for food on airlines is abysmal, continental breakfasts usually mean muffins and Danish, and hotel room service is outrageously overpriced. Oh, and good luck pulling something together while frantically looking for your car keys to make that flight. A protein shake solves all these problems!

**3. Always have lean high-protein snacks with you.** Beef, salmon, and turkey jerky are not only tasty but will keep you going for hours if you don't have access to food while traveling. Look for jerky from animals or fish raised without hormones, preservatives, MSG, or nitrates. I also like the aseptic packages of wild salmon. It doesn't get any easier!

**4. Have nutrients on hand.** When I'm on the go, I take a little extra vitamin C, and maybe a little extra zinc and probiotics. Vitamin C and zinc help avoid colds that crop up in close spaces like airplanes, and probiotics help make sure my tummy stays healthy as I navigate new environments.

**5. Powdered green drinks.** Drinking green vegetable powders detoxifies the liver, boosts energy levels, and provides valuable trace minerals to keep your blood sugar and mood stable. Pack your powders in a resealable plastic bag and bring a shake bottle with you to (really) dissolve the powder in water.

**6. Containers full of veggies.** Cut up raw vegetables the night before your trip and pop them into a plastic container or resealable bag. Wrap them in a damp paper towel before you stick them in the container, and they'll stay fresh for up to 12 hours. Vegetables are not only chock-full of antioxidants, they're also high-water foods that will help keep you hydrated. I especialy love jicama, carrots, and sliced red bell peppers.

**7. Bags of nuts.** Make your own trail mix! Nuts are nature's ultimate fast food— they contain an awesome balance of protein, carbs, and fats. Measure out ¼-cup, unsalted portions and put them in individual containers. Crunch your stress away with almonds and cashews...you'll be getting the benefits of zinc, magnesium, and balanced blood sugar and neurotransmitters. If nuts are a trigger food for you and you tend to overeat them, travel with only limited amounts.

Here's my Emergency Travel Food List. Refer to it when you want ideas for packing your own nourishing food to take along when you're on the move.

- ☑ Protein shake
- ☑ Nuts and seeds
- ☑ Nitrate-free jerky
- ☑ Aseptic-packed wild salmon
- ☑ Kale chips
- ☑ Virgin Diet Bars
- ☑ Individual packets of nut butters
- ☑ Freeze-dried fruit (you can add it to your shakes)
- ☑ Small boxes of So Delicious unsweetened coconut milk
- ☑ Mighty Maca Greens drink packets

## General Rules for Dining Out

Now, I'm going to go out on a limb and guess that you're not going to carry your own food with you to a restaurant (and I am guessing you would be quickly escorted to the door if you did), so let's dig in to ways you can enjoy your night out and still come away knowing you didn't become unhinged in the face of temptation. (By the way, for a great resource for finding healthy dining-out choices, check out cleanplates .com.)

- Never, ever assume anything. If you have the slightest bit of doubt, *ask*. It is far easier to over-ask in advance than to trouble your server to send something back.
- Remember that no restaurant experience is "ideal." You're better off preparing food yourself, where you can guarantee what goes into it. Even the most diligent cook, however, sometimes eats out. So do the best you can, which includes doing your homework before you go—review menus online, ask friends about their experience, and even call ahead if you still have questions.

- You will have a difficult time always finding grass-fed beef, wild fish, free-range poultry, and organic produce at restaurants. If you can find a restaurant that serves high-quality meat, frequent it and remind them that you are "voting" with your money.
- Most restaurant foods are cooked in soybean oil, which is ubiquitous and cheap. Avoid cooking with this and other omega-6-rich oils at home. At restaurants, do the best you can.
- GMOs are also a concern. Again, do the best you can.
- Many ethnic restaurants use sauces, MSG, gluten-containing spices, and other ingredients not compliant with the Virgin Diet. It is up to you to ask your server about these things before you order. Ignorance is never an excuse!
- Don't allow bread, chips, and other starters on your table. If your dining companions must have them, at least keep them away from you (look away!). Ask instead if you can have olives, guacamole with veggies, or something Virgin Diet–friendly to munch on. I often order one of the vegetable side dishes as a starter—try the grilled asparagus or roasted Brussels sprouts. Oh, and don't even *try* the three-bite rule with chips or bread unless you are a rock. Be real about your triggers and don't bring the enemy to the table!

## Cuisine-Based Menu Strategies

**Mexican**—*Best choice:* guacamole with raw veggies; chicken fajitas (see criteria below); tequila with fresh lime juice (if you drink). *Worst choice:* chips and salsa with a margarita to start and then a giant burrito topped with cheese and sour cream.

- Carne or chicken asada, shrimp diablo, snapper Veracruz
- If you're craving authentic Mexican, order fajitas:
  - Stick with lean meats, salsa, guacamole, onions/peppers, black beans.
  - Put this all on top of a big salad.
  - Skip the cheese, sour cream, rice, and tortillas.
- Ask for salsa to top dishes rather than sauces or sour cream.
- Gluten/corn–free tortillas—they're very hard to find, but it never hurts to ask!
- Black beans (if not, refried) or brown rice—the beans are the better choice here.
- Avocado and guacamole (ask for veggies to dip)

- Watch out for:
  - Anything breaded and/or deep-fried
  - Sugary, creamy sauces
  - Tortillas that aren't gluten-free
  - Chips (don't even let your server put them down!)

**Chinese**—*Best choice:* steamed chicken with broccoli and gluten-free brown rice. *Worst choice:* Orange chicken (I call this "chicken candy!").

- Beef, chicken, or vegetable skewers (skip the sauce)
- Steamed chicken, beef, pork, or fish
- Broccoli and other green veggies
- Small amount of gluten-free brown rice
- Keep in mind that Chinese food is easier to order after Cycle 1 because many dishes are cooked with soy sauce, cornstarch, and/or peanut oil.
- Watch out for:
  - Anything breaded and/or deep-fried
  - Sugary, syrupy sauces
  - MSG
  - Cornstarch thickener

**Fast food**—*Best choice:* grilled chicken breast on a salad. *Worst choice:* double bacon cheeseburger with fries.

- Many fast-food places like Chipotle offer customized salads. Ask for yours topped with chicken, avocado, salsa, veggies, tomatoes, cucumbers, black beans, and/or guacamole.
- Grilled chicken breast without the bun
- Burger without the bun—make sure it is 100 percent beef with no fillers.
- Green veggies (if they have them!)
- Watch out for:
  - Anything breaded and/or deep-fried
  - Sugary or creamy sauces

- Salad toppings—anything crunchy, creamy, or crispy is usually a red alert. Always ask, and tell your server exactly what you want.
- See "Oils and Healthy Fats" (pages 372–73). Most restaurants use inflammatory omega-6 oils that are reheated and become severely damaged. Always ask what oils your restaurant uses and, if possible, request olive oil for low-heat cooking.

**Thai**—*Best choice:* chicken coconut soup; chicken, scallops, or shrimp and veggies with red or green curry sauce. *Worst choice:* tofu pad thai.

- Chicken satays (no peanut sauce—get red or green curry sauce instead)
- Brown rice
- Coconut soup with shrimp or chicken
- Watch out for:
  - Anything breaded and/or deep-fried
  - Sugary or creamy sauces
  - Anything that comes with noodles—sometimes the menu does not alert you.
  - Peanut sauces

**French**—*Best choice:* Niçoise salad (no eggs); chicken Provençale. *Worst choice:* French onion soup, quiche.

- Grilled meat and/or veggies appetizer
- Salad—oil and vinegar dressing on the side
- Mussels or other steamed or grilled shellfish
- Grilled steak, chicken, or fish as entrée
- Legumes or non-gluten starchy carb
- Fresh berries for dessert
- Watch out for:
  - Anything breaded and/or deep-fried
  - Any kind of soufflé or other dish that includes egg
  - Sweet, creamy, or syrupy sauces
  - Dairy—especially butter

**Steakhouse**—*Best choice:* salad, filet mignon with steamed broccoli and half a sweet potato. *Worst choice:* steak drowned in sugary sauce with fries and battered onion rings.

- Salad with olive oil and vinegar dressing
- Shrimp cocktail (without the sauce)
- Grilled meat and/or vegetable appetizer
- Filet mignon or lean steak
- Broccoli, spinach, or other green vegetable
- Sweet potato
- Berries for dessert
- Watch out for:
  - Caesar and other salads with creamy dressings
  - Crunchy, crispy, and other "illegal" salad toppings
  - Anything breaded and/or deep fried
  - Dinner rolls (don't even let your server put them down!)
  - Breaded veggies and other "legal" foods (steakhouses love to fry anything for added appeal)

**American**—*Best choice:* salad; grilled chicken breast topped with peppers/onions/ mushrooms; steamed green vegetable; gluten-free healthy starch. *Worst choice:* bacon cheeseburger with fries and soda.

- Salad with olive oil and vinegar dressing
- Steamed veggies
- Grilled, broiled, or baked steak, chicken, pork, or seafood
- Large customized entrée salad
- High-fiber slow-release carbs like sweet potatoes, legumes, and quinoa
- Watch out for:
  - Anything crunchy and/or deep-fried
  - Salads with descriptions like "creamy" and "crunchy"
  - Anything breaded—always ask (I've seen breaded green beans, asparagus, and otherwise healthy foods on menus!)
  - Meats drowning in sugary, syrupy sauces

**Japanese**—*Best choice:* sashimi and cucumber salad. *Worst choice:* edamame, rolls with special sauce (usually mayonnaise).

- If sushi: Stick with sashimi and then half a roll (e.g., California roll) with gluten-free brown rice.
- Ask for (or bring your own) coconut aminos instead of soy sauce in Cycle 1.
- Hibachi grill: steak or chicken with steamed veggies, small amount of brown rice (they usually use only white rice, so ask for brown rice on the side or do double veggies)
- Miso soup if you are past Cycle 1; otherwise, do a side salad with ginger dressing.
- Watch out for:
  - Tempura and anything else crunchy, breaded, and/or deep-fried
  - Soy (tofu, etc., but also hidden sources)
  - Sugary, creamy sauces, including teriyaki sauce

**Italian**—*Best choice:* cioppino (fish stew); mussels; marinara. *Worst choice:* fettuccine Alfredo with garlic bread.

- Mussels
- Salad with tomatoes and olive oil drizzle
- Grilled or baked chicken, pork chop, or other dish
- Steamed veggies
- Watch out for:
  - Anything breaded and/or deep-fried
  - Pasta as a side dish (even with meat—some restaurants slide it in)
  - Sugary sauces
  - Garlic bread (don't even let them set it down!)

**Seafood**—*Best choice:* grilled salmon or halibut (wild if they have it); mixed veggies; scallop appetizer. *Worst choice:* fried shrimp with French fries.

- Salad with olive oil and vinegar
- Mussels or other shellfish appetizer

- Grilled seafood—salmon, shrimp; always look for lower-mercury fish and avoid shark, swordfish, and other larger fish.
- Steamed veggies
- Sweet potato or gluten-free starch
- Watch out for:
  - Anything breaded and/or deep-fried—always ask if your fish is breaded or battered in any way.
  - Sugary sauces or sauces with egg and other "illegal " ingredients (e.g., tartar sauce)
  - Drawn butter and other dipping sauces

**Mediterranean**—*Best choice:* roasted fish with bell peppers, artichokes, and lentils; and a glass of red wine. *Worst choice:* couscous.

- Lentils
- Fish
- Roasted peppers and artichokes
- Hummus
- Olives
- Red wine
- Watch out for:
  - Couscous
  - Pita
  - Feta
  - Pesto
  - Pasta

## Top Places for Allergy-Free Awareness/Menus★

Bonefish Grill

Burtons Grill

Chipotle Mexican Grill

Legal Sea Foods

★Thanks to AllergyEats.com: allergyeats.com/blog/index.php/the-most-allergy-friendly-restaurant-chains-in-america.

Longhorn Steakhouse
Outback Steakhouse
P.F. Chang's China Bistro
Papa Razzi
Red Robin Gourmet Burgers
Uno Chicago Grill

## My Favorite Places

I love trying new places, but when I want consistent, healthy, and satisfying meals, I always look for these favorites:

Chipotle
Lyfe Kitchen
Seasons 52
True Food Kitchen
Whole Foods Market

## *Specialty Foods*

### Artisan Bistro (thevirgindiet.com/artisanbistro)

Why am I resourcing premade dinners in a cookbook? Because you'll have days when you simply can't or don't want to make even the simple, time-efficient meals provided here. Rather than expensive takeout or unhealthy fast food, Artisan Bistro provides a delicious array of healthy heat-and-serve Virgin Diet–approved meals made with the highest-quality ingredients. For around $8 each you can enjoy meals like Wild Alaskan Salmon, Citrus Salsa Verde, and my favorite, Chicken Marsala. Conveniently delivered right to your door, Artisan Bistro makes a healthy meal as close as your freezer.

### Shirataki Noodles

*Shirataki* means "white waterfall," which describes the beautiful appearance of these thin low-carbohydrate Japanese noodles. Because they are mostly soluble fiber, shirataki noodles work perfectly into all cycles of the Virgin Diet. Most Asian markets sell dry and liquid-packaged shirataki noodles. Draining and dry-roasting the noodles gives them a more pasta-like consistency and removes any bitterness. Heads up: Look for traditional, *not* tofu, shirataki noodles. Most Asian markets sell shirataki noodles. You can also find them at amazon.com.

### Grassland Beef Jerky from U.S. Wellness Meats (grasslandbeef.com)

Jerky is such a healthy, portable snack. It's high in protein and good fats. But I skip commercial brands, which often contain sodium, gluten, and other additives. Grassland Beef, on the other hand, delivers low-heat-cooked grass-fed beef jerky cured in salt brine, with no nitrates or flavor additives.

Sometimes I like to mix things up by trying other flavors. U.S. Wellness Meats also sells high-quality, nitrate-free jerky made from bison, turkey, and wild salmon. It's great for whenever I need a quick, filling, delicious snack, whether I'm stranded at an airport or in the car.

### Fermented Black Beans

No, these aren't the black beans you find in Mexican restaurants. Fermented black beans are soybeans that have been dried and fermented with salt. You'll often find them in Cantonese cooking. Fermented black beans have a strong flavor and are frequently used with garlic and spicy foods. Most Asian markets and ethnic sections of grocery stores sell fermented black beans. You can also find them at amazon.com.

Note: Because they are soy (who knew!?), these are allowed only in Cycle 3 of the Virgin Diet.

### Andean Dream Quinoa Pasta (andeandream.com/OtherProducts.html)

Hankering for pasta on the Virgin Diet? No problem with Andean Dream Quinoa Pasta, the only quinoa pasta I know of that doesn't contain corn. Gluten-free and organic, Andean Dream Quinoa Pasta comes in traditional spaghetti as well as shells, macaroni, and fusilli for all your gluten-free pasta needs. Andean Dream is available at Whole Foods Markets and health food stores.

### Carolina Beef and Bison (carolinabison.com)

My top supplier for grass-fed beef and bison, delivered right to my door. Carolina Bison was founded by whole-health practitioner Dr. Frank J. King Jr. in 1985. They are located in the lush Blue Ridge Mountains of North Carolina, where their cows and bison are raised on top-quality grasses to yield the same pristine meats our Paleolithic ancestors once ate. When I order from Carolina Beef and Bison, I know I'm getting the highest-quality, nutrient-rich, grass-fed, free-range meats with no steroids, antibiotics, or any other nasty stuff found in conventionally raised meats.

### TruRoots Organic Sprouted Green Lentils (truroots.com)

TruRoots sprouts and dries the highest-quality green lentils, awakening their flavor and preserving healthful benefits. Sprouting is a traditional technique that boosts the lentils' nutritional profile—increasing vitamins and micronutrients and activating digestive enzymes.

### Vital Choice (vitalchoice.com)

By now you know that Vital Choice should be your trusted source for home delivery of the world's finest, freshest wild seafood harvested from well-managed wild fisheries and farms. They sustainably harvest Alaskan salmon and other Alaskan and northwest Pacific seafood by cleaning and flash-freezing it within hours of harvest. Vital Choice's wild seafood arrives at your door on dry ice to retain that fresh-caught flavor, texture, and nutritional benefit.

But Vital Choice sells far more than just seafood. They also provide high-quality macadamia nut oil and extra-virgin olive oil, vinegars, nuts, dried fruit, and my favorite, dark chocolate.

If you've never visited their website, prepare yourself for an amazing savory collection of wild seafood and so much more. And here's a huge bonus: Members of my tribe get 15 percent off their first order! Use gift code JJVIRGIN and this link to get the discount: thevirgindietcookbook.com/vitalchoice.

## Drinks

### Bulletproof Upgraded Coffee (bulletproofexec.com/category/coffee-2/)

What makes this coffee "bulletproof"? Well, Bulletproof Coffee is carefully produced and tested to yield the lowest toxin content with no pesticides or other chemicals. The beans are harvested from a single family–owned estate in Guatemala, located 1,250 meters above sea level (high enough to produce great coffee). I've kicked regular coffee to the curb in favor of fat-burning, flavorful Bulletproof Coffee. Once you try it, you'll never settle for plain coffee again.

### Hint Water (drinkhint.com)

Hint Water evolved when San Francisco native Kara Goldin couldn't find a delicious, refreshing drink for herself or her kids. What she wanted was simple: no sweeteners, sugars, fancy but useless additives, or ingredients you can't pronounce. Just plain, delicious pure springwater with a splash of natural flavor.

Sounds easy, right? It wasn't, which is why she created Hint Water.

When people tell me they don't like water or are trying to break their soda habit, I always recommend Hint Water in amazing flavors like raspberry-lime and strawberry-kiwi. Who says water has to be boring? You can have it shipped to your door from Amazon or pick it up at Whole Foods Market.

### So Delicious (sodeliciousdairyfree.com)

Cow's milk is so last-millennium! Trade the cow for coconut with So Delicious Unsweetened Coconut Milk Beverage. It provides a light coconut flavor that boosts your protein shakes and also makes a delicious stand-alone beverage. One cup contains just 50 calories and only 1 gram of sugar. So Delicious Unsweetened Coconut Milk Beverage provides medium-chain fatty acids (MCFAs), a healthy fat your body burns for energy rather than storing it. They have also just launched a line of culinary coconut milks to replace canned full-fat coconut milk in cooking.

If coconut milk isn't your thing, try So Delicious Unsweetened Almond Plus 5X Protein and my new favorite, Unsweetened Cashew Milk. So Delicious also provides a delicious selection of no-sugar-added coconut milk ice cream and cultured coconut milk. One bite of these delicious treats and you'll wonder why you ever fell for cow's milk. You can find So Delicious at health food stores and most major grocery stores nationwide.

## *Oils and Healthy Fats*

### Vital Choice Organic Extra Virgin Olive Oil (vitalchoice.com/shop/pc/viewPrd.asp?idproduct=198)

According to journalist Tom Mueller, 70 percent of the extra-virgin olive oil you buy is adulterated with cheaper oil. He even wrote a book about the problem.

Know your sources and don't settle for fake olive oil. Vital Choice Organic Extra Virgin Olive Oil is cold-pressed, unrefined, 100 percent organic extra-virgin olive oil (EVOO) from Spanish Picual olives, which give the oil its fruity, apple-like aroma and tangy flavor. I love drizzling this flavorful polyphenol-rich oil on salads, but don't cook with it because heat can damage the fragile fatty acids.

### Coconut Kefir Starter Mix

Yogurt fans: Check out coconut kefir. Its many benefits include probiotics for a healthy gut and better digestion. Kefir also boosts your immune system and is anti-aging. It's super-easy to make your own. I get the kefir starter from my brilliant pal Donna Gates at Body Ecology (bodyecology.com).

### Coconut Oil

I love cooking with coconut oil because it's stable even at very high temperatures. Vegetables like broccoli and spinach taste incredible with coconut oil, and the good fat helps you absorb the veggies' fat-soluble nutrients. Surely you've read about the medium-chain triglycerides (MCTs) in coconut oil, which your body burns for fuel rather than storing them. Coconut oil is also rich in beneficial fatty acids like immune-boosting lauric acid. My favorite is 365 Everyday Value brand.

### Coconut Secret Coconut Aminos (coconutsecret.com/aminos2.html)

I love sushi, but I avoid the soy sauce, which often has gluten and high sodium. Thankfully I have a fabulous substitute with coconut aminos: an organic, raw, gluten-free and soy-free sauce made from the nutrient-rich sap of coconut trees. Coconut aminos have a low glycemic index and come loaded with B vitamins, vitamin C, and minerals. It's my favorite sushi-dipping sauce, and it works well any time you would normally use soy sauce.

### Coconut Secret Coconut Flour (coconutsecret.com/flour2.html)

I love this gluten-free, low-carb flour for baking, cooking, thickening sauces, and any other time I need a flour substitute. Made from unheated coconut meat, Coconut Secret's raw coconut flour is unrefined and high in fiber. You can find coconut flour at health food stores and online.

## Malaysian Red Palm (Fruit) Oil Council (mpoc.org.my)

In addition to coconut oil, I love high-heat cooking with Malaysian red palm fruit oil. It's a rich source of vitamin D; tocotrienols (vitamin E); and pro–vitamin A carotenoids. It also tastes delicious and really brings out the flavor in vegetables and other foods. You can buy Malaysian red palm fruit oil at Whole Foods and local ethnic grocery stores.

A note about sustainability: Malaysia has pledged to follow sustainable practices, so always look for Malaysian red palm fruit oil.

## Grass-fed Organic Ghee from Pure Indian Foods (amazon .com/Grassfed-Organic-Ghee-7-8-Oz/dp/B0032RPLSY)

Ghee is clarified butter, meaning butter with the milk solids removed, so it's ideal for anyone sensitive to dairy. The Agarwal family has been in the ghee business for five generations (since 1889), so they're clearly doing something right! This amazing grass-fed, USDA-certified, 100 percent organic ghee comes from non-homogenized cow's milk. Unlike the waxy texture you sometimes find in other brands of ghee, this one has a nice grainy texture. Available at amazon.com.

## Kerrygold Pure Irish Butter (kerrygoldusa.com/products/butter/)

Sometimes you want the creaminess of pure butter. Kerrygold Pure Irish Butter is miles above regular butter because it comes from grass-fed cows whose milk is higher in nutrients like fat-burning conjugated linolenic acid (CLA) to yield the sweetest, richest butter in the world. You can find Kerrigold at most major grocery stores.

---

## FAVORITE BRANDS

### *365 Everyday Value brand (wholefoods.com)*

Far from being a generic brand, 365 Everyday Value provides high-quality GMO-free, organic frozen fruit, teas, non-irradiated spices, and much more, priced to compete against grocery store brands. When I'm not making my own in my Vitamix, I choose 365 Organic Smooth Almond Butter, which doesn't have added sugar, trans fat, or other junk found in many commercial nut butters. Also worth mentioning is 365 Everyday Value Natural Stevia Extract Powder. You get pure stevia without maltodextrin, dextrose, nebulous natural flavors, and other additives found in some commercial brands. You can grab my Virgin Diet–approved whole foods shopping list at http://thevirgindietcookbook.com/bonus.

## *Healthy Sweeteners*

### Monk Fruit BioVittoria (biovittoria.com/biovittoria)

BioVittoria calls itself "The Monk Fruit Company" for good reason. Their Fruit-Sweetness is a 100 percent natural powdered concentrate made from monk fruit (Chinese *luo han guo*) that's about 150 times sweeter than sugar. Unlike sugar, it doesn't raise your blood sugar levels, nor does it have the nasty characteristics of artificial sweeteners. All natural with zero calories, non-GMO, and fully water-soluble, Fruit-Sweetness is my go-to sweetener for green tea or whenever I need a healthy sweetener. You can find Fruit-Sweetness at health food stores.

### 365 Everyday Value Natural Stevia Extract Powder (wholefoods.com)

Stevia is a zero-calorie herb that sweetens without sugar's high glycemic index. In other words, unlike sugar, a little stevia in your green tea won't send your blood sugar levels all over the map. Safe for people with diabetes and on low-carb diets, 365 Everyday Value Natural Stevia Extract Powder is pure stevia without maltodetrixin, dextrose, artificial flavors, and other additives many stevia brands use. This container looks tiny, but be warned: A little, little dab will do you!

### The Ultimate Sweetener Xylitol (theultimatelife.net/CatSweet.htm)

Xylitol used to be my go-to sweetener because it still has some calories so it doesn't cause calorie disregulation like no-calorie sweeteners may do, sweetens like sugar, doesn't raise blood sugar levels like sugar does, and provides numerous benefits, from caries prevention to reducing candida to improving bone health.

Then I learned that most xylitol these days comes from corn, a highly reactive food that creates food intolerances. I was thrilled, then, to see that The Ultimate Life still uses 100 percent birch trees for their xylitol. Unlike some other brands, The Ultimate Sweetener contains no artificial sweeteners, sugars, potential food intolerances, or other additives—just pure birch tree–derived xylitol. Available on amazon.com or at your local health food store.

## *Green Drinks and Other Supplements*

### Mighty Maca Greens (mightymaca.com)

You know green powders can cover your vegetable base, but so many of them just taste gross. Mighty Maca Greens packs healthy greens like chlorella and spirulina with anti-inflammatory antioxidants like turmeric and grapeseed extract in a delicious, low-sugar, apple-flavored green powder. I love Mighty Maca Greens Double Shot Thin Sticks. No need to measure or sort: I just throw one in my bag, knowing I can just mix it with water to have a great-tasting, alkalinizing green drink wherever I go. This is available online.

### Thorne Research Supplements and Shakes (jjvirginstore.com)

This company is known and respected by health-care professionals for its purity and quality. I think of it as the "anti-magnesium stearate" company because Thorne Research has taken a stand to not use that or other flow agents that could impact nutrient absorption. These are the products I use personally, give to my family, and recommend to my clients. You can purchase Thorne Research supplements, protein powders, and organic skincare products on my website, where I have assembled my favorite specialty support packages for you as well. For products, descriptions, and ingredient information, visit thevirgindiet.com/store. You can also purchase Thorne Research products through health-care professionals.

## Healthy Ingredients

### Real Good Salt (get.realgoodsalt.com/thevirgindiet/)

Real Good Salt is nutrient-rich sea salt that comes from La Laguna de Cuyutlá (the same place where the Aztecs got their salt over 500 years ago). Traditional *salineros* (salt farmers) continue to harvest this salt using an organic, 100 percent renewable process (evaporated naturally by the sun) to protect the environment and wildlife. With your purchase, you are supporting this "small salt economy" of *salineros*, their families, and their way of salt harvesting. I wouldn't use any other salt with my food. Available only online.

### Bob's Red Mill (bobsredmill.com)

You've likely seen Bob's Red Mill in your health food store. This company has been around nearly forever (well, since 1978) and provides a wide variety of gluten-free oats and all-purpose flour as well as golden flaxseeds, chia seeds, and coconut flour. Bob's Red Mill remains the trusted leader in gluten-free flours, seeds, and other foods because they provide consistently superior products. You can find Bob's at most major grocery stores.

### Thai Kitchen (thaikitchen.com)

Besides high-quality fish sauce, red curry paste, organic coconut milk for cooking, and other ingredients for curries and other Thai dishes, Thai Kitchen provides clear information on their products about allergies and food intolerances. Unlike some brands, there's no guessing whether you're getting gluten, dairy, or any other highly reactive ingredients: It says so right on the label. Thai Kitchen products are available at most supermarkets.

### Navitas Naturals (navitasnaturals.com)

They aren't kidding when they call themselves "The Superfood Company": Navitas Naturals is a family-owned company that provides a wide array of organic, non-GMO, nutrient-rich raw cacao, flax, cashew, coconut, and other delicious foods. Among their "must try" products are raw cacao nibs and powder. You can find them online and at health food stores.

### Heintzman Farms Golden Flax (heintzmanfarms.com/)

Flaxseeds are one of my favorite foods because these tiny seeds are loaded with protein, fiber, lignans, and omega-3 fatty acids. If you follow my recipes, you know I often throw ground flaxseed into my protein smoothies.

I've been using Heintzman Farms flaxseeds for years because the company delivers fresh, whole, GMO-free Dakota Flax Gold flaxseeds right to my door. Their kit includes three 1-pound bags of seeds and a mini electric grinder so that you can grind the flaxseeds yourself. Toss them into your smoothie or other foods any time you need a fiber/nutrient boost.

## The Virgin Diet

### The Virgin Diet Coach (thevirgindietcoach.com)

Take your commitment to a whole new level with the Virgin Diet Coach, which allows you to engage in community forums, research and manage recipes, plan meals, determine whether you have leaky gut and other issues, and journal your success.

The Virgin Diet Coach divides your goals by cycle so you can track your weight, sleep, water intake, supplements, and daily activities to give you a better understanding of your health and habits.

The forum on the Virgin Diet Coach provides a caring, friendly community to engage with that helps create extra accountability and encourages you to meet your goals. My coaches also regularly answer your questions on the forum.

The Virgin Diet Coach provides all the tools to achieve and maintain long-term success on the Virgin Diet.

### The Virgin Diet One-on-One Coaching (jjvirgin.com/coaches)

Nearly everyone who excelled at something hired a coach at some point. Customize your food and nutrient plan with one of my rock-star wellness coaches whom I've personally trained. Based on your needs, preferences, budget, and other restrictions, they can develop a plan that works specifically for you to achieve and maintain your goals. They can also provide support and troubleshoot potential issues that arise along your journey. We offer several one-on-one packages at jjvirgin.com/coaches.

### The Virgin Diet Bars

When you want a healthy, delicious snack or mini-meal, reach for the Virgin Diet Bar. Made with fresh ingredients like organic cashew butter and chia seeds with no fractionated oils or other preservatives, the Virgin Diet Bar provides a low-sugar treat to curb your hunger and sweet tooth. Available in Cinnamon Cashew Crunch (Cycle 1) and Dark Chocolate Cherry (Cycle 3).

### All-in-One Shakes (jjvirginstore.com)

The Virgin Diet All-in-One Shake lives up to its name. Along with a great vegan protein blend, this premium powder contains optimal amounts of vitamins, minerals, enzymes, probiotics, whole food complexes (antioxidants), and fiber with only 5 grams of sugar. Start every morning with the Virgin Diet All-in-One Shake and you'll stay full, focused, and burning fat for hours. Available in chocolate, vanilla, or my favorite, chai.

## Virgin Diet Supplements (jjvirginstore.com)

### Extra Fiber

Virgin Diet Extra Fiber is a blend of plant-based, water-soluble fibers, formulated to promote regularity and healthy glycemic control, enhance nutrient absorption, and help maintain optimum digestive function. Virgin Diet Extra Fiber combines Sunfiber—a partially hydrolyzed guar gum fiber—with rice bran, larch arabinogalactan, apple pectin, prune powder, and green tea phytosome to provide an effective prebiotic fiber formula that is well-tolerated and easy to use. Because Virgin Diet Extra Fiber is tasteless, odorless, and dissolves readily in water, it can be easily mixed with a morning smoothie or any preferred beverage.

### Leaky Gut Support

Virgin Diet Leaky Gut Support provides nutrients, probiotics, and botanicals that nourish the intestinal tract and promote normal gut permeability. Glutamine nourishes and soothes intestinal mucosal cells, N-acetylglucosamine promotes a normal mucous layer in the gut and the growth of desirable Bifidobacterium bifidum; ginger provides antioxidant activity; and quercetin dampens histamine release. Lactobacillus sporogenes promotes beneficial gut flora; and Saccharomyces boulardii stimulates immune health in the gut.

### Digestive Enzymes

Virgin Diet Digestive Enzymes is a broad-spectrum enzyme formula that contains HCl, pepsin, pancreatin, and ox bile, which are important for those who need support for protein and carbohydrate digestion, as well as fat emulsification and absorption.

## Dairy-Free Resources

DairyFreeMarket.com: dairyfreemarket.com/
Go Dairy Free: godairyfree.org
Milk-Free Pantry: milkfreepantry.com

## *Organizations*

### Community Supported Agriculture (CSA)

Community Supported Agriculture (CSA) provides the perfect way to buy local, seasonal food directly from nearby farmers. Here's how it works: Your local farmers offer a number of "shares" to the public. You buy a share in the farm to support crop production and then receive fresh, seasonal produce as a thank-you. You get incredibly fresh, nutrient-rich foods harvested locally while teaching your kids and getting to know and support your local farmers. A win-win for everyone! To find a CSA near you: localharvest.org/csa/.

### Environmental Working Group (ewg.org)

The Environmental Working Group (EWG) is the nation's leading environmental health research and advocacy organization. They serve as a watchdog to see that you get clear, unbiased answers about healthier choices and a healthier environment.

From clean drinking water to food free of harmful chemicals, the EWG stays on top of the latest developments to protect you and your health. To learn how you can get involved: ewg.org/support-our-work/ways-to-donate.

Also visit the site to download their "Dirty Dozen" and "Clean Fifteen" lists, and to get the latest updates on the safest fish to eat.

### Institute for Responsible Technology (responsibletechnology.org/buy-non-gmo)

Expert Jeffrey Smith's site is loaded with great information, including your complete guide to avoid buying genetically modified foods.

## *Electronics and Other Gadgets*

### Kitchen Accessories

After well-stocked healthy food, nothing makes a good kitchen quite like premium-quality cookware, utensils, and other supplies. Among my favorite places to shop for kitchenware are Williams-Sonoma, Target, and amazon.com. They all offer a wide variety of fabulous pots, pans, utensils, and everything else I need, whether I want to host a lavish dinner party or just have a quiet meal for myself.

My go-to brands for kitchenware include:

- Oxo (oxo.com)—this company makes nearly every cool kitchen gadget you can imagine (and probably some you can't), from food storage to food scales.

- Analon (anolon.com)—the leader in built-to-last bronze, stainless steel, and other top-quality cookware.
- Oster (oster.com/index.aspx)—known for their blenders, Oster also has an excellent line of toaster ovens and even water dispensers.
- Farberware (farberware.com)—an affordable line for all your kitchen needs, from pots and pans to cutting boards, barware, and electronic appliances.
- Chicago Cutlery (worldkitchen.com/chicago-cutlery)—the leader in kitchen knives that stay sharp and handle any slicing, dicing, or other food preparation for years.
- Cuisinart (cuisinart.com/products.html)—far from just making the best food processors on the market, Cuisinart offers a varied line of coffeemakers, teakettles, grills, flatware, and just about anything else you can conceive of for your kitchen.
- Wüstof (www.wusthof.ca)—knives for the serious chef. You get what you pay for here, and Wüstof knives are an intelligent lifetime investment.
- Le Creuset (cookware.lecreuset.com)—I love the bold-colored enameled cast-iron skillets, braisers, kettles, and other kitchenware that lasts long after inferior-quality cookware falls apart.
- Rubbermaid (www.rubbermaid.com/Pages/Home.aspx)—the name is practically synonymous with affordable, sturdy kitchen gadgets, storage containers, and other BPA-free plastic kitchenware.

## Magic Bullet (buythebullet.com)

This portable, space-saving device is a great alternative to blenders and food processors. It also travels well. Find the product at the link above or at Bed Bath & Beyond and other retail stores. Honestly, I never travel without it!

## Nutribullet (nutribullet.com)

I'm not a big fan of juicing because when you strip away a juice's fiber, you're essentially left with nutrients (good) and sugar (bad). The Nutribullet extracts rather than juices or blends, so you get the nutrients in a fruit or vegetable in their most absorbable, healthiest form. Unlike bulky machines, the Nutribullet is compact and stores easily. Not that you'll need much storage space. If you're like me, you'll be using it about every day.

## Vitamix (thevirgindietcookbook.com/vitamix)

Comparing the Vitamix to a traditional blender is like comparing a Ferrari to a Toyota. Sure, both cars will get you where you want to go, but that Ferrari has unmatched horsepower. With the Vitamix I can whip up delicious nut butters, soups, and even coconut milk ice cream in just minutes, preserving all of the ingredients' fiber and delicate nutrients. The 64-ounce BPA-free pitcher is a cinch to clean. Vitamix blenders come with a 7-year warranty, which is peace of mind considering I use mine nearly every day!

### Gluten-Free Products

GF Harvest: glutenfreeoats.com
Amazon: amazon.com
GlutenFree.com: glutenfree.com/
The Gluten-Free Mall: glutenfreemall.com/

### Grass-Fed and Raw Dairy Products

A Campaign for Real Milk: realmilk.com/where03.html
Kerrygold: kerrygoldusa.com
Organic Pastures: organicpastures.com
Rocky Plains: rockyplains.com
Weston A. Price Foundation: westonaprice.org

### ShopNoGMO App

Look for it for your iPhone, iPad, or iPod Touch to help you shop GMO-free.

## Further Reading

Maybe *The Virgin Diet Book* and *The Virgin Diet Cookbook* have given you a whole new lease on life and you want to take that health commitment even further. These are some of my favorite books from my rock-star colleagues and friends to support you on that journey to a healthier, better you:

*Rich Food Poor Food* by Jayson and Mira Calton (absolute best grocery guide ever!)
*Nourishing Traditions* by Sally Fallon
*Practical Paleo* by Diane Sanfilippo
*The Healthy Gluten-Free Life: 200 Delicious Gluten-Free, Dairy-Free, Soy-Free & Egg-Free Recipes!* by Tammy Credicott
*The Omni Diet* by Tana Amen
*Wheat Belly* and *Wheat Belly Cookbook* by Dr. William Davis
*The Blood Sugar Solution Cookbook* by Dr. Mark Hyman
*The Body Ecology Diet* by Donna Gates
*The Hormone Cure* by Dr. Sara Gottfried

# Metric Conversion Chart

| Units | Teaspoons | Table-spoons | Fluid Ounces | Cups | Liquid Pints | Liquid Quarts | Mililiters | Liters |
|---|---|---|---|---|---|---|---|---|
| 1 Teaspoon (t) | - | ⅓ | ⅙ | - | - | - | 5 | - |
| 1 Table-spoon (T) | 3 | - | ½ | 1/16 | 1/32 | - | 15 | - |
| 1 Fluid Ounce (fl oz) | 6 | 2 | - | ⅛ | 1/16 | 1/32 | 30 | - |
| 1 Cup | 48 | 16 | 8 | - | ½ | ¼ | 240 (approx) | .24 |
| 1 Liquid Pint (liq pt) | - | - | 16 | 2 | - | ½ | 470 | .47 |
| 1 Liquid Quart (liq qt) | - | - | 32 | 4 | 2 | - | 950 | .95 |
| 1 Mililiter (mL) | ⅕ | - | - | - | - | - | | .001 |
| 1 Liter (L) | - | - | 34 | 4.2 | 2.1 | 1.06 | 1000 | - |

## Equivalence of Common Kitchen Volumes

**VOLUME**

1 quart = 2 pints = 32 fluid ounces = 946 milliliters

1 peck = 8 quarts = 8.8 liters

1 bushel = 4 pecks = 32 quarts = 35.23 liters

1 dry pint = 550 milliliters

1 dry quart = 1.1 liters

**WEIGHT**

1 ounce = 28.35 grams

1 pound = 16 ounces = 453.59 grams

# Index

# About the Author

## JJ Virgin, PhD, CNS, CHFS

> *Your body is not a bank account. It's a chemistry lab.*
>
> —JJ Virgin

Author JJ Virgin is a highly regarded fitness and nutrition expert, public speaker, and media personality. Her book *The Virgin Diet: Drop 7 Foods, Lose 7 Pounds, Just 7 Days* has appeared on numerous bestselling nonfiction lists, including the *New York Times*, *USA Today*, the *Chicago Tribune*, and the *Wall Street Journal*.

Internationally recognized as an expert in helping people overcome "weight loss resistance" (a term she uses to describe the condition of people who do everything right according to current dieting strategies but still can't lose weight), JJ has helped thousands of people achieve fast fat loss by addressing food allergies, food sensitivities, and other food intolerances. Clients feel better in days and achieve fast, lasting fat loss when they drop the 7 highly reactive foods she has identified.

JJ's recent media appearances include PBS, *Access Hollywood*, *Rachael Ray*, *The Doctors*, and *Today*. She is a frequent blogger for Livestrong.com, the *Huffington Post*, and *Prevention* magazine. JJ has been interviewed in numerous publications, including *Fox News Magazine*, *Women's World*, *Health*, *LA Weekly*, *Cosmopolitan*, and the *Los Angeles Times*.

High-performance athletes, CEOs, and A-list celebrities seek out JJ to deliver the results they need and expect. She has worked with Nicole Eggert, Tracie Thoms, and Tamara Johnson-George; and she helped Brandon Routh get in top physical form for *Superman Returns*.

For two years, JJ was the nutrition expert on the top-rated *Dr. Phil* show, and she spent two seasons as co-host of TLC's *Freaky Eaters*. She has one of the top pledge shows on PBS, *Drop 7 Foods, Feel Better Fast!* based on the Virgin Diet principles. She is also the bestselling author of *Six Weeks to Sleeveless and Sexy* and creator of the *4x4* workout series.

JJ is a lifelong learner and has completed forty graduate and doctoral courses in the areas of exercise science, nutrition, functional medicine, and psychology. She is a board-certified nutrition specialist through the American College of Nutrition, board certified in holistic nutrition, and a certified health and fitness specialist through the American College of Sports Medicine.

Most importantly, JJ is the mom of two amazing teenage boys. One of them survived a near fatal auto accident, and JJ used her knowledge, expertise, and peer network to take him from comatose to thriving. Every day JJ wakes up with gratitude to be able to spend another day with her children and to help more people live fuller lives by achieving better health.

For more information, please visit JJ at jjvirgin.com.